MORE THAN FLUENCY

The Social, Emotional, and Cognitive Dimensions of Stuttering

MORE THAN FLUENCY

The Social, Emotional, and Cognitive Dimensions of Stuttering

Barbara J. Amster, PhD, CCC-SLP, BCS-F
Evelyn R. Klein, PhD, CCC-SLP, BCS-CL

PLURAL PUBLISHING INC.

PLURAL PUBLISHING INC.

5521 Ruffin Road
San Diego, CA 92123

e-mail: info@pluralpublishing.com
website: http://www.pluralpublishing.com

FSC
www.fsc.org
MIX
Paper from responsible sources
FSC® C011935

Typeset in 11/13 Adobe Garamond by Flanagan's Publishing Services, Inc.
Printed in the United States of America by McNaughton & Gunn, Inc.

Library of Congress Cataloging-in-Publication Data

Names: Amster, Barbara J., editor. | Klein, Evelyn R., editor.
Title: More than fluency : the social, emotional, and cognitive dimensions of stuttering / [edited by] Barbara J. Amster, Evelyn R. Klein.
Description: San Diego, CA : Plural Publishing, [2018] | Includes bibliographical references and index.
Identifiers: LCCN 2018000652| ISBN 9781597569958 (alk. paper) | ISBN 159756995X (alk. paper)
Subjects: | MESH: Stuttering—psychology | Stuttering—therapy | Psychotherapy—methods | Sociological Factors
Classification: LCC RC424 | NLM WM 475.7 | DDC 616.85/54—dc23
LC record available at https://lccn.loc.gov/2018000652

Contents

Foreword

Let's be clear . . . there is an ever-increasing selection of stuttering textbooks on the market today. Most of the big sellers touch on the history of stuttering and stuttering theories, then progress to an introduction and explanation of traditional assessment strategies, followed by chapters on the traditions of stuttering therapy. With varying degrees, these texts introduce brain-imaging research, genetic research, epidemiology of stuttering, therapy research, and maybe a chapter on "other fluency disorders." Some texts break these assessment and treatment discussions into strategies for children, adolescents, and adults. Others simply treat these issues as general concepts that can be implemented across the age ranges. It's tough to publish and sell another book in this market.

When I was first asked to write the forward to this text, I agreed, and knew what I was expecting. Surprisingly, I found something different . . . and pleasantly so. Let me elaborate in the next few paragraphs.

An introduction and summary chapter written by the editors, Barbara Amster and Evelyn Klein, serve as bookends to a non-traditional textbook for stuttering intervention and understanding. Several years ago, a public discussion involving the main issues in stuttering treatment played out in *Language, Speech, and Hearing Services in Schools,* one of the profession's most widely read professional journals. The debate started with a Letter from the Editor (Nippold, 2011). This letter intended to address the lack of evidence in our field when treating school-age children who stutter. Nippold argued that there simply was not enough evidence to support anything but behavioral programs that treat stuttering in school-age children. The limited evidence that Nippold referred to was based upon one philosophy of evidence and one philosophy of what the dependent variable following stuttering treatment should be—that is, elimination of stuttering. On the surface (i.e., the "tip of the iceberg"), this is a reasonable view about how to judge stuttering. However, many thought that this was not the case. As a matter of fact, a response to Nippold's editorial (Yaruss, Coleman, & Quesal, 2012) was published the next year and was co-signed by over 100 speech-language pathologists who argued that Nippold's view of stuttering was too narrow and was focused on only the outcome of "no stuttering." In other words, these clinicians, researchers, and leaders in the field of stuttering thought that stuttering was "MORE THAN JUST FLUENCY." They argued that stuttering consists of more than the repetitions, prolongations, and blocks that we count as stuttering, but included the internal feelings of people who stutter (PWS) and the ways that they may avoid or try to escape from those external symptoms. They argued that the inner feelings of PWS and the environmental obstacles that face PWS are indeed part of this disorder/difference. They pointed to several successful treatment programs that targeted feelings and emotions associated with stuttering and argued that treating stuttering is treating *more than fluency.*

Full disclosure: I agree with Yaruss, Coleman, and Quesal and was one of the co-signers who supported the view that stuttering is *more than fluency*. Over the years, I came to appreciate this view from reviewing many papers on what really makes up the human condition and what constitutes stuttering. These ranged from readings within our field of speech-language pathology, including the "personal view" of stuttering promoted by researchers like William Perkins, to those by people in allied fields like psychology and sociology, such as George Kelly and Irving Goffman. Let me elaborate. Perkins' views led to the development of the neuropsycholinguistic theory of stuttering (Perkins, Kent, & Curlee, 1990). This view of stuttering included an explanation of the complexity of what it takes to produce connected speech and the "dyssynchrony" within this complex system that causes breakdowns in fluency. The important component that they added, however, was that the differences between stuttering and other, non-stuttering breakdowns in fluency had to do with internal time pressure. Breakdowns in fluency could be divided on the surface by specific rules for counting such behaviors (i.e., part-word repetitions, prolongations and blocks are *stuttering*; interjections, phrase repetitions, etc., are *disfluencies* [not stuttering]). But Perkins argued that the distinction between stuttering and other disfluencies was a result of internal time pressure to speak. I often wondered, how do we account for these internal factors? If stuttering was truly *more than fluency*, how can we count these behaviors? This point in itself leads many to believe that stuttering is just the observable blocks, prolongations, and repetitions that occur in the speech of those who stutter. However, speech and communication are far too complex to be counted so simply. This led Walt Manning to cite the British psychologist Don Bannister in the foreword of his 2010 textbook with the following quote, "Human beings are nonsensical unfit subjects for scientific inquiry." I interpret this to mean that stuttering is too complex to understand through something as simplistic as counting observable behaviors. Stuttering is complex, hard to study, and certainly *more than just fluency*.

I started to learn my lessons almost 20 years ago when I attended my first national conference of the National Stuttering Association. The National Stuttering Association is the largest self-help organization for PWS in the world and holds a national conference each year that attracts nearly 1,000 PWS, their family members, and a few rogue speech-language pathologists. I remember my first few National Stuttering Association conferences. I was not welcomed! I was an outsider! I was viewed as someone who did not understand the stuttering condition and who was still trying to "cure them" by eliminating all of their outward stuttering behaviors. I was seen as just another person who would tell them to "just slow down," "think about what you're saying," "your mouth is working faster than your brain," and "you could be fluent if you just tried harder." As a young academic in the field of stuttering, I clearly didn't "get it." I use this terminology because a few years ago, the best compliment I ever received professionally was from a PWS at a National Stuttering Association conference. He said to me, "For a person who does not stutter, YOU GET IT." What is it that I get? I'll go back to my previous statements relating to what I learned about stuttering from related professions.

Stuttering is far more than just obtaining fluency. George Kelly's classic writings on personal construct theory (Kelly, 1955) explained how people's experiences determine the way they view themselves and how they navigate the world. Those who build their personal construct as "stutterer" will allow that construct to influence how they face communication and communication challenges. One view might be that you have to change your "personal construct as a stutterer." However, another view argues that PWS "must accept their personal construct as a stutterer." Both views are explored in this text. Later, Irving Goffman (1963) studied and wrote about "stigma" and how it related to interpersonal communication and feelings of self. How people build their identities and how they stigmatize themselves or how they are stigmatized by others are important factors in human behavior. When these views are applied to stuttering, we can see that how a PWS sees himself and how others may see him can lead to public or personal stigma. If these are indeed results of stuttering, the people that we treat for stuttering must openly discuss *more than fluency*.

This text clearly reflects on *more than fluency* and provides important information to understand and treat PWS. It begins with some very important chapters making the case that stuttering is more than the outward behaviors exhibited by those who have fluency breakdowns. It then progresses to a very important chapter on the neurology of emotions. In this chapter, Jennifer Kleinow follows the trail of how emotions are exhibited in the brain and perceived by humans, and how these same emotions can affect physical performance. In many ways, speaking is a motor activity, but the generation of the message that needs to be communicated is equally, if not more, complex. Extra demands on the ability of the neurological system to complete this complex task draws resources from the entire system that can result in fluency breakdowns. Thus, stuttering is clearly *more than fluency*. Kleinow's explanation on the cortical and subcortical mechanisms of emotion are meaningfully explained in the context of stuttering.

In the following chapters, the authors explain concepts and mechanisms involved in stuttering and how to treat it. These chapters are consistent with the book's premise that stuttering is *more than fluency*. If this view wasn't taken, it would simply be another rehashing of fluency shaping and stuttering modification. This is not the case. The editors, authors, and I believe that it is more. Michael Boyle so clearly points this out in his chapter on self-efficacy and its relationship to stigma. His careful research studies are combined into a chapter that explains the burdens that society and the PWS place upon themselves making communication a barrier. However, he does not stop there; he goes on and offers sound advice. This information simply does not make it into many textbooks on stuttering today. It is clear in the research literature, but rarely makes it into the textbooks that students are using in the masters level courses or the textbooks that practicing clinicians purchase. I personally thank you for including this information in this text.

Boyle's chapter is followed by James Mancinelli's chapter on the social context of stuttering. He begins with several references to Goffman (e.g., 1963) but makes the case that stuttering (and communication) only takes place within social contexts. The way that a person negotiates this social context is crucial to understanding, and later, treating an individual who is navigating any social context. He wonderfully makes the case as to why a PWS may avoid certain situations or even fully withdraw from them. Once again, the case is made that stuttering is *more than fluency*.

The remaining chapters present varying views on how to treat stuttering. If you believe that stuttering is *more than fluency*, then you will relate to and agree with their premise. This is *not* a review of traditional stuttering therapies, but a collection of well-thought-out programs that help treat the whole person, not just her stuttering. Amster and Klein's chapter on *perfectionism* relates how maladaptive perfectionism (and the desire for perfect speech . . . or perfectly fluent speech) can lead to maladaptive behaviors. If PWS are not capable of *perfect fluency*, they may think they are destined for failure. In the next chapters, Klein and Amster, then Beilby and Yaruss review two of the areas that seem to be gaining steam in the understanding and treatment of stuttering. Cognitive Behavioral Therapy (CBT) and Acceptance and Commitment Therapy (ACT) have their roots in psychology and "mindfulness" and have been used as adjuncts to stuttering therapy for many years. However, both of these chapters now are looking to show exactly how CBT and ACT can benefit PWS and justify why speech-language pathologists who treat stuttering need to be aware of and consider these treatment methods.

Chapters 8 through 11 boast the benefits of Experiential Therapy for stuttering (Starkweather and Givens), Avoidance Reduction Therapy for stuttering (Sisskin), the power of augmentative strategies of self-help and support (Trichon and Raj), and community-centered intervention (Coleman). Although the implementation and even the basic philosophies of these methods vary greatly, the common factor running through each of them is that if speech-language pathologists are going to treat stuttering, they have to treat *more than fluency*. These methods include: viewing oneself as a PWS and understanding the experience; reducing the avoidance associated with stuttering; acknowledging the power of educating and being educated; and discussing stuttering with those in the community of a PWS. These can include the family and community of the PWS, as well as those with similar experiences, such as other PWS. The bottom line once more is this: Treating stuttering has to do with living with the condition, more than just treating the outward fluency. The power of treatment is in treating the entire condition, not just the fluency!

For many years, most speech-language pathologists owned a copy of the *Handbook of Speech Pathology*. The original version was published in 1957 with Lee Edward Travis serving as editor (as an aside, Travis is considered to be the first speech-language pathologist, earning his doctorate in psychology with an emphasis on speech correction from the University of Iowa in 1924). The text was viewed as an authoritative, encyclopedic collection of the basics of the profession. After many dormant years, a new version of the text was published in 2010 with new editors and a slightly new title, *The Handbook of Language and Speech Disorders*. The first chapter in the book, titled "The Social and Practical Considerations in Labeling" (Damico, Muller, & Ball, 2010), speaks to the social problems associated with labeling human beings and human conditions. The authors introduce a dichotomy of viewing disorders from a "medical model," which seeks to cure a condition, versus a "social model," which seeks to adapt to a condition. Amster and Klein's edited volume is clearly in line with the social model and helps us define how stuttering fits into this social model. From this viewpoint, stuttering and all of its characteristics must be considered whether they be clearly observed or are emotions and affective issues that are below the surface and cannot be readily observed. This text makes the case that all dimensions must be considered if we want to help the PWS who seeks our help. Treating stuttering, from this viewpoint, is treating *more than fluency*.

In conclusion, I reflected on how to use this textbook and who would use it. Before I was asked to review and write a foreword to *More than Fluency: The Social, Emotional, and Cognitive Dimensions of Fluency*, I asked the editors if I could share it with four of my doctoral students.[1] I was teaching a seminar in "stuttering treatment" and I thought that this edited volume could serve as a nice resource in addition to the many research articles that they read for this course. About halfway through the class, we completed reading the entire book and I asked for some comments. I let the four doctoral students specializing in fluency disorders know that they would be expected to teach a master's level course in fluency disor-

[1]The four doctoral students who read these chapters along with me and discussed them in a seminar on Fluency Treatment in the fall 2017 semester at the University of Louisiana–Lafayette are: Monica Johnson, Bornwell Katebe, Brittany Rutland, and Anne Williams. They are part of the next generation of academics in fluency disorders.

ders in the near future and asked them if they would use this book in their master's level class. One said, "No, because it did not cover the basics well enough." Another said, "It might serve as a nice adjunct to another textbook." Even I wondered if the master's students could handle this material and use it therapeutically without knowing ALL the basics first. Then, one brilliant doctoral student said, "It's our job to challenge students and make them think. I would use this textbook with my master's students." That comment really made me think. We may be underselling the ability of our students and "spoon-feeding" them along the way, rather than allowing them to indulge in a "full helping of thoughtful knowledge." When we think about today's clinicians, I hear many academics say that they "don't think enough" and that they "want a cookbook approach to therapy." This may be the case because that's what we train them to expect. *More than Fluency: The Social, Emotional, and Cognitive Dimensions of Stuttering* is anything but a cookbook approach! It introduces the reader to many concepts that force the practitioner to THINK. They will THINK about what their clients need, and what is involved in treating the person who stutters. Maybe we need to train the next generation of clinicians to think on their own and to make wise decisions about what determines success. If the next generation of therapists who treat PWS seek to do so and to treat the whole person, they will have to know that treating a PWS is "more than JUST fluency."

John A. Tetnowski, Ph.D., CCC-SLP, BCS-F, ASHA Fellow
Ben Blanco Endowed Professor of Communicative Disorders
University of Louisiana–Lafayette

REFERENCES

Damico, J. A., Muller, N. M. & Ball, M. J. (2010). Social and practical considerations in labeling. In J. S. Damico, N. M. Muller, & M. J. Ball (Eds.), *The handbook of language and speech disorders* (pp. 11–37). West Sussex, UK: Wiley-Blackwell.

Goffman, E. (1963). *Stigma: Notes on the management of spoiled identity*. Englewood Cliffs, NJ: Prentice-Hall.

Kelly, G. (1955). *The psychology of personal constructs*. New York, NY: W.W. Norton.

Manning, W. H. (2009). *Clinical decision making in fluency disorders* (3rd ed.). San Diego, CA: Singular.

Nippold, M. A. (2011). Stuttering in school-age children: A call for treatment research. *Language, Speech, and Hearing Services in Schools*, *42*, 99–101.

Perkins, W., Kent, R., & Curlee, R. (1991). A theory of neuropsycholinguistic function in stuttering. *Journal of Speech and Hearing Research*, *34*, 734–752.

Travis, L. E. (1957). *The handbook of speech pathology.* New York, NY: Appleton-Century-Crofts.

Yaruss, J. S., Coleman, C. E., & Quesal, R. W. (2012). Stuttering in school-age children: A comprehensive approach to treatment. *Language, Speech, and Hearing Services in Schools*, *43*, 536–548.

Acknowledgments

We would like to recognize Dr. Joseph Sheehan for his "stuttering Iceberg" analogy that served as the inspiration for our book cover. We also thank Ross Klein for his cover illustration that expertly captured our desire to bring the "stuttering Iceberg" to life. In addition, we want to thank several people who were instrumental in the development of this book. First of all, thank you to our chapter authors who generously shared their knowledge, experiences, and insights. What a wonderful group of colleagues! They made this project a pleasure! Additionally, we greatly appreciate Dr. John Tetnowski's insightful Foreword. Thank you also to our superb administrative assistant, Erica Nix, for her dedication and attention to detail. We were also fortunate to work with a talented editor, Kalie Koscielak, who was always available to answer our questions and provide guidance. Finally, we want to thank our husbands, Glenn and Dietrich, for their ongoing encouragement and support.

Contributors

Barbara J. Amster, PhD, CCC-SLP, BCS-F is founding Chair, founding Graduate Director, and Professor in the Department of Communication Sciences and Disorders at La Salle University where she teaches the graduate course in stuttering. She is a licensed and certified speech-language pathologist. She holds Board Specialty Certification in Fluency Disorders from the American Speech-Language-Hearing Association (ASHA). She is an ASHA Fellow and received Honors of the Pennsylvania Speech-Language-Hearing Association where she served as Vice President for Professional Preparation and Continuing Education. She was Pennsylvania's representative to the ASHA Advisory Council and served as Associate Coordinator for ASHA's Special Interest Group 4: Fluency and Fluency Disorders. Dr. Amster has investigated perfectionism in people who stutter (PWS) and has presented and published articles on perfectionism and the therapeutic use of cognitive behavioral therapy with PWS. She is also an editor and author of a book on children in the child welfare system.

Associate Professor **Janet M. Beilby** has been a lecturer, researcher and clinician in the field of stuttering for over 30 years. She has been a specialist advisor to Speech Pathology Australia on stuttering disorders and lectured on professional and medico-legal issues, speech-hearing sciences and the specialty area of stuttering disorders. Dr. Beilby is known internationally as a leader in speech pathology management and applied clinical treatment research. She has treated thousands of clients, and been awarded over half-a-million dollars in research funds. She has conducted integrated psychosocial resilience programs for stuttering disorders, pain, and spinal cord disabilities. She works in the School of Occupational Therapy, Social Work and Speech Pathology at Curtin University in Western Australia and is founder of the Curtin University Stuttering Treatment Clinic. She is a board member on the International Fluency Association Standards of Practice Committee and an advisory board member for the Speak-Easy Association of Australia.

Michael P. Boyle, PhD, CCC-SLP, is Assistant Professor of Communication Sciences and Disorders at Montclair State University. He is Director of the Fluency Disorders Laboratory in the Department. Dr. Boyle teaches undergraduate and graduate courses in stuttering in addition to research methods, and anatomy and physiology. He is an active researcher who studies psychosocial aspects of stuttering including stigma and empowerment experienced by people who stutter. He is the author of numerous peer-reviewed research articles and book chapters related to stuttering and psychosocial aspects of communication disorders. Dr. Boyle has presented his research findings at local, national, and international conferences. In addition, Dr. Boyle is a certified clinical speech-language pathologist focused on assessing and treating individuals who stutter.

Craig Coleman, MA, CCC-SLP, BCS-F is an Assistant Professor at Marshall University and a Board-Certified Specialist in Fluency Disorders. He has given over 200 presentations at local, national, and international conferences. In addition, he has published more than 10 journal articles on stuttering. He has published three children's books on stuttering, and was a contributing author of the School-Age and Teen versions of the *Overall Assessment of the Speaker's Experience of Stuttering* (OASES). He is a former two-term President of the Pennsylvania Speech-Language-Hearing Association and Coordinator of the American Speech-Language-Hearing Association Special Interest Group 4: Fluency Disorders. Prior to joining the faculty at Marshall University, he was the Clinical Coordinator and Co-Director of the Stuttering Center of Western Pennsylvania at Children's Hospital of Pittsburgh.

Janet Givens received her MA in sociology and, after a 25-year career in fundraising, graduated from the Pennsylvania Gestalt Center as a certified Gestalt psychotherapist. Along with Woody Starkweather, she wrote the book *Stuttering* and has provided workshops around the world for people who stutter and for the speech-language pathologists who treat them. Then, in 2004, they joined the Peace Corps and were placed in Kazakhstan. Based on her experiences there, she wrote an award-winning memoir, *At Home on the Kazakh Steppe*, now in its fifth edition, and lectures widely on her experience in Kazakhstan. Her weekly blog, *And So It Goes*, explores cultural differences and the value of civility and curiosity in our lives. She is working on her next book, a memoir focused on her stuttering story.

Evelyn R. Klein, PhD, CCC-SLP, BCS-CL is a Professor of Communication Sciences and Disorders at La Salle University and a licensed and certified speech-language pathologist and licensed psychologist with post-doctoral training in neuropsychology. She holds Board Specialty Certification in Child Language from the American Speech-Language-Hearing Association. She is an ASHA Fellow. Dr. Klein has conducted research using cognitive behavioral therapy (CBT) with people who stutter and has presented and published on this topic. She is also an author of the textbook *Acquired Language Disorders: A Case-Based Approach.* She is also on the Scientific Advisory Board of the Selective Mutism Association and is a consultant for the Selective Mutism Research Institute. She received the Lindback Award for Distinguished Teaching from La Salle University and the Pennsylvania Clinical Achievement Award from the Pennsylvania Speech-Language-Hearing Association. As a practicing clinician, Dr. Klein evaluates and treats individuals with communication disorders including people who stutter.

Jennifer Kleinow, PhD, CCC-SLP, is a Professor in the Department of Communication Sciences and Disorders at La Salle University. Dr. Kleinow's research focuses on various topics in speech motor control (how the brain coordinates and executes the movements required for fluent speech) in both typical and disordered speakers. Her current laboratory projects include examining new techniques for the measurement and recording of human speech, and documenting the relationship between cognitive-linguistic and emotional processing and speech motor control. She has recently served as Professional Development Manager for the American Speech-Language-Hearing Association's Special Interest Group 4: Fluency and Fluency Disorders and as Vice President for Professional Preparation and Continuing Education of the Pennsylvania Speech-Language-Hearing Association.

James M. Mancinelli, PhD, CCC-SLP is Assistant Professor and Director of Clinical Education at La Salle University's Department of Communication Sciences and Disorders. Dr. Mancinelli has 20 years experience in medical speech-language pathology in acute care, rehabilitation, long-term care, outpatient, and home care settings. He is also an author of the textbook *Acquired Language*

Disorders: A Case-Based Approach. His interest in fluency emerged out of working with adults who stutter and hearing their narratives about the social history of their stuttering. He appreciated the role of social interaction in communicative events for adults who stutter; grounded in social identity, stigmatization, and each client's social history. His recent research investigated the effects of self-disclosure on the conversational interaction with a normally fluent speaker.

Erik X. Raj, PhD, CCC-SLP is an Assistant Professor and Clinical Supervisor in the Department of Speech-Language Pathology at Monmouth University. Dr. Raj works daily with school-age children and adolescents with various communication difficulties. In addition to developing numerous top-ranking educational iPad apps for children with communication difficulties, he regularly presents interactive workshops demonstrating how speech-language pathologists can use Internet and digital technologies to motivate and teach students. His research focuses on exploring Internet and digital technologies and its implementation to speech-language therapy and education.

Vivian Sisskin, MS, CCC-SLP, BCS-F is a Clinical Professor at the University of Maryland, an ASHA Fellow, and Board Certified Specialist in Fluency. She received the Excellence in Teaching Award from the University of Maryland, and ASHA's Media Champion Award. She was named Speech-Language Pathologist of the Year by the National Stuttering Association. Ms. Sisskin served as Coordinator for ASHA's Special Interest Group (Fluency), and on the Boards of Directors of the National Stuttering Association and The American Board on Fluency and Fluency Disorders. She is on the Professional Advisory Board of the Stuttering Foundation, and a faculty member for the Foundation's Mid-Atlantic and University Instructors Workshops. She is the book review editor for the Journal of Fluency Disorders. Her articles and workshops cover treatment for stuttering, atypical speech fluency disorders, and communication strategies in autism. She is the owner of the Sisskin Stuttering Center in the Washington DC area.

C. Woodruff Starkweather, PhD, a Fellow of ASHA, has been a lifelong lover of words—spoken, written, or sung. He taught at the City University of New York and most recently at Temple University where he is Professor Emeritus. His research on stuttering and its treatment, led to the publication of over 50 articles and monographs and nine books. One book, *Stuttering,* written with Janet Givens, was listed in Choice Magazine's *Best Textbooks of 1997*, a first in the speech pathology profession. He was named Speech Pathologist of the Year by the National Stuttering Association in 1999 and received the Malcolm Fraser Award from ASHA's Special Interest Division for lifetime achievement in the stuttering field in 2009. In 2017, the *Woody Starkweather Intensive Stuttering Treatment Center* at Children's Hospital of Philadelphia was named in his honor. He has also published two novels and a book of short stories.

Mitchell Trichon, PhD, CCC-SLP, is a cofounder of Stutter Social, an Internet-based videoconferencing community and private social network community for people who stutter. As a faculty member at La Salle University and prior to that at St. John's University, he taught classes in fluency disorders. He also supervised graduate students who were treating clients who stutter. He has 10 peer-reviewed publications and over 50 professional presentations at international, national, and regional conferences. His primary research focuses on self-help activities for people who stutter. Dr. Trichon is currently a Board Member of the International Stuttering Association

(ISA). As a Board Member of the National Stuttering Association, he co-led the national network of adult support groups. Dr. Trichon has a private practice and will be a keynote speaker at the Inaugural Joint World Congress of the ISA, International Fluency Association, and the International Cluttering Association in Japan in 2018.

J. Scott Yaruss, PhD, CCC-SLP, is an ASHA Fellow and a board-certified specialist in fluency disorders. After 19 years at the University of Pittsburgh, Dr. Yaruss joined the faculty of Michigan State University as Professor of Communicative Sciences and Disorders. He has published approximately 70 peer-reviewed manuscripts, more than 115 other papers on stuttering, and several resources including the *Overall Assessment of the Speaker's Experience of Stuttering* (OASES), *Early Childhood Stuttering Therapy: A Practical Guide, School-Age Stuttering Therapy: A Practical Guide,* and the *Minimizing Bullying for Children Who Stutter Program.* Dr. Yaruss has been named SLP of the Year by the National Stuttering Association and received the University of Pittsburgh SHRS Dean's Distinguished Teaching Award. He teaches classes on stuttering and counseling methods for SLPs and frequently conducts workshops around the world designed to help clinicians improve their ability to work with individuals who stutter.

Reviewers

Plural Publishing, Inc. and the authors would like to thank the following reviewers for taking the time to provide their valuable feedback during the development process:

Angela M. Medina, PhD, CCC-SLP
Assistant Professor
Communication Sciences and Disorders
Florida International University
Miami, Florida

Charlie Osborne, MA, CCC-SLP
Clinical Associate Professor
Communication Sciences and Disorders
University of Wisconsin-Stevens Point
Stevens Point, Wisconsin

Jean Sawyer, PhD, CCC-SLP
Associate Professor
Communication Sciences and Disorders
Illinois State University
Normal, Illinois

Ying-Chiao Tsao, PhD, CCC-SLP, BCS-F
Associate Professor
Communicative Disorders
California State University-Fullerton
Fullerton, California

We dedicate this book to those who stutter.
Thank you for your courage, sharing your stories, and teaching us what matters.

CHAPTER 1

Introduction

The Importance of the Social, Emotional, and Cognitive Dimensions of Stuttering

Barbara J. Amster and Evelyn R. Klein

"[N]ot everything that can be counted counts, and not everything that counts can be counted."

—William Bruce Cameron, *Informal Sociology: A Casual Introduction to Sociological Thinking* (1963, p. 13)

The genesis for this book came from listening to both our clients and our graduate students in speech-language pathology. Our clients all had a story to tell and wanted to tell it. They wanted to tell us about their experiences as people who stutter (PWS), what they thought caused the problem, their challenges, thoughts, emotions, and difficulties with social interactions, while relying on a speech system that did not always work for them. They often started the therapeutic process looking for a quick fix, a magic bullet toward fluency, but soon circled back to these other concerns.

Our graduate students, who did not have a course in fluency and stuttering until their final semester, expressed their fears about dealing with the emotional and social issues of their clients who stuttered. They were not sure if they were up to the task and were worried that in attempts to help, they may be doing harm. We did not often hear these concerns when the students were working with other clients, only those who stuttered. These feelings of discomfort are echoed by many working speech-language pathologists (Cooper & Cooper, 1985, 1996; Quesal & Yaruss, 2000), who feel unprepared in working with people who stutter (PWS). Surveys have shown that speech-language pathologists are most uncomfortable treating people who stutter and often feel unprepared to work with this population, especially regarding social, emotional, and cognitive aspects of the disorder. These areas are often overlooked in more traditional behavioral treatments (St. Louis & Durrenberger, 1993; Yaruss & Quesal, 2002).

A 2009 survey conducted by the National Stuttering Association found that therapeutic interventions that focus on changing attitudes were more successful than those that focus on changing speech patterns (NSA, 2009). Yet speech-language pathologists often feel ill-equipped to address the more psychologically focused areas of attitudinal change. It seems that their discomfort with the emotional and social issues, those very issues of concern to our clients, was triggering a sense of uneasiness.

Frustration with typical stuttering treatment was also expressed by an eloquent mother of a child who stutters. Doreen Lenz Holte (2011), who in her book, *Voice Unearthed,* for parents of children who stutter, urges a change of emphasis away from fluency toward comfort in communicating in an effort to help prevent the social, emotional, and cognitive consequences of stuttering that are often the most troubling parts of the disorder for the child or adult who stutters.

Our interests as professors, authors, and editors of this book have guided us to the importance in helping speech-language pathologists incorporate counseling and psychotherapeutic principles into treatment to help change the attitudes PWS have about themselves and stuttering. Therefore, the goal of this text is to provide a broader framework for speech-language pathologists when working with PWS.

We feel very strongly that these areas should be incorporated into an effective treatment plan for PWS. It can be within the speech-language pathologists' scope of practice to work with the social, emotional, and cognitive dimensions of stuttering. ASHA's Preferred Practice Patterns for Fluency Intervention (ASHA, 2004) are in agreement. The following three bullet points are part of ASHA's clinical guidelines for fluency intervention:

- Assisting the person who stutters to communicate in educational, vocational, and social situations in ways that optimize activity/participation.
- Reduction of attitudes, beliefs, and thought processes that interfere with fluent speech production or that hinder activity/participation.
- Reduction of emotional reactions to specific stimuli when they have a negative impact on stuttering-like disfluencies, attempts to modify stuttering behavior, and/or activity/participation.

Because speech-language pathologists have the knowledge and skills to understand stuttering, we are the right people to help. A word of caution is necessary, as some individuals will present with issues beyond our training and scope of practice, such as depression/anxiety, marital problems, personality disorders, chemical dependency, and suicidal ideation, among others. A referral to an appropriate professional such as a licensed clinical psychologist or psychiatrist may be in order. We have often worked in collaboration with these professionals to best treat our patients, and a responsible speech-language pathologist must know his/her limits. We also feel strongly that graduate speech-language pathology programs should offer courses in counseling for our profession.

Speech-language pathologists must also be mindful of cultural influences, as they can affect the course of treatment. This is certainly true when working with people who stutter, as cultural beliefs can influence therapeutic progress (Manning & DiLollo, 2018). Further, Manning and DiLollo (2018) encourage clinicians to explore PWS's beliefs and expectations about stuttering so that they can be discussed as they may relate to the social, emotional, and cognitive dimensions of treatment.

Traditional stuttering treatment often focuses on teaching techniques to increase fluency, yet PWS may feel stigmatized and defeated in their attempts at obtaining the often elusive goal of fluency (Boyle, 2013). We focus on the social, emotional, and cognitive realms of this disorder and offer new insights and applications based on research in the field.

The current consensus about stuttering is that it is a multifactorial, dynamic, epigenetic, neurodevelopmental disorder (Smith, 1999; Smith & Weber, 2016, 2017; Weber-Fox & Smith, 2014) that unfolds with brain development. This view of stuttering considers that there are "cognitive, linguistic, emotional, and motor factors in the etiology of stuttering." (Smith, 1999, p. 32). With the average age of onset in the preschool years, the child is mastering language learning which places demands on the developing speech-motor system. Many young children go through a period of disfluency, but most recover. Estimates of recovery vary but are as high as 80% (Yairi & Ambrose, 1992). The preschool years are also a time of change for the child in psychosocial growth. Children's experiences including interactions with others, their thoughts, beliefs, and feelings all contribute in various ways to their recovery or persistence in stuttering.

Similarly, when stuttering becomes chronic, it is often fueled by interactions with others. The thoughts, beliefs, and feelings of PWS result in what Starkweather (1987) called *the reactive features of stuttering* such as avoidance and fear, which make stuttering more debilitating.

This book contributes a broadened scope to treating PWS. It offers extensive theoretical discussion of how the social, emotional, and cognitive dimensions influence stuttering and provides practical application-based strategies for intervention. The authors present a strategic conceptualization underlying stuttering. We begin with the chapter by Kleinow involving physiological influences on stuttering and how the brain influences the motor, social, emotional, and cognitive aspects. In this chapter, a straightforward explanation of the complex neural systems involved in human emotion is introduced. In reviewing the literature, she reinforces the notion that stuttering is a multifactorial disorder. Kleinow explains how these neural emotional systems bridge with motor control systems to offer implications for multifactorial treatment.

Boyle discusses the importance of self-efficacy, which has great relevance for stuttering because it involves the belief that one can change one's own behavior. Boyle reviews self-efficacy, why it is important, its theoretical relevance to stuttering, and how PWS can benefit from the belief that they can succeed at meeting their goals. Boyle also discusses how self-efficacy is empirically linked with certain psychosocial areas of stuttering, such as stigma. In addition, he discusses locus of control and causal attribution and reviews treatment studies that include aspects of increasing self-efficacy in PWS. We believe that enhancing a sense of self-efficacy is an important part of effective treatment.

Mancinelli discusses stuttering from a social interaction perspective. The social context is extremely important for PWS, as stuttering rarely occurs when talking to animals or babies when the social consequences are reduced. He discusses that stuttering is a stigmatizing disorder that emerges in a social context. Using a sociological framework, he describes the type of talking, the flow of the interactions, and the ramifications of avoidance or disclosure. Mancinelli offers suggestions in bridging the gap between theory and practice by formulating strategies to help clients analyze social contexts and how they affect one's speech.

Amster and Klein explore the clinical implications of maladaptive perfectionism and its potential impact on stuttering. Heightened concern about mistakes is a central feature of maladaptive perfectionism. Perfectionists are often self-critical when their unrealistic standards are not met. The authors discuss that having this personal characteristic may have implications for stuttering development and maintenance and offer practical suggestions for intervention.

Subsequent chapters in this text offer a variety of therapeutic interventions and techniques to address social, emotional, and cognitive issues. The authors discuss interventions that have been designed to alleviate distress in those who stutter and offer practical guidelines. Klein and Amster introduce Cognitive Behavioral Therapy (CBT), a well-established therapeutic intervention, as a problem-solving method to analyze distressful feelings and automatic thoughts that can color perceptions and affect one's sense of well-being. Basic principles of CBT are reviewed along with a novel educational model for incorporating CBT for people who stutter.

Beilby and Yaruss present another well-established treatment approach, Acceptance and Commitment Therapy (ACT) to reduce frustration through acceptance and mindfulness. Their chapter offers valuable insights encouraging PWS to focus on the positives in their lives through acceptance rather than trying to hide their stuttering or focus on attempts to be fluent. They offer useful guidance for incorporating the core ACT processes for people who stutter.

Starkweather and Givens present their novel treatment approach, Experiential Therapy for adults who stutter. This approach considers stuttering from the inside out. They discuss how stuttering can be more than just a behavior. It is an experience, beginning in simple frustration but often developing into a complex amalgam of behavioral adaptation, shame, humiliation, anger, grief, and fear. In response, they developed this treatment and offer case scenarios for application.

Sisskin developed another innovative approach, Avoidance and Reduction Therapy for Stuttering (ARTS®). ARTS was designed to help PWS reduce struggle, confront fear, reduce shame, and change avoidance behaviors. This approach aims to eliminate efforts to control stuttering that paradoxically perpetuate it. Sisskin gives guidance on ARTS implementation, discussing concepts of control, concealment, change, and connection.

The final two chapters provide important information on the advantages of peer support and community involvement related to intervention. Trichon and Raj discuss the history, benefits, and evolution of peer support. They describe national and regional organizations for those who stutter, including face-to-face and online communities. These groups offer identification and socialization which can be both empowering and comforting, leading to greater acceptance.

Finally, Coleman discusses the importance of community-centered assessment and treatment for children who stutter. He describes a model for incorporating important people into the child's life to help enhance the therapeutic process when working on the social, emotional, and cognitive aspects of stuttering. This broader focus expands the therapeutic environment and experiences, encouraging acceptance. Emphasizing this community approach provides a natural way to increase comfort and generalization.

As the reader may note, the interventions discussed differ in approach, each offering their own roadmap to support and empower people who stutter. All of the chapters provide information that we believe can help those who stutter lead a more authentic and satisfying life.

REFERENCES

ASHA. (2004). Fluency intervention. *Preferred practice patterns for the profession of speech-language pathology, 31.* Retrieved from http://www.asha.org/policy/PP2004-00191.htm#sec1.3.31

Boyle, M. P. (2013). Assessment of stigma associated with stuttering: Development and evaluation of the Self-Stigma of Stuttering Scale (4S). *Journal of Speech, Language, and Hearing Research, 56,* 1517–1529.

Cooper, E., & Cooper, C. S. (1985). Clinician attitudes towards stuttering: A decade of change (1973–1983). *Journal of Fluency Disorders, 10,* 19–35.

Cooper, E., & Cooper, C. S. (1996). Clinician attitudes towards stuttering: Two decades of change. *Journal of Fluency Disorders, 21*, 119–136.

Holte, D. L. (2011). *Voice unearthed: Hope, help, and a wake-up call for the parents of children who stutter*. n.p.: Author.

Manning, W. H., & DiLollo, A. (2018). *Clinical decision making in fluency disorders* (4th ed.). San Diego, CA: Plural.

National Stuttering Association. (2009). *The experience of people who stutter. A survey by the National Stuttering Association.* Retrieved from http://98.129.102.154:8888/opencms/opencms/nsa/stutteringInformation/NSA_Survey_Results.html

Quesal, R. W., & Yaruss, J., S. (2000). Historical perspectives on stuttering treatment: Dean Williams. *Contemporary Issues in Communication Science and Disorders, 27*, 178–187.

Smith, A. (1999). Stuttering: A unified approach to a multifactorial, dynamic disorder. In N. Bernstein Ratner & E. C. Healey (Eds.), *Stuttering research and practice: Bridging the gap* (pp. 27–44). Mahwah, NJ: Erlbaum.

Smith, A., & Weber, C. (2016). Childhood stuttering: Where are we and where are we going? *Seminars in Speech and Language, 37*, 291–297.

Smith, A., & Weber, C. (2017). How stuttering develops: The multifactorial dynamic pathways theory. *Journal of Speech, Language, and Hearing Research, 60*, 2483–2505.

St. Louis, K. O., & Durrenberger, C. H. (1993). What communication disorders do experienced clinicians prefer to manage? *ASHA, 35*, 23–31.

Starkweather, C. W. (1987). *Fluency and stuttering*. Englewood Cliffs, NJ: Prentice-Hall.

Yaruss, J. S., & Quesal, R.W. (2002) Academic and clinical education in fluency disorders: An update. *Journal of Fluency Disorders, 27*, 43–63.

Weber-Fox, C., & Smith, A. (2014, Summer). Update from Purdue. *Stuttering Foundation of America Newsletter.* Retrieved from http://www.stutteringhelp.org/update-purdue

Yairi, E., & Ambrose, N. (1992). A longitudinal study of stuttering in children: A preliminary report. *Journal of Speech and Hearing Research, 35*, 755–760.

CHAPTER 2

How the Brain Influences the Cognitive, Emotional, and Motor Aspects of Stuttering

Jennifer Kleinow

"Movement is both how we move and what moves us. Movement is the look in our eyes, the tensions and the tone in our muscles, our breathing, our thinking, our longings and fears."
—Keith Bain, *The Principles of Movement*

Stuttering theorists have long included emotional factors as having predisposing and moderating roles in stuttering (Bloodstein & Bernstein Ratner, 2008). For example, early theories correlated stuttering with classically conditioned negative speaking responses (Brutten & Shoemaker, 1971), while current theories posit that emotional activity is one factor among many that contribute to the disorder (Arenas, 2016; Conture et al., 2006; Smith, 1999; Smith & Weber, 2017). Examining the role of emotion in stuttering has been a challenge for generations of researchers and clinicians. While stuttering treatments that include emotional components continue to gain acceptance, it is surprisingly difficult to find simple answers to pivotal questions such as:

- How are emotions generated?
- Is it possible that emotion could affect speech processes, and if so how? What is the role of emotion in stuttering?
- Should improvements in fluency be expected when therapy focuses on emotion? Why or why not?

While clear-cut answers to these questions might not presently exist, a deep study of how emotion might affect all aspects of fluency seems to be a timely and paramount task. The purpose of this chapter is to begin this conversation—to describe the complex neural systems involved in human emotion, to theorize about the potential role of emotion in the onset and maintenance of stuttering, and to discuss how knowledge of this intricate relationship may contribute to successful models for improved treatment outcomes.

CLASSIC EMOTION THEORIES CAN INFORM THERAPY

How are emotions generated? General theories of emotion have long linked awareness of feelings with non-voluntary changes in physical activity. Although most introductory psychology books present general theories of emotion thoroughly (e.g., Gazzaniga, Ivry, & Mangun,

2014), I believe that introducing these theories is the best place to start when attempting to connect one complex neural behavior (emotion) to another (stuttering). In fact, no chapter concerning human emotion would be complete without introducing William James, the nineteenth-century philosopher, physician, and psychologist who articulated one of the first theories of emotional processing in humans. Rather than restate conventional wisdom that human feelings trigger physiological responses (e.g., a man feels scared, and then his heart begins to race), James proposed the converse: Emotion arises only after the sensation of physiological responses. He elaborated that emotion is the product of three distinct events. First, a person perceives an emotional stimulus, which is then followed by a physiological reaction. Finally, the cognitive system detects the physiological reactions and responds with feelings of fear, happiness, anger, and so forth (James, 1884). Lange, an intellectual peer, proposed a similar theory and together these ideas became known as the James-Lange theory of emotion. Using their model, James and Lange concluded that an emotion requires information generated by somatic activity, and would not occur without it.

Cannon and his colleague Bard criticized the James-Lange theory on two counts. First, they believed that physiological reactions were too generalized to be interpreted as specific emotions. Heart rate, for example, could increase if a person saw a snake, got into an argument, or fell in love. Second, they believed that emotions could be experienced even without awareness of bodily reactions. They supported their theory with studies documenting that decerebrate animals (in which connections to the cortex are severed, prohibiting awareness of physiologic reactions) still exhibited rage responses when provoked (Bard, 1934). While they did not dispute the idea that emotions are a product of three events (stimulus perception, physical reaction, cognitive appraisal), they proposed that the physical reaction and cognitive appraisal could occur concurrently instead of serially as James and Lange had proposed.

These theories were modified still by Schacter and Singer (1962), who famously administered adrenaline to three groups of research participants to test how people assign emotions to perceived changes in physical state. The researchers informed one group that they had taken adrenaline and to expect secondary physiological symptoms such as a racing heart. Another group was told that they had been given adrenaline and to expect only vague side effects, and a third group was told that they had received vitamins. A fourth group received a placebo and served as a control. After placebo or drug administration, all groups then interacted with confederates who displayed either joy or anger. Participants who knew the reason for their physical symptoms were not affected by the scene, but the experimental groups attributed their sudden racing heart to their joyful or angry environment. Schacter and Singer essentially qualified a condition in the work of Cannon and Bard—not only do physiological signals of the body get simultaneously appraised by the cognitive system, but the way we appraise the physiological signals is by actively interpreting our environmental cues. Barrett (2006) adds that language, culture, and previous life experiences also influence emotion appraisal.

Working within these classic theories, we might already be able to see their utility in fluency therapy. For example, it might be important to explain any physiological changes a client notices during speech production, so the speaker does not associate the physiological responses with a negative emotion. We could also examine environments that might lead to misattribution of emotional cues during speaking.

Recently developed theories of emotions can highlight even more interesting perspectives on stuttering development and treatment. Not only can cognitive neuroscientists further refine traditional models of emotion, but now new models can be explored and tested using neuroimaging and other brain research techniques. Joseph LeDoux and colleagues, for example, have been studying the neural systems for emotion, primarily fear, from a cognitive science perspective for decades. LeDoux and Brown (2017) put forward the hypothesis that the human emotional system is not one but two distinct neural systems. The first system, which LeDoux and Brown now refer to as a survival system, is innately hardwired to allow all animals to quickly avoid or approach stimuli in a way that is evolutionarily beneficial. The second system functions much more slowly as it creates a rich cognitive appraisal of the stimulus and generates conscious feelings. To illustrate, we have probably all jumped back in fear after seeing a large insect in our path, and then breathed a sigh of relief when we realized the "insect" was nothing more than a stone. Jumping back with a racing heart was the safest, most life-protective action until we became consciously aware that the situation contained no real risks, and that *both* emotional systems functioned as intended in that event.

LeDoux and Brown (2017) elaborate that the conscious emotional system employs general cognitive systems such as attention and memory to construct conscious feelings. One interesting aspect of this view is that emotions can be generated in the absence of bodily sensations if only the conscious emotional system is activated. The conscious emotional system can generate feelings in the absence of emotional stimuli, such as when people express worry about things that have not happened, or about the impossible-to-be-known thoughts of other people. This hypothesis has important implications for stuttering treatments such as Cognitive-Behavioral Therapy, which may help ameliorate self-constructed worries.

CAN EMOTIONS AFFECT SPEECH PRODUCTION? A LOOK AT NEURAL PATHWAYS

Common to all general theories of emotion is the perception of an emotional stimulus, which generates a physical response and a feeling. But can a feeling affect physical movements? Can feelings affect speech production? For emotional processing to affect speech production generally and stuttering specifically, the brain's emotional system and motor system must be able to interact in some predictable way. To explore potential links between systems, I will present a simplified description of the emotional system circuitry, followed by the motor system circuitry. Finally, I will compare the two systems and highlight any areas of neural overlap.

First, some preliminary vocabulary terms may clarify the study of the emotional neural circuitry. The human brain has three primary divisions, the hindbrain, midbrain, and forebrain. The hindbrain controls the involuntary, basic functions of life such as breathing and blood circulation. The midbrain is responsible for arousal and wakefulness, and the forebrain is responsible for the most complex of human behaviors, including much of the processing for speech and language production. The forebrain can be divided further into cortical and subcortical structures. Regarding cortical structures, the outermost layer of the cortex, or neocortex, is the convoluted orb of gyri and sulci that is probably the first thing that comes to mind when imagining a human brain. If one separates the two hemispheres and peers internally at a sagittal section of the brain, the medial cortex, which hugs the internal border of the hemispheres, becomes visible. Subcortical areas are simply those that lie inferiorly to the cortex. Another common reference in neuroscience is the term "nucleus," which refers to a grouping of cell bodies that share processing function and connectivity. A nucleus is a busy processing center for cells that have similar functions, and many brain structures contain "nucleus" as part of their name.

After the perception of an emotional stimulus, emotional processing has two distinct outcomes: a physical response and a conscious feeling. The neural circuits involved in both components connect heavily to other systems (notably, attention and memory; Duncan & Barrett, 2007). To produce a physical response, we activate an evolutionarily beneficial system which responds to environmental stimuli in ways that will maintain an organism's well-being. Subcortical structures such as the amygdala, hypothalamus, and brainstem are the key players in this system, and their activation triggers simple, stereotyped responses to an emotional environmental signal.

Our sensory receptors begin this process by detecting environmental stimuli and then sending that information to the thalamus. In the fast, survival emotional system, the signals from the thalamus are routed directly to the amygdala. The amygdala is a complex structure with many distinct functional nuclei. The lateral nucleus coordinates emotional learning (LeDoux, 1992; Maren, 1999). The central nucleus is responsible for physiological reactivity such as autonomic arousal, hormonal secretion, and, in the case of fear, freezing and avoidance behaviors (Critchley, Mathias, & Dolan, 2002). Because of its premier role in emotional learning and behavioral response, many researchers devote book chapters to the examination of the amygdala's central role in fear conditioning. Finally, the amygdala can send signals downstream to the brainstem and hypothalamus (Critchley, Mathias, & Dolan, 2002). The hypothalamus coordinates somatic, visceral, and endocrine responses, while the brainstem coordinates simple rhythmic or stereotyped behaviors such as chewing, walking, and producing facial expression.

While we might imagine that most physiological changes are specific and localized (e.g., increased sweating in the palms, dilated pupils), activation of the survival circuit can also induce global changes in brain functioning. Heightened autonomic arousal, for example, increases alertness, vigilance, and sensitivity to other relevant stimuli and decreases other, non-related motivational behaviors (Lang, Bradley, & Cuthbert, 1997).

The pathway outlined above is quick and unconscious and provides only crude information about the nature of the stimulus and the actions the person must take to cope with it. A second emotional pathway also exists—one that involves the generation of emotion as a conscious experience. This pathway centers on the reciprocal connections between the amygdala and the cortex. In this pathway, both the thalamus and the amygdala project signals to the sensory cortex, potentially affecting perception and attention. The amygdala also projects to the lateral prefrontal cortex, anterior cingulate cortex, and orbital cortex, which all function in working memory and executive functioning. The prefrontal cortex appears to send signals back to the amygdala, providing the amygdala with updated information about the current environment (Phelps, Delgado, Nearing, & LeDoux, 2004). In other words, the brain can rely on knowledge of the current environment as well as memories of past experiences to generate a conscious feeling. The conscious emotional pathways share resources with other cognitive processes, such as attention, working memory, reinforcement, and motivation—leading LeDoux and Brown (2017) to conclude that emotional states are processed by a general cognitive processor, a higher-order brain system that creates consciousness for emotional and non-emotional states alike.

Finally, one brain structure that might be of theoretical and clinical importance in stuttering is the anterior cingulate cortex (ACC), which also receives signals from the amygdala. The cingulate gyrus sits atop the white curve of the corpus callosum, and the aptly named ACC is the most anterior portion of that gyrus. The functions of the ACC appear to be complex and varied, but it has demonstrable roles in cognition, emotional processing, and (summarized in the next section) motor control. Interestingly, the ACC functions in error detection (i.e., signaling when you make a mistake), response selection, selective attention, and motor planning (Paus, 2001). Most importantly, Bush, Luu, and Posner (2000), after conducting a meta-analysis of 64 functional neuroimaging studies, suggested that the ACC is a unique brain area likely to provide an interface between cognition and emotion.

NEURAL PATHWAYS FOR MOTOR CONTROL

Now that I have outlined the general neural pathways for emotion, I will describe the pathways involved in motor control. If one were to imagine the steps involved in voluntary movement, the routine might proceed in the following way. One needs to have the motivation to move as well as a motor plan before initiating a movement. Next, there must be some form of coordinated muscle contractions which result in the body movement. Additionally, the brain should make assurances that the movement is accurate and efficient. These procedural steps map onto neural structures and pathways and are relatively simple to outline.

The supplementary motor and premotor areas are responsible for planning and preparing complex movement sequences. The supplementary motor area is active even before electrical activity in muscles can be observed (Tanji, Taniguichi, & Saga, 1980). The premotor area is appropriately named, as it structurally sits anteriorly to the motor area and its activity precedes that of the motor area. Mirror neurons in this region respond to the observation of movements, possibly indicating a role in social behavior and communication (Rizzolatti & Arbib, 1998). Both the supplementary motor and premotor areas receive modifying input from the prefrontal cortex, which, as indicated in the previous section, is believed to be involved in planning, attention, working memory, decision making, and emotional processing. The ACC has regions that are involved in attention and emotional regulation, but posterior regions control and plan movements, especially complex or novel behaviors that require cognitive control (Paus, Petrides, Evans, & Meyer, 1993). The ACC also appears to have a pivotal role in response selection (Milham et al., 2001) and error detection (Carter et al., 1998).

The supplementary area, premotor area, and ACC project to the primary motor cortex, which generates simple movement commands. These movement commands are modified by the cerebellum and basal ganglia to produce smooth, accurate movements. Descending pathways ultimately connect motor neurons to muscle fibers, activation of which results in muscle contraction.

CAN EMOTIONS AFFECT SPEECH PRODUCTION? FINDING COMMON GROUND

It seems intuitive that emotion can affect voluntary behaviors. A star athlete who chokes at the free throw line, a person of poor physique who suddenly runs quickly to the aid of a stranger, an artist who gestures wildly in front of an audience—all are anecdotal evidence of emotions changing (or being expressed in) action. But how are emotions and motor behaviors linked? Could emotions be related to stuttering, and, if so, by what mechanism? Zhu and Thagard (2002) speculate that the neural interface between emotion and motor control takes place in the brain regions that are common to both circuits. In other words, which brain structures are common to both the emotional system and the motor system? Certainly, there could be neural "cross talk" in those areas.

Outlining these interactions, if they exist, would require much more intellectual devotion than one book chapter could provide. But I would like to discuss two examples, one from the emotional survival circuit and one from the conscious cortical emotional circuit, to theorize about how the human brain might facilitate the potential interactions between emotional and motor circuits during speaking.

Evidence from the Survival Circuit: Arousal and Motor Control

Extrapolating from the literature on general motor control, one might expect that increases in arousal affect speech motor control, possibly secondary to changes in muscle activation (Coombes, Cauraugh, & Janelle, 2006) and other movement parameters (Hälbig et al., 2011). To infer effects of arousal on the speech motor system, we need to measure autonomic nervous system (ANS) activity simultaneously with speech behavior observations. We do know that simply the act of speaking is associated with increased autonomic responses (Baldwin & Clevenger, 1980; Brondolo, Karlin, Alexander, Bobrow, & Schwartz, 1999; Friedmann, Thomas, Kulick-Ciuffo, Lynch, & Suginohara, 1982; Long, Lynch, Machiran, Thomas, & Malinow, 1982; Lynch et al., 1980). Arnold, MacPherson, and Smith (2014) reported that both children and adults demonstrated higher arousal for speech compared with non-speech tasks, with boys showing higher arousal than girls during narrative tasks. While speaking can produce increases in arousal, increases in arousal can modify speech movements in typical speakers. For example, Kleinow and Smith (2006) found that lip movement kinematics were more variable in both adults and children under experimental conditions designed to increase autonomic arousal during speech production.

Researchers have also explored the role of autonomic arousal in stuttering. In a study of 24 adults who stutter and 24 matched typically fluent controls, Peters and Hulstijn (1984) investigated possible differences between adults who do and do not stutter during the anticipatory period before the performance of motor, cognitive, and speech tasks. All participants performed four tasks: reading, conversation, mirror writing, and a task from an intelligence test. They collected arousal measures (electrodermal activity, digital pulse volume, heart rate) during task anticipation, performance, and recovery. Regarding autonomic variables, adults who do and do not stutter did not show autonomic differences during rest, task anticipation, task performance, or immediately following the tasks. Both groups of speakers showed higher heart rate, pulse volume, and electrodermal activity before and during speech tasks than the cognitive and motor tasks.

Weber and Smith (1990) observed similar results. They measured several autonomic variables in 19 adults who stutter and 19 matched controls. All participants were asked to perform non-speech jaw movements, a Valsalva maneuver (holding breath forcefully), reading, and spontaneous speech. Blood pulse volume, skin conductance response, and heart rate were recorded before, during, and after the performance of each task. None of the autonomic measures showed group effects during the baseline or the various intervals around the experimental tasks. For adults who stutter, larger increases in autonomic responses were observed before, during, and after disfluent speech. Like Peters and Hulstijn (1984), Weber and Smith (1990) concluded that speaking is associated with relatively large increases in autonomic activity for both adults who do and do not stutter and that people who stutter did not have overall higher levels of ANS activity compared with their typically fluent peers. They suggested that adults who stutter, however, might be vulnerable to breakdowns in motor processes because speech production typically increases sympathetic arousal.

Zengin-Bolatkale, Conture, and Walden (2015) recorded somewhat similar results in preschool children. Overall, preschool children who stutter did not differ significantly from preschoolers who do not stutter in baseline skin conductance levels. Both groups of children showed increased skin conductance activity during a rapid picture naming task, and there were no overall group effects of picture naming on skin conductance level. When broken down by age group, only the youngest preschoolers who stutter (3-year-olds) showed skin conductance levels higher than their peers on the picture naming task. Taking these results broadly, we may conclude that speech production produces increases in autonomic activity in both children and adults, and that speech production can be affected by arousal. However, adults and children who stutter do not seem to exhibit autonomic response level ranges that are different from their matched peers.

Evidence from the Conscious Cognitive Circuit: Anterior Cingulate Cortex and Motor Control

The subcortical survival circuit carries the largest responsibility for activating the autonomic nervous system, which increases arousal. Although arousal levels do not appear to be different in people who stutter compared with their typically fluent peers, as discussed in the previous section, we can look to higher-order brain areas/circuits that might be more fruitful in establishing an emotion/motor control link. Parallel to choosing arousal as one example from the survival circuit as in the previous section, I'll provide an example from the conscious cognitive circuit to study: the ACC.

As previously mentioned, the anterior cingulate cortex is activated by emotional, attentional, error detection, behavioral regulation, and motor functions (see Allman, Hakeem, Erwin, Nimchinsky, & Hof, 2001 for review). Regarding speech production, studies of ACC activation during speech have led to fascinating results. For example, Fu et al. (2002) conducted a functional (f)MRI study in which healthy volunteers were asked to perform a word generation task. Each participant was given a letter and asked to produce a word out loud that began with that letter. The researchers had categorized the letters as "easy" or "difficult" based on verbal fluency performance in previous studies. The researchers found that participants made more mistakes in word fluency during the difficult letter prompt task and that the ACC was more active in the difficult task. The authors suggested that ACC activity was correlated with likelihood to retrieve inappropriate verbal responses. Likewise, Thothathiri, Rattinger, and Trivedi (2017) found the ACC to be more active in sentence compared with word generation, and to be more active under conditions of greater phonological competition.

Many imaging studies implicate the ACC in stuttering, including at least one meta-analysis (Brown, Ingham, Ingham, Laird, & Fox, 2005). Results from this meta-analysis indicated that the disfluent speech of adults who stutter was associated with increased brain activation in motor areas, including the ACC, when compared with the fluent speech of adults who do not stutter. The meta-analysis included the work of De Nil, Kroll, Kapur, and Houle (2000), who found increased activation of the left ACC in adults who stutter during silent reading and single word production. Additionally, Braun et al. (1997) observed changes in lateralization of

ACC activity between adults who stutter and fluent controls. Using a different approach and level of analysis, Arnstein, Lakey, Compton, and Kleinow (2011) measured evoked response potentials in adults who do and do not stutter in a cognitively challenging word rhyming task designed to induce frequent error responses. They found that adults who stutter exhibited a larger amplitude of error-related negativity, generated by the ACC, in rhyming tasks even in the absence of overt errors. Using MRI, Liu et al. (2014) also found differences in ACC activity between adults who do and do not stutter. Chang et al. (2017) aggregated 224 high-quality resting state fMRI scans from 22 children who stutter and an equal number of typically fluent controls and found differences in connectivity patterns in children who stutter in brain regions referred to as the default mode network, which includes the posterior cingulate cortex. These researchers found widespread connectivity differences between children who do and do not stutter. Finally, O'Neil et al. (2017), using proton magnetic resonance spectroscopy to trace chemical uptakes in the brain, found similar results. Their study also revealed brain differences for adults who stutter in speech motor, default mode networks, and emotional memory networks. Across all of these studies, we can conclude that situational, affective, and attentional factors contribute to the onset and maintenance of stuttering.

SHOULD WE EXPECT FLUENCY GAINS WHEN THERAPY FOCUSES ON EMOTION?

When I think about evidence-based practice, I naturally look to published studies of treatment efficacy, as well as to the informed clinical opinions of my colleagues and personal experience reports from clients. Ultimately, though, I strive to find practice techniques that make theoretical sense. The big question, then, is whether it makes sense to work on emotional aspects of stuttering as a therapeutic target. Can this (at least theoretically) help improve speech production? How can theories of emotion generation and knowledge of emotional/motor neural systems be used clinically?

Based on the findings presented in this chapter, there does seem to be evidence that emotional processing can affect speech motor control. But when comparing the two emotional circuits (survival versus cognitive conscious), at least from the limited examples I have provided, it appears more likely that emotion affects fluent speech production through the workings of the conscious cognitive circuit than through the lower survival circuits. Recent work by Choi, Conture, Walden, Jones, and Kim (2016) supports this theory. These researchers studied 47 young children who stutter and compared emotional reactivity, tonic skin conductance level, and disfluency rates after neutral, positive, and negative emotional movie clips. While positive emotional reactivity (most likely related to higher cortical emotional structures) was related to disfluency measures across all tasks, tonic skin conductance level (most likely related to survival circuits) was not predictive of stuttering. I speculate that treatment approaches that deal with the more cognitive aspects of emotion (including, but not limited to, Acceptance and Commitment Therapy, Cognitive Behavioral Therapy, etc.) may prove to have better outcomes on reducing the motor load in people who stutter than therapies strictly focused on reducing autonomic responses.

It would be theoretically interesting to test how cognitive appraisals of one's speaking environment are manifest in neural changes, particularly in both emotion and motor systems. Not only do the motor system and conscious cortical systems share brain circuitry, but at least one area of study (the ACC) has been shown to have functional differences in adults who stutter during speaking and linguistic tasks. This is not to say that stuttering "resides in" or is caused by the ACC. Rather, the ACC is part of a highly connected neural network that provides an interface between conscious emotion and motor control. Other overlapping pathways may prove to be equally interesting in the development of stuttering in children (Smith & Weber, 2017).

Because the ACC also has roles in executive functioning, attention, behavior regulation, and error monitoring, it becomes even more compelling to view stuttering as a multifactorial disorder. It becomes clear that each contributing factor presented in the various multifactorial models is expressly testable as it relates to fluency. But, more importantly, observed links between the conscious emotional system and fluency document the call for multifactorial treatment designs, including all treatment approaches that include a cognitive, social, and emotional component. Finally, I should also stress that this chapter focuses on the relationship between emotions and motor control specifically. Research and clinical treatments that focus on the relationship between emotions and overall communicative success, or overall well-being, are also incredibly important. Many upcoming chapters in this volume speak to cognitive, social, and emotional stuttering treatments—all positive communication approaches which would be supported based on current research studies connecting higher-level emotion centers to stuttering.

REFERENCES

Allman, J. M., Hakeem, A., Erwin, J. M., Nimchinsky, E., & Hof, P. (2001). The anterior cingulate cortex. *Annals of the New York Academy of Sciences*, *935*(1), 107–117.

Arenas, R. M. (2016). Conceptualizing and investigating the contextual variability of stuttering: The Speech and Monitoring Interaction (SAMI) framework. *Speech, Language and Hearing*, *20*, 1–14.

Arnold, H. S., MacPherson, M. K., & Smith, A. (2014). Autonomic correlates of speech versus nonspeech tasks in children and adults. *Journal of Speech, Language, and Hearing Research*, *57*, 1296–1307.

Arnstein, D., Lakey, B., Compton, R. J., & Kleinow, J. (2011). Preverbal error-monitoring in stutterers and fluent speakers. *Brain and Language*, *116*, 105–115.

Baldwin, S. F., & Clevenger, T. (1980). Effect of speakers' sex and size of audience on heart-rate changes during short impromptu speeches. *Psychological Reports*, *46*, 123–130.

Bard, P. (1934). On emotional expression after decortication with some remarks on certain theoretical views: Part I. *Psychological Review*, *41*(4), 309–329.

Barrett, L. F. (2006). Solving the emotion paradox: Categorization and the experience of emotion. *Personality and Social Psychology Review*, *10*, 20–46.

Bloodstein, O., & Bernstein Ratner, N. (2008). *A handbook on stuttering* (6th ed.). Clifton Park, NY: Thomson-Delmar.

Braun, A. R., Varga, M., Stager, S., Schulz, G., Selbie, S., Maisog, J. M., . . . & Ludlow, C. L. (1997). Altered patterns of cerebral activity during speech and language production in developmental stuttering. An H_2 (^{15}) O positron emission tomography study. *Brain*, *120*(5), 761–784.

Brondolo, E., Karlin, W., Alexander, K., Bobrow, A., & Schwartz, J. (1999). Workday communication and ambulatory blood pressure: Implications for the reactivity hypothesis. *Psychophysiology*, *36*, 86–94.

Brown, S., Ingham, R. J., Ingham, J. C., Laird, A. R., & Fox, P. T. (2005). Stuttered and fluent speech production: An ALE meta-analysis of functional neuroimaging studies. *Human Brain Mapping*, *25*(1), 105–117.

Brutten, G. J., & Shoemaker, D. J. (1971). A two-factor learning theory of stuttering. In L. E. Travis (Ed.), *Handbook of speech pathology and audiology* (pp. 1035–1072). New York, NY: Appleton-Century-Crofts.

Bush, G., Luu, P., & Posner, M. I. (2000). Cognitive and emotional influences in anterior cingulate cortex. *Trends in Cognitive Sciences, 4*(6), 215–222.

Carter, C. S., Braver, T. S., Barch, D. M., Botvinick, M. M., Noll, D., & Cohen, J. D. (1998). Anterior cingulate cortex, error detection, and the online monitoring of performance. *Science, 280*(5364), 747–749.

Chang, S. E., Angstadt, M., Chow, H., Etchell, A. C., Garnett, E. O., Choo, A., . . . Sripada, C. (2017). Anomalous network architecture of the resting brain in children who stutter. *Journal of Fluency Disorders*. Advance online publication. doi:10.1016/j.jfludis.2017.01.002

Choi, D., Conture, E. G., Walden, T. A., Jones, R. M., & Kim, H. (2016). Emotional diathesis, emotional stress, and childhood stuttering. *Journal of Speech, Language, and Hearing Research, 59*(4), 616–630.

Conture, E. G., Walden, T., Graham, C., Arnold, H., Hartfield, H., & Karrass, J. (2006). Communication-emotional model of stuttering. In N. Bernstein Ratner & J. Tetnowski (Eds.), *Stuttering research and practice: Contemporary issues and approaches* (pp. 17–46). Mahwah, NJ: Erlbaum.

Coombes, S. A., Cauraugh, J. H., & Janelle, C. M. (2006). Emotion and movement: Activation of defensive circuitry alters the magnitude of a sustained muscle contraction. *Neuroscience Letters, 396*(3), 192–196.

Critchley H. D., Mathias C. J., & Dolan R. J. (2002). Fear conditioning in humans: The influence of awareness and autonomic arousal on functional neuroanatomy. *Neuron, 33*, 653–663.

De Nil, L. F., Kroll, R. M., Kapur, S., & Houle, S. (2000). A positron emission tomography study of silent and oral single word reading in stuttering and nonstuttering adults. *Journal of Speech, Language, and Hearing Research, 43*, 1038–1053.

Duncan, S., & Barrett, L. F. (2007). Affect is a form of cognition: A neurobiological analysis. *Cognition and Emotion, 21*(6), 1184–1211.

Friedmann, E., Thomas, S. A., Kulick-Ciuffo, D., Lynch, J. J., & Suginohara, M. (1982). The effects of normal and rapid speech on blood pressure. *Psychosomatic Medicine, 44*, 545–553.

Fu, C. H., Morgan, K., Suckling, J., Williams, S. C., Andrew, C., Vythelingum, G. N., & Mc-Guire, P. K. (2002). A functional magnetic resonance imaging study of overt letter verbal fluency using a clustered acquisition sequence: Greater anterior cingulate activation with increased task demand. *Neuroimage, 17*(2), 871–879.

Gazzaniga, M. S., Ivry, R. B., & Mangun, G. R. (2014). *Cognitive neuroscience: The biology of the mind* (4th ed.). New York, NY: W. W. Norton.

Hälbig, T. D., Borod, J. C., Frisina, P. G., Tse, W., Voustianiouk, A., Olanow, C. W., & Gracies, J. M. (2011). Emotional processing affects movement speed. *Journal of Neural Transmission, 118*(9), 1319–1322.

James, W. (1884). What is an emotion? *Mind, 9*, 188–205.

Kleinow, J., & Smith, A. (2006). Potential interactions among linguistic, autonomic, and motor factors in speech. *Developmental Psychobiology, 48*(4), 275–287.

Lang, P. J., Bradley, M. M., & Cuthbert, B. N. (1997). Motivated attention: Affect, activation, and action. In P. Lang, R. Simons, & M. Balaban (Eds.), *Attention and orienting: Sensory and motivational processes* (pp. 97–135). Hillsdale, NJ: Erlbaum.

LeDoux, J. E. (1992). Brain mechanisms of emotion and emotional learning. *Current Opinion in Neurobiology, 2*(2), 191–197.

LeDoux, J. E., & Brown, R. (2017). A higher-order theory of emotional consciousness. *Proceedings of the National Academy of Sciences, 114*(10), E2016–E2025.

Liu, J., Wang, Z., Huo, Y., Davidson, S. M., Klahr, K., Herder, C. L., . . . & Peterson, B. S. (2014). A functional imaging study of self-regulatory capacities in persons who stutter. *PloS One, 9*(2), e89891.

Long, J. M., Lynch, J. J., Machiran, N. M., Thomas, S. A., & Malinow, K. L. (1982). The effect of status on blood pressure during verbal communication. *Journal of Behavioral Medicine, 5*, 165–172.

Lynch, J. J., Thomas, S. A., Long, J. M., Malinow, K. L, Chickadonz, G., & Katcher, A. H. (1980). Human speech and blood pressure. *Journal of Nervous and Mental Disease, 168*, 526–534.

Maren, S. (1999). Long-term potentiation in the amygdala: A mechanism for emotional learning and memory. *Trends in Neurosciences, 22*(12), 561–567.

Milham, M. P., Banich, M. T., Webb, A., Barad, V., Cohen, N. J., Wszalek, T., & Kramer, A. F. (2001). The relative involvement of anterior cingulate and prefrontal cortex in attentional control depends on nature of conflict. *Cognitive Brain Research, 12*, 467–473.

O'Neill, J., Dong, Z., Bansal, R., Ivanov, I., Hao, X., Desai, J., . . . Peterson, B. S. (2017). Proton chemical shift imaging of the brain in pediatric and adult developmental stuttering. *JAMA Psychiatry, 74*(1), 85–94.

Paus, T. (2001). Primate anterior cingulate cortex: Where motor control, drive and cognition interface. *Nature Reviews Neuroscience, 2*(6), 417–424.

Paus, T., Petrides, M., Evas, A. C., & Meyer, E. (1993). Role of the human anterior cingulate cortex in the control of oculomotor, manual, and speech responses: A positron emission tomography study. *Journal of Neurophysiology, 70*, 1–18.

Peters, H. F. M., & Hulstijn, W. (1984). Stuttering and anxiety: The difference between stutterers and nonstutterers in verbal apprehension and physiologic arousal during the anticipation of speech and non-speech tasks. *Journal of Fluency Disorders, 9*, 67–84.

Phelps, E. A., Delgado, M. R., Nearing, K. I., & LeDoux, J. E. (2004). Extinction learning in humans: Role of the amygdala and vmPFC. *Neuron, 43*(6), 897–905.

Rizzolatti, G., & Arbib, M. A. (1998). Language within our grasp. *Trends in Neurosciences, 21*, 188–194.

Schachter, S., & Singer, J. (1962). Cognitive, social, and physiological determinants of emotional state. *Psychological Review, 69*(5), 379–399.

Smith, A. (1999). Stuttering: A unified approach to a multifactorial, dynamic disorder. In N. Bernstein Ratner & E. C. Healey (Eds.), *Stuttering research and practice: Bridging the gap* (pp. 27–44). Mahwah, NJ: Erlbaum.

Smith, A., & Weber, C. (2017). How stuttering develops: The multifactorial dynamic pathways theory. *Journal of Speech, Language, and Hearing Research, 60*, 2483–2505.

Tanji, J., Taniguchi, K., & Saga, T. (1980). Supplementary motor area: Neuronal response to motor instructions. *Journal of Neurophysiology, 43*, 60–68.

Thothathiri, M., Rattinger, M., & Trivedi, B. (2017). Cognitive control during sentence generation. *Cognitive Neuroscience, 8*(1), 39–49.

Weber, C. M., & Smith, A. (1990). Autonomic correlates of stuttering and speech assessed in a range of experimental tasks. *Journal of Speech and Hearing Research, 33*, 690–706.

Zengin-Bolatkale, H., Conture, E. G., & Walden, T. A. (2015). Sympathetic arousal of young children who stutter during a stressful picture naming task. *Journal of Fluency Disorders, 46*, 24–40.

Zhu, J., & Thagard, P. (2002). Emotion and action. *Philosophical Psychology, 15*(1), 19–36.

CHAPTER 3

The Importance of Self-Efficacy for Individuals Who Stutter

Michael P. Boyle

INTRODUCTION

Self-efficacy theory has been and continues to be one of the most heavily documented and discussed concepts in the field of psychology. The principle of self-efficacy was developed as part of a larger theory, called Social Cognitive Theory, and presents a model in which human behavior is shaped by environmental and personal factors. The essence of self-efficacy theory is that personal agency plays an important role in determining behavior and that individuals can exercise power over life events, rather than viewing human behavior as being totally shaped by one's environment and external reinforcement or punishment. The concept of self-efficacy is extremely relevant to a discussion of the nature, evaluation, and treatment of the communication disorder of stuttering. This is because a stuttering disorder is a complex multidimensional disorder with physical, behavioral, social, cognitive, and affective elements. An integrative and interactional model is necessary to account for the complexity of stuttering and its clinical management, and self-efficacy theory provides a suitable lens through which the disorder can be examined. This chapter discusses the relevance of self-efficacy to the disorder of stuttering and its clinical management. I first review the construct of self-efficacy and its place in social cognitive theory in detail. I believe that it will be beneficial for the reader to have a nuanced understanding of the construct of self-efficacy before proceeding to descriptions of how it is relevant for people who stutter (PWS), which is why I spend the first third of this chapter explaining it in depth. Then, I discuss the relevance of self-efficacy in the understanding and management of a stuttering disorder, including a review of empirical research on the topic. I conclude with recommendations for integrating aspects of self-efficacy theory with the assessment and treatment of stuttering.

OVERVIEW OF SELF-EFFICACY AND SOCIAL COGNITIVE THEORY

Self-efficacy is one of the most extensively researched principles in the field of psychology. It is a concept that has impacted many areas of study across the world. The prominent psychologist Albert Bandura is credited with developing a comprehensive theory of self-efficacy and documenting it as a major influence in human behavior. Bandura explained that "perceived self-efficacy refers to beliefs in one's capabilities to organize and execute the courses of action required to manage prospective situations" (1995, p. 2). In essence, self-efficacy refers to people's beliefs that they are important agents for determining life circumstances and outcomes. Perceived ability to control valued outcomes has advantages in many areas of life. Conversely, perceived inability to control adverse events contributes to negative psychological states. According to Bandura, the need for individuals to feel like they have some control over their functioning and circumstances provides a strong rationale for the discussion of how human beings can develop and exercise personal control and efficacy.

The notion of self-efficacy was presented by Bandura (1977a) as part of a larger theory, called social-cognitive theory (SCT), which attempted to explain the various factors that influence human functioning and goal attainment. This theory was presented by Bandura to address perceived limitations in psychoanalytic and behavioral models. Bandura believed that pure behaviorism, with its emphasis on unidirectional environmental determinism, was limited in its explanatory power. The psychoanalytic approach, on the other hand, appeared to place all emphasis on personal factors to the exclusion of relevant environmental influences. Bandura's SCT addressed these limitations by proposing an interactional model which describes the effects of cognitive, behavioral, personal, and environmental factors on human behavior and goal attainment. Figure 3–1 provides an illustration of these concepts. A simple illustration of this model is to consider the example of how academic performance (behavioral factors) is influenced by how students are impacted cognitively and affectively (personal factors) by school conditions and instructional strategies of teachers (environmental factors).

In his SCT, Bandura explained that behavior change and goal attainment are not just accomplished through sheer will power,

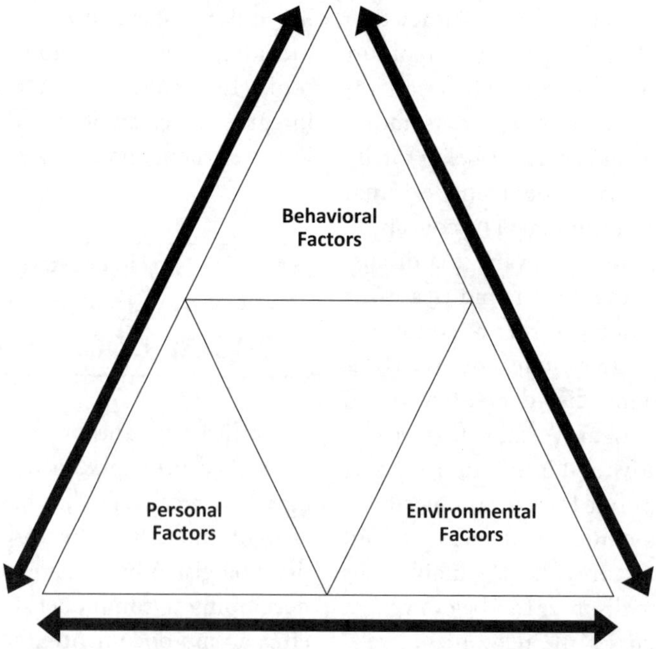

Figure 3–1. Bandura's model of triadic reciprocal determinism for human functioning. *Source:* Adapted from Bandura (1997).

but rather through several self-regulatory skills including self-observation, self-evaluation, self-reaction, and self-efficacy. In other words, to achieve durable and meaningful behavior change, individuals need to monitor and observe the behaviors to be changed, set achievable goals that would guide and motivate them to change, and enlist the help of social supports to motivate and sustain their efforts. Importantly, a sense of efficacy is needed in this process because individuals who obtain skills but do not have a strong belief in their ability to change will be more likely to abandon those skills when faced with challenges or when desired results are not obtained quickly. According to Bandura, SCT improved upon psychoanalytic and behavioral theories by increasing the need for client action as one of the most powerful determinants of personal change. Individuals need to develop skills that would enable them to influence their own behaviors and motivations. SCT represents the accumulation and integration of various health promotion models that have been developed over the years. The informational model of behavior change, which focused on imparting knowledge and changing attitudes, was later augmented by self-regulatory skills to increase personal efficacy, and then expanded further to discuss enlisting social supports in one's community as vital for personal change. Bandura's SCT attempts to integrate these various factors and demonstrate that human behavior and goal attainment can be influenced by various combinations of behavioral, personal, and environmental factors.

Before proceeding further, it is important to clarify that self-efficacy is not the same thing as self-esteem, although the two may be closely related. Self-esteem refers to global feelings of self-worth (i.e., how a person feels about him/herself in general), whereas self-efficacy is thought to be task or behavior specific. Surely, feelings of personal self-efficacy in certain tasks can contribute to overall feelings of positive self-esteem. However, the two can indeed operate separately. For example, an individual may have a very high sense of self-efficacy for a task that carries very little personal meaning or fulfillment, and therefore this would not contribute to a higher sense of self-esteem. In addition, a person can have beliefs of low self-efficacy for certain tasks that are not highly valued by the person subjectively, and still maintain an overall positive sense of self-esteem. It is also important to distinguish between self-efficacy and outcome expectancy. Outcome expectations are beliefs that certain behaviors will lead to certain outcomes. Efficacy expectations are beliefs that one can successfully execute behaviors that will result in particular outcomes. These two concepts need to be differentiated because individuals may recognize that given behaviors lead to certain expected outcomes; however, if they have serious doubts about their abilities to perform those behaviors, they will not be as motivated to modify that behavior. If self-efficacy belief and outcome expectation differ, it is likely that self-efficacy belief will have a greater impact on behavior.

Bandura (1977b) also specified several dimensions of self-efficacy that could have important implications for performance. Efficacy expectations can vary in *magnitude*, that is, efficacy may be high in certain individuals for only simple tasks, whereas in other individuals they can extend to the most difficult tasks. Efficacy expectations can also vary in *generality*, meaning that some experiences engender a more generalized sense of efficacy, whereas others may produce more situation-specific effects. Also, expectancies can vary depending on *strength*, meaning that some individuals may have weak expectations of success which are easily attenuated in the face of challenges, whereas strong expectations will be more likely to last in the face of adversity. Bandura (1977b) also acknowledges that efficacy expectation is not the sole cause of behavior. For example, expectation without acquisition of requisite skills will not produce desired performance. Also, individuals with skills and efficacy beliefs may not perform certain behaviors if they lack the motivation or desire to do so. Still, Bandura's theory emphasizes that when appropriate skills and incentives are acquired, self-efficacy beliefs can be a major contributor to decisions regarding what activities to pursue, how much effort will be expended in pursuit of those activities, and how long people will persist in their efforts when facing adverse circumstances and life stresses.

Sources of Perceived Self-Efficacy

There are several information sources in one's environment that contribute to a sense of self-efficacy. Bandura (1994) describes these sources as mastery experiences, vicarious experiences, social persuasion, and physiological and emotional states. Importantly, certain methods or modes of treatment for creating behavior change can expose an individual to these sources of information, whereas other methods are more limited in the opportunities they provide for acquiring information about self-efficacy. In addition, these different sources can be related and combined so that they enhance the other aspects.

Mastery experiences, sometimes called *performance accomplishments*, are the single most influential in behavior change because they are based on personal experiences. Success begets success. People who have been successful in certain endeavors will develop a strong sense of efficacy in those activities. Conversely, failures will undermine that sense of efficacy. This is especially true if the failures occur before a strong sense of efficacy has been established through earlier successes. However, failures will not always lead to reduced self-efficacy. In fact, persevering and succeeding after experiencing failures can actually increase perceived self-efficacy and resilience by demonstrating that individuals have what it takes to succeed even in the face of adversity. In contrast, if individuals experience only easy and quick successes, they might be more discouraged by a later failure. Hence, the effect of success and failure on perceptions of efficacy depend on many factors, including the timing of these events and the context in which they are experienced. In general, however, if individuals have performed a task well in the past, they expect that they can perform well in the future. This belief can also generalize to other situations and activities. In stuttering therapy, for example, it is incredibly important for clients who stutter to have experienced several instances of success in achieving a particular goal for increased self-efficacy and their belief that they can be successful at that task in the future.

The second source of information that can affect perceived self-efficacy is *vicarious experience*. Seeing other people perform activities and succeeding without experiencing feared consequences can lead people to believe that they can also perform those activities required to succeed. An observer may begin to believe "If he can do it, so can I." On the other hand, observing others fail despite high effort can decrease observers' judgments of self-efficacy. Vicarious experiences are thought to be less powerful than mastery experiences in which individuals achieve performance outcomes, and it would not be ideal for them to be used in isolation without mastery experiences. There are several variables that appear to enhance the effect of modeling behaviors. The more similar the model is to the observer, the more persuasive the model's successes or failure are perceived to be because of the perceived increased relevance of the information. Also, observers acquire more powerful efficacy beliefs if the model overcomes difficulties through determined and sustained effort, rather than if models appear highly naturally skilled and perform with ease. This is true because if models deal with temporary distress and anxiety and still overcome the problem, observers will feel that they can persevere as well. Modeling behaviors can provide the observer with a standard for comparison regarding skills and capabilities. Modeling can extend beyond behavior, however. A model who demonstrates the competencies that one aspires to can transfer ways of thinking and responding to external stressors. The observer can learn from the model's attitudes and values even if these were never intentionally transmitted. Of course, this means that clinician modeling is of critical importance in stuttering therapy. Clinicians can model the way they would like the client to behave, and how they view and react to environmental demands. Other PWS, whether they are fellow clients, friends, or support group members, can also model more adaptive ways of responding to stuttering.

Another way of strengthening people's self-efficacy beliefs is through *social persuasion*, also referred to as *verbal persuasion*. People who are persuaded verbally that they have what it takes to succeed in various activities are more likely to put forth sustained effort to achieve success and will not be as easily deterred by difficulties encountered. In raising people's efforts to try hard to accomplish a goal and succeed, self-efficacy can be promoted. These verbal persuasions can shift attention away from self-doubts or perceived deficiencies and therefore help individuals perform. Verbal persuasion is used frequently because it is relatively easy to provide. Still, it is not considered as influential as mastery experiences that provide evidence of one's own accomplishments. In fact, it is considered difficult to raise perceptions of self-efficacy with verbal persuasion alone. This is because efficacy expectations stemming from suggestions alone, especially if unrealistic, are quickly undermined by disconfirming experiences and lead to disappointment. Negative verbal persuasion (e.g., convincing people that they lack the capabilities and competencies to achieve a desired goal) results in the avoidance of that activity or the proclivity to give up quickly when faced with difficulties. Bandura (1994) stated that it is more difficult to instill beliefs of efficacy through verbal persuasion alone than it would be to undermine perceptions of efficacy through negative persuasion. Bandura emphasized that to develop efficacy in another person, more than verbal persuasions need to be used. Instead, it is of the utmost importance that situations are structured so that people can achieve successes and avoid situations in which they experience repeated failure. It is relatively simple to see how these principles would apply in stuttering therapy. It is critical for the clinician to verbally encourage the client and structure activities so that the client can experience success.

The last source of information that influences how people judge their capabilities is *somatic and emotional states*, also referred to as *emotional arousal*, or *physiological feedback*. People use how they feel physiologically and emotionally to gauge their capabilities in various situations. From a physiological standpoint, stress reactions and physical feelings of tension are often interpreted to mean that one will have difficulty performing successfully. Mood and emotions also impact perceptions of self-efficacy. Judgments of personal efficacy are increased with positive and optimistic moods; however, they are decreased in states of dejection or sadness. It is difficult for individuals to expect success when they are highly and aversively physiologically aroused and emotionally agitated. Therefore, beliefs of self-efficacy can also be altered by altering stress reactions, and more importantly, by changing how people interpret their physiological stress reactions. There have been many methods in the field of psychology that have been detailed for the purposes of lowering negative emotional reactions, including counterconditioning (replacing unhelpful emotional responses with more adaptive ones), extinction (weakening a conditioned response), discrimination learning (gaining awareness of cues that produce certain behaviors), and social imitation (imitation of someone else's behavior) (see Bandura, 1961, for a full review). The overarching goal in these types of approaches is to interrupt the cycle of negative emotions which generate negative thoughts and ultimately contribute to lack of competency in behavioral outcomes. This can be done using methods that focus on physical relaxation, or adjusting how individuals interpret or perceive physical or emotional states. For example, affective arousal can be perceived as debilitating or energizing, and therefore people can choose meanings that are conducive to successful performances. Addressing this domain is critical because increasing the belief that people can cope successfully in threatening situations is a very important aspect of self-efficacy. In stuttering therapy, there are many methods available for changing stress responses, increasing physical relaxation, and adjusting how clients interpret certain environmental stressors. These will be detailed later in the chapter.

Mechanisms of Change Related to Self-Efficacy

The preceding section discussed sources of self-efficacy; however, it is important to also discuss how that information is processed and transformed by individuals to shape beliefs of self-efficacy that regulate human functioning. Bandura (1995) described how efficacy beliefs are regulated through four major types of psychological processes, including cognitive, motivational, affective, and selection processes. Self-efficacy beliefs affect *cognitive processes* in a variety of ways. Much of human behavior is purposeful and based on pre-established goals that are motivated by personal values. Goal setting, however, is influenced by our self-appraisal of our own capabilities. If individuals have higher perceived self-efficacy, they will select more challenging goals and have a stronger sense of commitment to achieving them. In addition, many actions that individuals perform are preceded by thought patterns. People's efficacy beliefs influence how they visualize the action playing out. If efficacy beliefs are high, people anticipate successful scenarios, and if efficacy beliefs are low, people can dwell on the possibility of failure and things going wrong. Self-doubt can make it very difficult to achieve successful performance. Self-efficacy, then, helps in achieving the type of analytical thinking that contributes to successful performance. When people are faced with accomplishing tasks in the context of stressors or demanding circumstances, experiencing self-doubt can limit the quality of analytic thinking needed to complete the task. They in turn may lower their aspirations and a subsequent deterioration in performance results. On the other hand, if beliefs in self-efficacy are high, the person can remain task oriented in the face of stressful situations and use analytical thinking that will help in performance.

Motivational processes are also relevant because self-efficacy beliefs are very important for the regulation of motivation. People use forethought to motivate themselves, guide their actions, and form beliefs about what they can do. Setting goals, planning actions to achieve those goals, and gathering necessary resources for goal achievement are cognitive motivators. Self-efficacy influences causal attributions, as individuals with high self-efficacy tend to attribute failure to lack of effort or situational conditions, whereas those with low self-efficacy attribute failure to low personal ability. Beliefs about self-efficacy help determine whether certain actions are performed to attain desirable outcomes. Even if people know that a certain course of action will lead to a positive and desired outcome, they will likely not undertake that action if they believe they do not have the capability to perform that action. Motivation is also sustained through the development of explicit challenging goals and the evaluation of whether performance has met personal standards for goal achievement. Making satisfaction contingent on reaching a certain standard motivates people and helps them persevere until the goal is reached. Individuals are certainly motivated by the satisfaction they gain from fulfilling valued goals, and their efforts can therefore increase if they perceive that they are not performing well enough. In summary, Bandura (1995) explains that efficacy beliefs influence motivation by the goals people set for themselves, how much effort they put forth to achieve those goals, their level of persistence in the face of difficulties, and their sense of resilience to failure.

People's judgments about their self-efficacy also affect their emotions and physiological states, and therefore *affective processes* are critical to consider. People experience stress and negative emotional states when facing situations in which they feel they are challenged beyond their ability to cope successfully. Therefore, the perception of having control over stressors is important for reducing stress and negative affective states. If threats are viewed as unmanageable, people tend to focus on potential dangers in the environment and dwell on perceived coping deficiencies. This almost exclusive focus on the worst case scenario occurring causes psychological and emotional distress and reduced ability to function. In contrast, individuals who are confident in their ability to cope with and exercise control over possible stressors in their environment do not focus on these threats and experience reduced negative thoughts and emotions. This coping and exercise of control over stressors can be thought of in terms of coping behaviors as well as cognitive reframing. People's beliefs about their ability to control negative thoughts is related to the amount of anxiety they feel. If a person believes that negative thoughts can be either "turned off," reframed, or viewed from a different context, it is likely that the person will not react as negatively to them. The implications of this are that if individuals with strong emotional or phobic reactions can come to believe that they demonstrate control over stressors, they will experience less autonomic arousal and emotional distress. If these individuals do not believe in their coping efficacy, however, anxiety and emotional reactions will intensify. Related to stuttering, many cognitive-behavioral therapies aim to help clients' abilities to alter unhelpful thinking patterns or view them from a different context, and can also reduce negative emotions experienced by clients.

Efficacy beliefs also affect coping behavior that can alter threatening environments. The stronger a person's efficacy, the more likely the person will enter into challenging or stressful situations and handle them successfully, thereby continuing to strengthen perceived efficacy. This is critical because fears and deficits in behavior are interdependent. Avoidance of stressful or challenging activities or environments thwarts the development of coping skills and perceived competency. This lack of competency then serves as a contributor to further escalation of fear. There are many other ways that self-efficacy can help mood and affect. People who believe they have high levels of efficacy in developing and maintaining supportive social relationships are more likely to establish a network of social support which can buffer negative effects of stress and depression.

People are impacted greatly by their environment and there are many *selection processes* regarding the activities and environments they choose to spend time in that may have an effect on self-efficacy. Individuals are in part a product of their environment, and decisions about what situations, activities, and environments people choose can play a large role in shaping life courses of individuals. People tend to avoid situations and activities in which they believe they have low self-efficacy, but they approach those they perceive themselves as capable of handling. What environments and activities people choose then influence their cultivation of the values, goals, interests, competencies, and social networks that shape their lives. An example of this is that self-efficacy influences career choices (and the educational pursuits people undertake to prepare themselves for their occupations), which comprise a large part of people's lives and contribute to their personal growth and the development of their social network.

Benefits of Enhanced Self-Efficacy Beliefs

There are many setbacks and adversities that people face when trying to accomplish goals in life, and a robust sense of self-efficacy helps individuals' well-being and ability to accomplish goals. Individuals with high self-efficacy view challenging goals as mastery opportunities, rather than dangers to be avoided. They have a strong sense of commitment and resilience in the face of difficulties or failures. If they do experience failures they recover rapidly and focus on increasing their effort, knowledge, or skills to master the situation. They approach challenging situations with the belief that they can exhibit control over stressful environmental events. Innovators require high self-efficacy because new proposals that counter traditional methods are often met with resistance by others. In order to persist in their beliefs, innovators need to be resilient in the face of early rejections. Bandura (1994) stated that an overestimation of one's abilities can be very beneficial in certain situations. He stated that realists can adapt well to current situations and realities; however, they may have difficulty seizing opportunities that lay out of their immediate grasp. In contrast, individuals who overestimate their capabilities are more likely to change their current realities. It is also important to note that although the discussion on self-efficacy thus far in this chapter has been related to an individual sense of self-efficacy, the collective sense of efficacy in groups of people is very much related to their success and ability to accomplish goals as well.

This personal belief in high self-efficacy can enhance well-being in a variety of ways. Bandura (1997) reviews literature that has found that a high sense of self-efficacy allows individuals to accomplish personal goals, reduces physiological and emotional stress levels, and helps to buffer against anxiety and depression. Self-efficacy can help in any life endeavor. For example, it has been documented that self-efficacy plays an important role in family issues such as marital relationships, parenting and raising children, and balancing work and family life. Self-efficacy is relevant in the intellectual and educational realm in order to increase students' beliefs of their own capacity to learn and regulate their own thinking and behavior to succeed academically and socially, teachers' beliefs in their instructional skills, as well as the collective school efficacy needed to create environments that are conducive to student learning. Self-efficacy influences the vocational realm in many ways, including the choices people make regarding the career they choose to pursue, the range of options they believe they have, and the development of their skills, knowledge, and innovation in order to be productive in their work. Self-efficacy is also relevant for promoting health, through influencing healthy life style habits and environmental practices, and the ability to modify biological stress reactions and cope successfully with stressful events and situations that could cause physically deteriorating effects (e.g., immune system weakening, anxiety, depression).

Different stages of life call for certain types of functioning to meet changing environmental demands. The type of self-efficacy needed for various life stages changes throughout the lifespan. It is possible for a person to exhibit high self-efficacy beliefs in certain stages of life, but not in others. Newborns gradually acquire a sense of personal agency as they develop and perceive that they can effectively manipulate their environment to meet their needs. Young children continually develop physical, social, cognitive, and linguistic capabilities through play and school as they mature, and they are constantly comparing their capacities to those of their peers. This process continues throughout the school-age and adolescent years. Adolescents are in a stage of life where they are taking increased responsibility for themselves, acting more independently, and transitioning into the role of the adult and the increased amount of environmental demands and stressors that come with adulthood. Young adulthood requires learning to cope with many new demands, including long-lasting or marital relationships, parenthood, and establishment and development of a career. In the middle years of life, people often reach a point of relatively stable personal efficacy beliefs in family and occupational areas of life. However, life situations do not remain static and adults need to continually adapt to changing environmental circumstances and technological developments. In their jobs, adults may be challenged by younger competitors to be promoted or to keep their jobs. The elderly must contend with declining physical, and sometimes cognitive, abilities, as well as lowered societal expectations of their functioning and contribution. Major life events such as retirement, relocations, loss of loved ones, and reduced social network can tax the individual's ability to cope. New opportunities and challenging activities can become decreased in old age. In all of these life phases, a strong sense of self-efficacy is very important for increasing people's ability to overcome obstacles and positively shape people's lives so that they can be healthy and productive.

THE RELEVANCE OF SELF-EFFICACY TO A STUTTERING DISORDER

Stuttering can be experienced as a loss of control over volitional speech production, and self-efficacy has to do with perceived ability to control. Therefore, it is not surprising that many PWS experience low levels of self-efficacy regarding their speech production ability. There are data suggesting that adolescents (Bray, Kehle, Lawless, & Theodore, 2003) and adults who stutter (Ornstein & Manning, 1985) demonstrate lower self-efficacy for speaking than fluent controls; however, adults who stutter have higher overall generalized self-efficacy compared with normative data (Boyle, 2013b). Because this loss of control can be frustrating and cause negative emotional and behavioral reactions, a large part of stuttering management includes helping a person establish a sense of control, either in producing speech a different way (fluency shaping), modifying moments of stuttering when they occur to be less tense and atypical (stuttering modification), influencing the environment to receive appropriate accommodations (increasing assertiveness, disclosing, etc.), or controlling negative thinking or emotional patterns that would typically inhibit the person (improved cognitive/affective adjustment). Treatment studies in the area of stuttering have documented that gains in self-efficacy are possible with approaches that address these various components of stuttering. It is clear that self-efficacious beliefs can increase as a result of appropriate therapy that addresses behavioral, cognitive, affective, and social factors, as many treatment studies have documented (Blood, 1995a, 1995b; Fry, Millard, & Botterill, 2014; Ladouceur & Saint-Laurent, 1986; Lee, Manning, & Herder, 2015).

It should be stressed that self-efficacy for PWS is not just focused on improving efficacious beliefs in the ability to produce fluent speech, but also the ability to manage social environment and cognitive emotional states so that the overall efficacy beliefs in communicating effectively can increase. One can continue to stutter and still have high self-efficacy in communicating and getting one's message across. Therefore, in this chapter's discussion of the connections between stuttering and self-efficacy, the reader should keep in mind that although speech change is often a component of increasing perceptions of efficacy in communication, there are many other methods related to modification of cognitive, affective, and social realms that are critical to consider. The following sections describe how self-efficacy is related to behavioral, cognitive/affective, and social components of a stuttering disorder.

Behavioral Aspects of Stuttering

Behavioral methods for speech modification in PWS have a well-documented history and the majority of treatment studies in the area focus on behavioral approaches. Williams stressed the notion that stuttering is something one does rather than something that "just happens." Although Williams' (1957) beliefs seem to conflict with current research that does demonstrate neurological and genetic differences in PWS (e.g., Chang & Zhu, 2013; Kang et al., 2010), his idea of instilling a sense of personal efficacy in speech production still resonates today. He reasoned that if PWS believe that stuttering just happens to them, there would be no real incentive to try to make speech change. In order for speech change to occur, clients need to believe that they have some control over their speech mechanism (Williams, 1957). Boyle (2016a) examined the beliefs of 348 adults who stutter and found that higher ratings of general self-efficacy were related to significantly higher levels of belief in personal control over the cause of stuttering. Boyle (2015) also found that lower ratings of self-efficacy were related to significantly higher ratings of self-reported speech disruption severity in a sample of 249 adults who stutter. Ladouceur, Caron, and Caron (1989) found that self-efficacy perceptions predicted behavioral improvements in speech modification among nine adults who stutter. Craig (1998) noted that maintenance of speech gains following stuttering therapy can be predicted by increased feelings of control combined with speech mastery skills and positive attitudes toward speaking. These findings seem to support the notion that a sense of control is relevant for helping PWS to effectively manage the speech disruptions associated with stuttering.

How can PWS achieve a feeling of control over their stuttering? There are many methods commonly used by speech-language pathologists to increase clients' perceptions that they do have the ability to manipulate their speech production. Discussing the speech production process with the client is often a good first step in therapy. Basic processes such as respiration, phonation, and articulation can be described in lay terms so that the client understands the foundation of speech production. For example, it can be explained that air exhaled from the lungs passes through the larynx and can then be turned into voice which is ultimately shaped and modified by the articulators. Then, it can be discussed that there are several things that can be done physically to obstruct the flow of air or voice, such as tension at the larynx or articulators. Basic exercises can be demonstrated, such as producing voiced and voiceless sounds to detect vocal fold vibration, making sounds with certain articulatory movements, or voluntarily producing sounds with too much tension, to help the client understand that speech is a product of one's actions and the speech mechanism can be altered in several kinds of ways. The important idea to get across is that not only can speech be altered in many ways, but it is the client who is manipulating it.

One of the most well-known approaches for behavioral modification in stuttering is fluency shaping. Fluency shaping is focused on teaching the client to generate smoother and more fluent speech. This is also called deliberate or controlled fluency because clients actively use a different way of speech production to achieve these aims. Because this method can feel unnatural for the speaker, it may be difficult to use in all situations. However, the important point in fluency shaping approaches is to instill in clients the belief that there is a method of speech production that will result in more fluent speech and the client can use that method to speak more smoothly. Clients can switch into this mode of speaking if they choose rather than feeling like there is nothing that can be done to control their speech production. There are many strategies contained within the fluency shaping approach, including easy voice onsets, light articulatory contacts, slower rate of speech (achieved through vowel stretching or pausing more frequently with fewer words per utterance), and focusing on continuous voicing rather than choppiness. Even though these approaches can sound unnatural and somewhat slow initially, the ultimate goal is for clients to gradually achieve smoother speech with a nearly typical rate and intonation. Although some therapy programs may target this new way of speech production all of the time, other approaches acknowledge that this new, deliberate way of speaking can be used when desired. The main idea is that the client can improve perceptions of self-efficacy regarding communication by realizing that speech production does not have to be left to chance, but can be switched into another mode. An analogy is that clients can shift gears in speech just like shifting gears in a car, once they know that they have the ability to do so and that other gears do exist. There is lots of evidence suggesting that these behavioral fluency shaping methods do in fact increase fluent speech production (Herder, Howard, Nye, & Vanryckeghem, 2006; Nye et al., 2013).

Another common behavioral approach for stuttering is called stuttering modification, or easier stuttering. Stuttering modification is quite different from fluency shaping because clients can continue to talk as they normally do; however, when a moment of harder stuttering occurs they are able to catch it and modify it. This is a very difficult process because speaking, and stuttering, is so habitual that very often clients do not pay much attention to it. Or, it is possible that the stresses associated with stuttering lead clients to disassociate from the moment of stuttering, or mentally "check out" while it is occurring. Often, emotional arousal makes it difficult for clients to become behaviorally aware of what it is exactly that they are doing as they are stuttering. The goal of the stuttering modification approach is really to increase behavioral awareness and reduce emotional reaction for the purpose of altering stuttering to an easier form. This process often begins with the clients exploring what they do when they stutter so that they have a clearer idea of what they will ultimately need to change. Then, a more systematic identification phase begins in which clients identify stuttering in others (e.g., the clinician) and then ultimately in themselves (both on tape and in real time). Identification is a critical stage because in order to modify the moment of stuttering, the client needs to become adept at sensing when it is occurring and what is happening in that moment. Then, a series of strategies including cancellations, pull-outs, and preparatory sets can be taught which aim for clients to modify hard stuttering moments after they occur, while they occur, and before they occur, respectively.

Stuttering modification approaches are designed to increase clients' beliefs in self-efficacy regarding their ability to produce speech and communicate effectively. Clients can realize that they are not prisoners of habitual responses, but that the moments of stuttering, which appear so frightening and stressful, can actually be modified, even as they are occurring. Although fluency shaping and stuttering modification approaches appear quite different, clients can in fact use both. For example, a client may increase a sense of self-efficacy by implementing certain fluency facilitating strategies. However, even if clients are unable to change how they talk, or if they don't desire to use those strategies in certain contexts, they can still feel like they have control over stuttering when it does occur using stuttering modification techniques.

All of the approaches described above, whether fluency shaping or stuttering modification, can be perceived not only as behavioral but also psychological. Because PWS often have many life experiences built up in which communication has been challenging and frustrating, it can be very difficult to begin to trust that another way of speaking is possible. Therefore, considerable practice and experience using those tools is traditionally needed for mastery. This is not only because a new way of speaking can be physically and mentally taxing, but also because clients need to demonstrate to themselves repeatedly that they can in fact alter their default way of speaking (Yairi & Seery, 2015). This is why repeated practice is so critical with these behavioral methods. Clients need the repetition to demonstrate that they are not in fact helpless to alter their speech production. Therefore, increasing a client's perceived self-efficacy for their capacity to manipulate their speech production is a major goal of the behavioral stuttering treatments discussed above.

Cognitive and Affective Aspects of Stuttering

Some PWS may not want to modify their speech, and instead be free from the need to constantly worry about their stuttering (Venkatagiri, 2009). Others may desire to speak more fluently or with less tension, but their feelings and beliefs may be preventing them from fully achieving these goals. Therefore, the internal aspect of stuttering, namely, thoughts and emotions, are very relevant when discussing the scope of a stuttering disorder. The external demands of stressful speaking situations (e.g., facing time pressure or the judgments of others) can increase tension and speech disruption. Even if clients can use the behavioral techniques described in the previous section very well in therapy, or in low stress settings, it can be very difficult to use them when the pressure level is high. Because these environmental pressures are filtered through the individual and produce thoughts and feelings which can either detract from or contribute to optimal performance, it is critical that therapy also focus on perceptions of efficacy for managing cognitive and affective features of stuttering.

Studies have found that self-efficacy is linked to a variety of psychological benefits in PWS. Craig, Blumgart, and Tran (2015) found that self-efficacy was a protective influence in reducing the impact of negative mood states such as anxiety and depression in 200 adults who stutter. Craig, Blumgart, and Tran (2011) reported that self-efficacy predicted psychological resilience that could buffer the negative effects of stuttering in the same sample. Boyle (2016a) found that increased beliefs in personal control over the cause of stuttering were related to significantly lower levels of self-stigma, anxiety, depression, and significantly higher levels of self-esteem and hope, controlling for self-reported severity of speech disruption in a study involving 348 adults who stutter. Boyle (2015) also reported that after controlling for demographic and stuttering-related factors, including self-reported severity of speech disruption, self-efficacy was a significant predictor of quality of life in a sample of 249 adults who stutter. These findings emphasize the importance of self-efficacy for the psychological experiences of PWS.

Persons' desire to change their way of speaking may be outweighed by their fear of stuttering. In essence, people may not even attempt to make speech change if they believe that it leaves them vulnerable to experiencing a difficult moment of stuttering and therefore being unable to complete their message. This fear and apprehension can obviously make it even more challenging, if not impossible, to complete the demanding task of speech modification. It is therefore critical that PWS have methods for managing their thoughts and emotions so as not to be overtaken by them during times of discomfort or stress. There are several methods that have been mentioned extensively in the stuttering literature that seek to decrease the emotional arousal associated with stuttering so that PWS feel like they have more control over their stuttering as well as the environmental stressors that exacerbate it.

Increasing efficacy beliefs in the ability to cope with stuttering when it occurs involves strengthening the belief that emotional upheaval does not need to occur in the moment of stuttering. For example, clients can be taught to hold on to the moment of stuttering as it is occurring. This toleration of stuttering, sometimes called freezing, can help reduce the emotionality associated with stuttering as well as increase behavioral awareness of what is occurring physically during stuttering events. This is a desensitization method that parallels exposure therapy for individuals with phobias where the goal is for these persons to be calm in the presence of what frightens them. Charles Van Riper used to twiddle his thumbs, massage his face, and do other relaxing acts during a moment of freezing a stutter to demonstrate the point that it is not necessary for the loss of control that is experienced with stuttering to be reacted to with fear and tension (Stuttering Foundation, 2005). It is a critical point that even if attempts at speech change are not successfully executed, people can still demonstrate efficacious beliefs about their communication by believing that they can successfully cope with stuttering when it occurs.

Another common method for increasing beliefs in ability to cope with stuttering is the use of voluntary stuttering. The client is asked to feign stuttering on non-feared words by either using easy sound or syllable repetitions (bounces) or sound prolongations (stretches). Voluntary stuttering can help weaken the link between stuttering moments and feelings of distress. If stuttering is done voluntarily and in an easier manner, it does not seem as scary. Real stuttering moments may then lose some of their power. Being able to manipulate a moment of voluntary stuttering can be a very helpful precursor to being able to manipulate real moments of stuttering as well. Another major benefit of voluntary stuttering is that fear can often be reduced through clients acknowledging that their speech is different at the beginning of interactions. If PWS are no longer worrying about what will happen if they stutter, they can go ahead with communicating. Treatments that utilize these strategies have resulted in reduced struggle, avoidance, and expectancy related to stuttering (Blomgren, Roy, Callister, & Merrill, 2005). Many PWS also report that voluntary stuttering is particularly beneficial when it closely matches their actual stuttering and when it is used outside of the therapy room (Byrd, Gkalitsiou, Donaher, & Stergiou, 2016). Strategies like voluntary stuttering increase the ability of PWS to cope with their stuttering and the loss of control that comes with it. If PWS are experiencing intense negative emotional reactions, it will be much more difficult to focus on the message or employ speech modification strategies. So, the ability of PWS to increase efficacy in their ability to cope with stuttering is of the utmost importance.

There may be situations where direct discussion of thoughts and feelings of clients is needed. Some clients might exhibit negative and automatic self-defeating thoughts that can interfere with their ability to communicate. These clients may exhibit intense emotional and physiological reactions that can make effective communication extremely difficult. Without addressing the cognitive and affective domains explicitly, some clients may have trouble making lasting changes to their communication. Several methods can be used to address negative thoughts and feelings in therapy so that clients can feel like they have more control over these components of their stuttering. Clients can learn about the cognitive model, which demonstrates how behaviors are shaped by our physiology, emotions, and thoughts. Importantly, all of these elements are interconnected so that modifications made in one area modify the others. For example, if a person is not willing to talk to a store clerk to request an item, feelings (e.g., fear), physiological reactions (e.g., nervous stomach), and thoughts (e.g., "he will think I'm stupid") associated with that behavior can be uncovered. Uncovering these underlying negative thoughts is important because it sets the foundation for clients to be able to identify and recognize these thoughts and feelings as they occur. Once they are brought into consciousness, they can also be challenged and replaced with more empowering thoughts, essentially enabling clients to "talk back" to disempowering thoughts.

Once clients become adept at identifying their own negative thoughts related to stuttering, they can conduct behavioral experiments to test the validity of their beliefs. If the client's hypothesis is that the store clerk will laugh when stuttering is seen, this can be tested. To do so, the client will need to talk to the clerk and study his or her reactions to stuttering to see if the negative assumption was true. At first, these experiments do not need to be conducted by the client, but the clinician can do these things as the client evaluates the listener reaction. Then, the client can be the one acting. These types of activities help to reduce avoidance in people who stutter. What the clients find from doing these experiments may help them to check their disempowering assumptions and beliefs. Clients may in fact find that listener responses were not as negative as was previously assumed.

Working on coping skills can also be effective in stuttering treatment. Making speech changes can be scary and so clients need to become resilient and courageous in the face of stressful situations. Clients can be taught how to manage negative emotions (e.g., fear, panic, dread, anxiety) and physiological reactions (e.g., increased heart rate, shallow breath, sweating) when they occur. Because it is hard to communicate or modify speech production when one is very emotionally or physiologically upset, it is useful for clients to have several ways of regulating their physiology and emotional states. It can be useful to rate clients' level of worry or anxiety on a scale from no anxiety to very high anxiety. Brainstorming with clients regarding things that can be done to reduce negative emotions related to stuttering can be very helpful. Things like taking slow, deep diaphragmatic breaths and implementing positive self-talk can be highlighted so that when clients become emotionally upset in a stressful situation, they can use the worry as a cue to implement the coping strategies. This type of activity can be done with more than just worry—any emotion (discomfort, frustration, anger, disappointment, etc.) can be discussed and coping options that are stress reducing for each specific emotion can be identified by the client and utilized in future situations in which those emotions arise.

The strategies discussed in the previous paragraphs are utilized in the psychological treatment Cognitive Behavioral Therapy (CBT), and this approach has been used successfully with individuals who stutter. Menzies, O'Brian, Onslow, Packman, St. Clare, and Block (2008) tested the effects of a CBT program including cognitive restructuring, gradual exposure to previously avoided situations, and behavioral experiments in a group of 30 adults who stutter. The group of PWS who received CBT in conjunction with speech therapy demonstrated significantly higher psychological functioning, less anxiety and avoidance, and significantly more willingness to enter into feared speaking situations compared with a group that received speech therapy without CBT. Helgadottir, Menzies, Onslow, Packman, and O'Brian (2014) completed a phase I study of the effects of a CBT program taken online called CBTPsych. The study was a pretest-posttest single group design with 13 participants. After the intervention the participants demonstrated reduced fear of negative evaluation and social phobia, reduced unhelpful thoughts and beliefs about stuttering, and reduced life impact and improved quality of life as shown by scores on the Overall Assessment of the Speaker's Experience of Stuttering (OASES) (Yaruss & Quesal, 2006). Menzies, O'Brian, Lowe, Packman, and Onslow (2016) found similar positive results in a sample of 267 adults who stutter using the same online program, even without participant contact with clinicians or researchers. For a review of using CBT for PWS, see Chapter 6 in this book.

Another method for giving clients increased efficacy beliefs in their ability to manage their thoughts and emotions is using mindfulness-based approaches. In these approaches, clients learn how to view their thoughts from a different context (i.e., that thoughts are mental events that do not necessarily reflect reality accurately). Mindfulness approaches emphasize behavioral exposure to stressors, awareness of internal (e.g., thoughts, feelings, physical bodily sensations) and external (e.g., sights, sounds) phenomena, and increased acceptance. De Veer, Brouwers, Evers, and Tomic (2009) compared 37 adults who who had completed an eight-week Mindfulness Based Stress Reduction with participants on a waitlist and found that treated participants demonstrated less stress and less anxiety about speech situations, as well as increased self-efficacy for approaching speaking situations, locus of control, problem-oriented coping, and positive attitudes toward speech situations immediately after therapy and at one month follow-up. Mindfulness is also a component of an increasingly popular treatment in the area of stuttering called Acceptance and Commitment Therapy (ACT), which focuses on self-concept, acceptance of thoughts and emotions, mindfulness skills, noticing thoughts as thoughts and not facts, clarifying personal values, and implementing value-directed action. Beilby, Byrnes, and Yaruss (2012) examined the effects of ACT combined with speech therapy on 20 adults who stutter and found improvements on all sections of the OASES indicating reduced negative emotions about stuttering, less avoidance tactics, negative thoughts; less difficulty communicating, and less negative life impact of stuttering. In summary, approaches for modifying cognitive and affective dimensions of stuttering are important for increasing the efficacious beliefs of PWS that they can manage their minds and emotions in order to optimize their communication performance. If clients feel as if they have power over these internal aspects of themselves, they will feel much more empowered to communicate without fear and therefore increase their communicative participation and quality of life by entering previously avoided situations. For a review of using ACT for PWS, see Chapter 7 in this book.

Social Aspects of Stuttering

Stuttering manifests in the social realm and can clearly lead to social uneasiness. Many studies have reported that PWS exhibit higher levels of social anxiety than people who do not stutter (Iverach & Rapee, 2014). This is to be expected because the public does not often understand stuttering, and as a result PWS can face stigmatization including negative stereotypes, prejudiced emotional reactions, and discriminatory behaviors or intentions (Boyle & Blood, 2015). PWS are very much aware of these negative public perceptions (Boyle, 2013a) and this awareness is linked to internalization of stigma, as well as increased anxiety and depression (Boyle, 2015). Facing constant fear of negative listener perceptions naturally elevates social anxiety. As a result, PWS might avoid saying certain sounds or words, or entire speaking situations. Some may even try to pass as a fluent speaker to avoid negative listener reactions. This pattern of avoidance can eventually drastically restrict one's social functioning, communicative participation, and achievement of life goals.

If PWS restrict themselves socially due to fear of negative evaluation from others, substantial problems can arise regarding basic social skills and functioning. These individuals may not give themselves many opportunities to develop or improve such basic social skills as turn taking and maintaining eye contact with a listener. As a result, they may have low beliefs in their own efficacy for being able to establish and maintain social relationships. Lacking supportive social networks and relationships can be very detrimental to one's overall sense of well-being and quality of life and can leave people more vulnerable to the negative effects of stress. Therefore, strategies in therapy aimed at improving efficacy for social skills and establishing or strengthening social relationships can be a crucial activity. Clients can become adept at using behavioral or cognitive/affective strategies to manage their stuttering, but if they continue to operate in a social environment that is not supportive of their goals, the use of these skills is not likely to persist.

There are many strategies that are useful to increase clients' efficacy in social functioning. First, it is important to help clients feel more comfortable talking about their stuttering. This can be with the clinician, and then family, friends, acquaintances, and even strangers. Talking about stuttering openly can be very destigmatizing for the PWS as it signals to others that the person possesses some level of comfort with stuttering. Once that happens, others can then be more comfortable with the individual who stutters. PWS can be shown how to explain what stuttering is if they are asked or if someone says something inappropriate. PWS can learn to summarize what they are doing in therapy and why. This type of disclosure helps the client feel more comfortable in transferring what is being learned in therapy to outside situations, and makes listeners feel more comfortable. Disclosing one's stuttering by stuttering openly or talking about the fact that the speaker is a PWS can help reduce discomfort and put the speaker and others at ease. For example, many PWS use disclosure of stuttering at the beginning of a talk or when meeting someone new. Some PWS use lighthearted comments or jokes to break the ice. Increased disclosure and openness about stuttering has been linked to significantly increased levels of quality of life and self-empowerment and lower levels of self-stigma and anxiety in adults who stutter (Boyle, 2014, 2016b).

Disclosure and openness about stuttering has beneficial effects for the speaker (Plexico, Manning, & DiLollo, 2005) but it also can have the effect of reducing public stigma. Boyle, Dioguardi, and Pate (2016) found that watching a contact video with a PWS sharing personal stories about stuttering increases affirming attitudes about PWS more than other stigma reduction approaches (education and protest) among members of the public and that these attitude changes persist over time. Those authors have also identified key ingredients in contact-based anti-stigma programs that lead to positive attitude change. These include discussing daily challenges associated with stuttering, an "on-the-way-up story" that highlights resilience in the face of stuttering, achievement of goals demonstrating that stuttering does not need to hold one back, and an affirming goal statement of what the speaker would like the listener to gain from the presentation. Therefore, it seems that disclosure and openness regarding stuttering can have a double effect, public and private stigma reduction and an increase in empowering perceptions of both members of the public and of PWS.

Increasing assertiveness in PWS is also helpful for increasing efficacy beliefs regarding social interactions. Because of stuttering, many PWS might prefer to avoid speaking up if they feel they have been treated unfairly. However, clients can learn that they can actually make requests of their communication partners to change their behaviors. For example, PWS can express their needs directly, request respectful behavior from others (e.g., "allow me to finish my point"), share how they want listeners to respond (e.g., "please maintain eye contact with me during a block"), and appropriately respond to listener reactions (e.g., knowing how to respond assertively but respectfully to the question, "Why do you talk like that?"). All of these things can be perceived by the client as helping the listener because the listener likely does not understand stuttering and needs help about how to best respond. Also, it can be helpful to focus on instilling basic social skills, if these are lacking in the client, such as maintaining eye contact when talking, turn-taking, and listening.

Establishing or strengthening the social network and relationships of PWS is also an important aspect of increasing self-efficacy beliefs in the social realm. It is important to identify supportive people who can help PWS during difficult times. A support network that the client feels comfortable with comprising family, friends, teachers, co-workers, and others can be an incredibly powerful buffer against the negative influence of stresses associated with stuttering. This social network should be examined carefully with names written down. The individuals on this list should be people that the client can seek out to talk about problems, or share successes. These individuals can also be the people that the client first tries transferring therapy skills with and establishing behavioral activation. That is, transfer of therapy tools (e.g., speech modification skills) to daily life situations is one of the most problematic and difficult aspects of stuttering treatment. So, it can be beneficial for clients to first attempt the transfer activities with people they feel comfortable with and who understand what the client is doing.

Boyle (2015) found that increased perceived social support (from friends, family, and significant others) in PWS was related to significantly higher levels of self-efficacy in a sample of 354 adults who stutter. The same study showed that self-efficacy in PWS was significantly correlated to many important social variables, including community activism, participation in self-help or support group meetings, consistency of attendance at self-help meetings, and group identification with other individuals who stutter. Importantly, social support for PWS is also available from self-help organizations such as the National Stuttering Association (NSA) in the

United States. Trichon and Tetnowski (2011) have also documented that there are many benefits for PWS in attending annual conferences that bring together hundreds of PWS. These benefits include increased socialization opportunities and feelings of affiliation, as well as increased disclosure about stuttering after the conference.

Note that the social strategies mentioned in the preceding paragraphs do not necessitate any speech change whatsoever. They can be used separately from, or in conjunction with, the other behavioral and cognitive/affective strategies mentioned in the previous sections. Although modification of speech behaviors has a long history in the area of stuttering, there is a growing emphasis on social models of disability that emphasize alteration of environment for improving the quality of life of individuals who stutter (Boyle, Daniels, Hughes, & Buhr, 2016; Constantino & Alpern, 2016; Simpson & Everard, 2015). For example, instead of viewing a communication breakdown as being due solely to PWS disfluencies, it can be realized that the communication partner who interrupts or attempts to finish a word is also disrupting the communication exchange. These social models are sometimes criticized as giving personal power away to individuals in one's environment. However, it can also be viewed that addressing social issues and environmental barriers is in fact very self-empowering. This is because PWS can realize that they have some control not only over their own behavior, but they can in fact manipulate their environment and get others to act in certain ways to meet their goals.

To summarize, there are many domains of a stuttering disorder that PWS can gain increased control over, perhaps more than they ever imagined. Normally, clients come to stuttering therapy assuming that speech change will be the primary goal. Although this is usually an important component of stuttering therapy, it can be a surprise for clients to learn that they actually do have options that extend beyond the speech domain. It is therefore crucial that clinicians communicate these issues to clients to increase their options for managing stuttering in any given situation. Learning that one can gain footholds of control in cognitive, affective, and social realms of experience can be empowering because of the variety of options that have been added to the management plan. Clients can realize that there are many ways to increase self-efficacy in the ability to communicate effectively. Behavioral treatment objectives can give clients the feeling that there is something concrete they can do to modify how they speak to make the process more efficient, natural, and less stressful. Cognitive and affective objectives can change how PWS think and feel in relation to stuttering and communication and increase their perceived self-efficacy in their management of their own thoughts and emotions. Finally, social objectives can empower clients to feel like they can modify their environment in their favor and benefit from the support of others. When clients possess efficacious beliefs in the multiple dimensions of a stuttering disorder (behavioral, cognitive/affective, social), they will become more resilient and confident in their ability to communicate effectively and achieve their goals.

THE INTEGRATION OF SELF-EFFICACY PRINCIPLES WITH THE CLINICAL MANAGEMENT OF STUTTERING

This section will discuss how the self-efficacy principles outlined in this chapter so far can be applied to the assessment and treatment of stuttering. Although the previous section described the relevance of self-efficacy to a variety of domains in a stuttering disorder, this section will provide concrete recommendations for integrating self-efficacy into clinical work with people who stutter, regardless of the therapeutic approach taken. The basic principles described in this section can be applied by all therapists regardless of what the client's individualized therapy program looks like, and are not dependent on the use of one particular strategy.

Assessment of Self-Efficacy

As demonstrated by the previous section, which established the relevance of self-efficacy in the understanding and management of a stuttering disorder, it is important to take this variable into account clinically when working with a PWS. It seems clear that improvements in self-efficacy are an important outcome measure because efficacy beliefs are predictive of behavioral changes. However, clinicians cannot hope to manage a variable that they cannot measure and document empirically. Therefore, it is important that self-efficacy is documented in the assessment process with PWS. There are several kinds of assessments, including global (i.e., general) self-efficacy measures, as well as domain-specific measures. Although there are many specific self-efficacy scales that intend to measure perceptions of a variety of behaviors, this discussion will mostly focus on those that are specifically related to beliefs about speaking behaviors.

Scales have been developed that attempt to measure global or general levels of perceived self-efficacy. For example, the General Self-Efficacy Scale (GSES), developed by Schwarzer and Jerusalem (1995), assesses self-efficacy from a broad perspective that primarily focuses on ability to cope with daily hassles and adapt to a variety of stressful life experiences. The scale contains 10 items (e.g., "I am confident that I could deal efficiently with unexpected events"). A four-point response scale is used for each question (1 = not at all true, 2 = hardly true, 3 = moderately true, 4 = exactly true). Individual items are summed yielding an overall score that ranges from 10 to 40, with higher scores representing higher levels of general self-efficacy. This scale has been used extensively in a variety of research studies across several countries and has been translated into 33 different languages (Luszczynska, Guiterrez-Dona, & Schwarzer, 2004).

Despite the potential importance of measuring general levels of self-efficacy, Bandura (2006) indicates that it is usually more useful to focus on domain-specific self-efficacy. This is due to the fact that it is unrealistic to expect that one can have mastery in all domains of life. Different people focus on different life areas in which to develop efficacy, and therefore a general measure becomes problematic. Bandura warns against use of a "one-size-fits-all" assessment because the items in such a scale are unlikely to tap into the specific domains of interest, and the generality of the scale leads to ambiguity about what precisely is being measured. This distinction between domain-specific and general measures of self-efficacy likely explains why previous studies found that although PWS have lower self-efficacy for speaking compared with the non-stuttering population (Bray et al., 2003; Ornstein & Manning, 1985), PWS have been found to have higher levels of general self-efficacy compared with normative data (Boyle, 2013b). Clinicians need to consider whether they want to administer a more general self-efficacy scale, such as the GSES, or a more focused scale targeting speech production or communication.

Bandura (1997) discussed that because self-efficacy varies in terms of magnitude, generality, and strength of efficacy expectations, an adequate analysis and assessment will examine these domains in detail. For example, this means efficacy beliefs should be obtained for a variety of experiences (easy, moderate, and difficult) for magnitude because efficacy expectations likely differ depending on the difficulty level of the task. The impediments to performance need to be carefully considered and constructed based on determining the variety of challenges faced by the group to be assessed. In addition, the degree to which people believe they can do something, or the strength of their efficacy beliefs, is important to document. A person with weak expectations of success is not as likely to persevere in the face of challenging situations compared with someone with a strong belief. Response options for these scales should include options ranging from "cannot do" to "moderately certain can do" to "highly certain can do" or some variation of those responses. This is normally done on a unipolar scale from 0 to 10 or 0 to 100, where zero represents complete incapability. These scales should measure what people believe they can do presently, not what they anticipate they might be able to do in the future, or what their potential is.

To measure self-efficacy for PWS specifically, Ornstein and Manning (1985) developed the Self-Efficacy Scale for Adult Stutterers (SESAS) based on the work of Bandura (1977b). This scale presents 40 different speaking situations that vary in their difficulty, and participants are asked to report whether they would enter certain situations and how confident they would be (e.g., call up a friend on the phone, ask a policeman for directions, talk with a family member during a meal). First, participants are asked to check off which situations they can do, and for those items they checked, they report their confidence in their belief that they would enter that situation (with response options ranging from 10 = quite uncertain, to 50–60 = moderately certain, to 100 = very certain). The higher the percentages given, the more likely the client is to enter a particular speaking situation. The strengths of the SESAS are that it captures a variety of speaking situations that differ in the magnitude of difficulty and challenges presented, and it allows for clear differentiation between clients using a sensitive 10 to 100 scale. There are some limitations in the SESAS, however, including that the instructions ask only how confident clients are that they would enter a situation, not whether they could complete the task successfully. The instructions also ask clients how they think they would perform rather than what participants can do presently. In addition, the different steps of checking off what the participants think they can do, and then rating their confidence level, may not be necessary. The check box for "can do" could be replaced by a single unipolar response option that ranges from "0" = cannot do, to "100" = very certain can do. This would allow for easier scoring by keeping all data continuous. Finally, self-efficacy beliefs are relevant for a variety of other areas besides behavior, including regulation of emotional states, thought processes, or one's social environmental conditions (Bandura, 2006), and the SESAS solely focuses on confidence in entering speaking situations.

Practically speaking, clinicians and researchers can use pre-existing scales to measure general (e.g., GSES) or domain-specific (e.g., SESAS) areas in their clients or participants who stutter. Using pre-existing scales is certainly easier and time saving; however, there can be advantages to developing specific self-efficacy scales that meet the needs of the specific researcher or clinician. This takes more effort and time; however, the results can be more precise in the information obtained. If new scales are developed, it is recommended that a variety of speaking situations that vary in their demands and difficulty are presented, and the response options should be on a scale with many steps so that the scale can be highly sensitive to differences between individuals, and changes in individuals over time. Depending on what needs to be assessed, instructions could vary but should ask participants what they can do at the present moment. The domain of functioning to be assessed (i.e., what domains of efficacy are being measured) should be clearly specified in the instructions as well. There are many options for domains of efficacy that can be relevant for a person's management of stuttering (e.g., entering speaking situations, communicating one's message in those situations, employing speech modification strategies, modifying moments of stuttering, regulating affect, managing thoughts). For example, if negative emotional reactions trigger more severe stuttering, it is relevant to measure efficacy in managing emotions and thoughts. Importantly, factors should only be measured in which the person can have some control and can be expected to have some effect on the quality of performance in the domain of functioning. Whether professionals use preexisting measures or create their own, efficacy expectations should be assessed before therapy begins and then repeated at various intervals throughout the change process in order to determine if efficacy beliefs are changing along with other behavioral objectives. In short, self-efficacy beliefs should be monitored over time so that not just performance, but also belief in ability to perform is documented.

Treatment Considerations to Increase Self-Efficacy

Although different components of therapy outlined in previous sections (e.g., fluency shaping, modifying stuttering, regulating emotional and cognitive processes) can all help increase clients' self-efficacy, this section will focus on specific principles that would be included in a therapy program to increase clients' perceptions of self-efficacy. First, the most important thing that a clinician can do to improve feelings of self-efficacy in a client is to provide abundant mastery experiences for the client to achieve success. Failure undermines self-efficacy, especially if the failure occurs before feelings of self-efficacy are established. Therefore, the clinician must be very careful to structure therapy and goal setting so that it is incremental, taking one step at a time rather than starting with a very difficult task. It is important to define what success means in therapy and then take small steps to achieve that success. For example, success may be defined as just entering into a speaking situation that one previously avoided, or just speaking in that situation regardless of fluency. Other goals might define use of stuttering modification, maintaining eye contact during speaking, or using fluency techniques as a measure of success. However, speech modification goals should be realistic in their expectations. For example, if success is defined as clients using their techniques all of the time, in every situation outside therapy, failure in achieving this unrealistic goal will make the client feel like a failure and reduce feelings of self-efficacy. Therefore, realistic goals should be generated with the client based on what the client feels is realistically accomplishable at a given time. An example might be using a certain technique for one minute of an interaction, or on one sentence with specific people. These manageable goals help generate success, which improves perceptions of efficacy.

Some clients experience such negative emotional reactions related to their stuttering that they begin to avoid sounds, words, people, or speaking situations entirely. It can be very difficult for these clients to do what they fear, namely, talk. Therefore, a therapeutic environment needs to be created where individuals can succeed despite their intense emotional reactions. Bandura (1994) discusses how a variety of mastery aids can be used for this purpose, including: clinician modeling of the feared activity, breaking coping tasks into easily mastered subtasks, performing feared activities with the clinician rather than independently, and making threatening tasks short in duration at first. After the client's coping efficacy increases, mastery aids can be withdrawn and the client can enter more difficult situations independently in order to test coping abilities.

Vicarious experiences provided by social models are another way to increase self-efficacy. Therefore, it is of the utmost importance that clinicians model the behaviors and modes of thinking that their clients aspire to demonstrate. Clinician modeling of successfully attaining goals can instill a feeling in clients that they too can achieve these goals. It is more beneficial when people observe models overcoming obstacles with determination and effort than observing a seemingly effortless performance put on by a highly skilled model. Observing a model who encounters temporary difficulty and succeeds in spite of it better helps instill in clients the feeling that success can come even if one is anxious and encountering challenges (Bandura, 1977b). The implications are that clinicians should not only model fluent speech, but also model disfluencies and how to work out of them in a productive way. Clinician modeling can provide not only a social standard of comparison for the client, but also a means of learning strategies related to managing cognitive processes, emotions, and environmental demands. Models can be even more effective when they come from someone perceived by clients to be similar to themselves. Therefore, introducing the client to other individuals similar to themselves in a variety of characteristics, including age and gender, through group therapy or self-help support groups may be beneficial.

Modeling target behaviors is a key aspect of self-efficacy, and the more similar the model is in age and gender, the more influence it will have on the client. Therefore, it can be reasoned that a self-model could provide the most impact because it is a model that provides clear evidence of mastery of certain tasks. In self-modeling, a client is videotaped demonstrating a target behavior. In this way clients can see and reflect on being successful and completing mastery experiences, which will engender future successes and help them visualize future successes on the same task. Bray and Kehle (1996, 1998, 2001) conducted a series of research studies analyzing video modeling with seven children and adolescents who stutter which demonstrated that this approach can reduce stuttering frequency and for some children benefits can last over time. Typically these videos were 2 to 4 minutes and were shown to clients about six to eight times over the course of about a month. It should be noted that in the studies conducted by Bray and Kehle, speech fluency was the target behavior, although it seems quite possible that this type of approach could be utilized with other therapy goals (e.g., voluntary stuttering, stuttering modification).

Another way to boost a client's self-efficacy is through social persuasion, or telling clients that they have what it takes to succeed, and they know how to succeed. The clinician can empower clients with the self-assurance that they can achieve their goals. Certainly, it would be very detrimental to clients' self-efficacy if they were told that they lack the capability to succeed. Clinicians can also praise clients for their effort and completing challenging tasks, and provide positive feedback after tasks are performed. They can also reflect with the client on past successes. Constructive feedback can help clients overcome feelings of doubt in their abilities. Although it is true that encouragement from the clinician can usually boost self-efficacy to a certain extent, that encouragement and persuasion can easily be undermined by repeated failures. Therefore, it is essential that clients are set up for success in achievable increments of difficulty to ensure that success is consistently experienced, as discussed above.

Another important way to improve self-efficacy is to be able to alter physiological states. If one is in a stressed and fearful physiological or emotional state, perceptions of efficacy decrease. Negative thoughts and feelings can generate physical stress, and so it becomes important to teach strategies for reducing physiological and emotional tension when working with a client who experiences impaired performance due to emotional reactions. This can include desensitization activities, relaxation activities, mindfulness exercises, and therapies that address analyzing thoughts and feelings. As mentioned previously, therapies like Cognitive Behavioral Therapy (Menzies et al., 2008; Menzies, Onslow, Packman, & O'Brian, 2009), mindfulness-based stress reduction (Boyle, 2011; De Veer et al., 2009), and Acceptance and Commitment Therapy (Beilby et al., 2012) are being documented as effective for decreasing negative emotions, thoughts, and avoidances related to stuttering. Again, the goal in this case would not be to eliminate negative thoughts or emotions, but rather instill a way for clients to interpret these experiences in a more empowering way. Once clients feel that they are no longer controlled by compulsive thought patterns or helpless when experiencing negative emotional reactions, they can change these processes and therefore their own physiology and perceptions of self-efficacy.

The personal characteristics of clinicians and how they interact with clients are also very important to consider in this discussion. For example, although modeling, allowing opportunities for mastery experiences, and verbal persuasion might be powerful ways to increase self-efficacy, clients are unlikely to want to imitate models that they do not like personally. Therefore, clinicians should come across as caring individuals who will permit clients to express themselves in an accepting manner, even when that involves difficult emotions or thoughts. Clinicians should not be disapproving, critical, or disinterested when the client discusses difficult topics or emotions. This allowance for discussion of anxiety-producing thoughts in itself can help with desensitization by elimination of negative feedback in response to the anxiety-producing thoughts (i.e., extinction) (Bandura, 1961). Plexico, Manning, and DiLollo (2010) reported on a qualitative analysis of key aspects of therapeutic alliance between client and clinician reported by PWS. It was found that clinicians demonstrating an understanding of stuttering and caring to develop a strong client–clinician alliance were associated with beneficial therapy.

Another aspect of self-efficacy in stuttering management goes beyond individual therapy and could be associated with groups of individuals who stutter working to achieve goals directed at societal change. For example, common goals of self-help support groups for stuttering involve educating the public, dispelling common myths, and sharing information with others about stuttering. This is critical, as it has been documented consistently that stuttering is a stigmatized disorder (St. Louis, 2015). The National Stuttering Association (NSA) has chapters across the United States, but the groups vary substantially in terms of number of attendees and group leaders. It is an interesting area of future research to consider the sense of collective group efficacy in PWS. It is quite possible that some groups and their leaders possess a greater sense of collective efficacy in their ability to bring societal change than others, and it could be possible to describe what contributes to feelings of group efficacy. Social reform requires mobilization of many individuals in a collective effort, and so this can be more complex than personal self-efficacy. Social reform is a long and tiring process in which progress is incremental over long periods of time. Often, social reformers do not obtain their ultimate goals, even if important progress is made. Transforming current social systems is a large task, and so it is critical that social reformers and leaders of collective groups possess a certain level of unreasonableness, even an overestimation of their abilities to enact change. Bandura (1994) argues that if reformers were entirely realistic, they would not sustain the effort needed to make large social changes. He stated that realists can adapt well to existing realities, but individuals with relentless self-efficacy are more likely to change current realities.

CONCLUSION

In summary, self-efficacy is an important variable for professionals to consider when working clinically with PWS. Clients' sense of self-efficacy can be predictive of ability to make and sustain behavioral changes that are often targeted in stuttering therapy. There are specific ways to assess and measure perceived self-efficacy in clients that should be analyzed before therapy in order to develop treatment goals, as well as monitoring changes over the course of therapy. Many of the clinical strategies that are commonly used in stuttering help to build self-efficacy, and this chapter sought to highlight these and provide specific recommendations for fostering the growth of self-efficacy for communication among clients who stutter.

REFERENCES

Bandura, A. (1961). Psychotherapy as a learning process. *Psychological Bulletin, 58*(2), 143–159.

Bandura, A. (1977a). *Social learning theory.* Upper Saddle River, NJ: Prentice Hall.

Bandura, A. (1977b). Self-efficacy: Toward a unifying theory of behavioral change. *Psychological Review, 84*(2), 191–215.

Bandura, A. (1994). Self-efficacy. In V. S. Ramachandren (Ed.), *Encyclopedia of human behavior* (Vol. 4, pp. 71–81). New York, NY: Academic Press.

Bandura, A. (Ed.). (1995). *Self-efficacy in changing societies.* Cambridge, UK: Cambridge University Press.

Bandura, A. (1997). *Self-efficacy: The exercise of control.* New York, NY: W. H. Freeman.

Bandura, A. (2006). Guide for creating self-efficacy scales. In F. Pajares & T. Urdan (Eds.), *Self-efficacy beliefs of adolescents* (pp. 307–337). Greenwich, CT: Information Age.

Beilby, J. M., Byrnes, M. L., & Yaruss, J. S. (2012). Acceptance and Commitment Therapy for adults who stutter: Psychosocial adjustment and speech fluency. *Journal of Fluency Disorders, 37*(4), 289–299.

Blomgren, M., Roy, N., Callister, T., & Merrill, R. M. (2005). Intensive stuttering modification therapy: A multidimensional assessment of treatment outcomes. *Journal of Speech, Language, and Hearing Research, 48*(3), 509–523.

Blood, G. W. (1995a). A behavioral-cognitive therapy program for adults who stutter: Computers and counseling. *Journal of Communication Disorders, 28*(2), 165–180.

Blood, G. W. (1995b). POWER^2: Relapse management with adolescents who stutter. *Language, Speech, and Hearing Services in Schools, 26*(2), 169–179.

Boyle, M. P. (2011). Mindfulness training in stuttering therapy: A tutorial for speech-language pathologists. *Journal of Fluency Disorders, 36*(2), 122–129.

Boyle, M. P. (2013a). Assessment of stigma associated with stuttering: Development and evaluation of the Self-Stigma of Stuttering Scale (4S). *Journal of Speech, Language, and Hearing Research, 56*(5), 1517–1529.

Boyle, M. P. (2013b). Psychological characteristics and perceptions of stuttering of adults who stutter with and without support group experience. *Journal of Fluency Disorders, 38*, 368–381.

Boyle, M. P. (2014, November). *Relations between stuttering disclosure and quality of life, anxiety, and stigma in adults who stutter*. Poster presented at the American Speech-Language-Hearing Association annual convention, Orlando, FL.

Boyle, M. P. (2015). Identifying correlates of self-stigma in adults who stutter: Further establishing the construct validity of the Self-Stigma of Stuttering Scale (4S). *Journal of Fluency Disorders, 43*, 17–27.

Boyle, M. (2016a). Relations between causal attributions for stuttering and psychological well-being in adults who stutter. *International Journal of Speech-Language Pathology, 18*(1), 1–10.

Boyle, M. P. (2016b, November). *Relations between stuttering disclosure and self-empowerment in adults who stutter*. Poster presented at the American Speech-Language-Hearing Association annual convention, Philadelphia, PA.

Boyle, M. P., & Blood, G. W. (2015). Stigma and stuttering: Conceptualizations, applications, and coping. In K. O. St. Louis (Ed.), *Stuttering meets stereotype, stigma, and discrimination: An overview of attitude research* (pp. 43–70). Morgantown, WV: West Virginia University Press.

Boyle, M. P., Daniels, D., Hughes, C., & Buhr, A. (2016). Considering disability culture for culturally competent interactions with individuals who stutter. *Contemporary Issues in Communication Sciences and Disorders, 43*, 11–22.

Boyle, M. P., Dioguardi, L., & Pate, J. E. (2016). A comparison of three strategies for reducing the public stigma associated with stuttering. *Journal of Fluency Disorders, 50*, 44–58.

Bray, M. A., & Kehle, T. J. (1996). Self-modeling as an intervention for stuttering. *School Psychology Review, 25*(3), 358–369.

Bray, M. A., & Kehle, T. J. (1998). Self-modeling as an intervention for stuttering. *School Psychology Review, 27*(4), 587.

Bray, M. A., & Kehle, T. J. (2001). Long-term follow-up of self-modeling as an intervention for stuttering. *School Psychology Review, 30*(1), 135–141.

Bray, M. A., Kehle, T. J., Lawless, K. A., & Theodore, L. A. (2003). The relationship of self-efficacy and depression to stuttering. *American Journal of Speech-Language Pathology, 12*(4), 425–431.

Byrd, C. T., Gkalitsiou, Z., Donaher, J., & Stergiou, E. (2016). The client's perspective on voluntary stuttering. *American Journal of Speech-Language Pathology, 25*, 290–305.

Chang, S., & Zhu, D. C. (2013). Neural network connectivity differences in children who stutter. *Brain: A Journal of Neurology, 136*, 3709–3726.

Constantino, C., & Alpern, E. (2016, July). *Self-empowerment and solidarity*. Paper presented at the annual convention of the National Stuttering Association, Atlanta, GA.

Craig, A. (1998). Relapse following treatment for stuttering: A critical review and corrective data. *Journal of Fluency Disorders, 23*(1), 1–30.

Craig, A., Blumgart, E., & Tran, Y. (2011). Resilience and stuttering: Factors that protect people from the adversity of chronic stuttering. *Journal of Speech, Language, and Hearing Research, 54*, 1485–1496.

Craig, A., Blumgart, E., & Tran, Y. (2015). A model clarifying the role of mediators in the variability of mood states over time in people who stutter. *Journal of Fluency Disorders, 44*, 63–73.

De Veer, S., Brouwers, A., Evers, W., & Tomic, W. (2009). A pilot study of the psychological impact of the mindfulness-based stress-reduction program on people who stutter. *European Psychotherapy, 9*, 39–56.

Fry, J., Millard, S., & Botterill, W. (2014). Effectiveness of intensive, group therapy for teenagers who stutter. *International Journal of Language & Communication Disorders, 49*(1), 113–126.

Helgadóttir, F. D., Menzies, R. G., Onslow, M., Packman, A., & O'Brian, S. (2014). A standalone Internet cognitive behavior therapy treatment for social anxiety in adults who stutter: CBTpsych. *Journal of Fluency Disorders, 41*, 47–54.

Herder, C., Howard, C., Nye, C., & Vanryckeghem, M. (2006). Effectiveness of behavioral stuttering treatment: A systematic review and meta-analysis. *Contemporary Issues in Communication Science and Disorders, 33*, 61–73.

Iverach, L., & Rapee, R. M. (2014). Social anxiety disorder and stuttering: Current status and future directions. *Journal of Fluency Disorders, 40*, 69–82.

Kang, C., Riazuddin, S., Mundorff, J., Krasnewich, D., Friedman, P., Mullikin, J., & Drayna, D. (2010). Mutations in the lysosomal enzyme-targeting pathway and persistent stuttering. *New England Journal of Medicine, 362*, 677–685.

Ladouceur, R., Caron, C., & Caron, G. (1989). Stuttering severity and treatment outcome. *Journal of Behavior Therapy and Experimental Psychiatry, 20*(1), 49–56.

Ladouceur, R., & Saint-Laurent, L. (1986). Stuttering: A multidimensional treatment and evaluation package. *Journal of Fluency Disorders, 11*(2), 93–103.

Lee, K., Manning, W. H., & Herder, C. (2015). Origin and pawn scaling for adults who do and do not stutter: A preliminary comparison. *Journal of Fluency Disorders, 45*, 73–81.

Luszczynska, A., Gutierrez-Dona, B., & Schwarzer, R. (2004). General self-efficacy in various domains of human functioning: Evidence from five countries. *International Journal of Psychology, 139*, 439–457.

Menzies, R., O'Brian, S., Lowe, R., Packman, A., & Onslow, M. (2016). International phase II clinical trial of CBTPsych: A standalone internet social anxiety treatment for adults who stutter. *Journal of Fluency Disorders, 48*, 35–43.

Menzies, R. G., O'Brian, S., Onslow, M., Packman, A., St Clare, T., & Block, S. (2008). An experimental clinical trial of a cognitive-behavior therapy package for chronic stuttering. *Journal of Speech, Language, and Hearing Research, 51*(6), 1451–1464.

Menzies, R. G., Onslow, M., Packman, A., & O'Brian, S. (2009). Cognitive behavior therapy for adults who stutter: A tutorial for speech-language pathologists. *Journal of Fluency Disorders, 34*(3), 187–200.

Nye, C., Vanryckeghem, M., Schwartz, J. B., Herder, C., Turner, H. I., & Howard, C. (2013). Behavioral stuttering interventions for children and adolescents: A systematic review and meta-analysis. *Journal of Speech, Language, and Hearing Research, 56*(3), 921–932.

Ornstein, A. F., & Manning, W. H. (1985). Self-efficacy scaling by adult stutterers. *Journal of Communication Disorders, 18*(4), 313–320.

Plexico, L., Manning, W. H., & DiLollo, A. (2005). A phenomenological understanding of successful stuttering management. *Journal of Fluency Disorders, 30*, 1–22.

Plexico, L. W., Manning, W. H., & DiLollo, A. (2010). Client perceptions of effective and ineffective therapeutic alliances during treatment for stuttering. *Journal of Fluency Disorders, 35*(4), 333–354.

Schwarzer, R., & Jerusalem, M. (1995). Generalized Self-Efficacy Scale. In J. Weinman, S. Wright, & M. Johnston (Eds.), *Measures in health psychology: A user's portfolio* (pp. 35–37). Windsor, UK: Nfer-Nelson.

Simpson, S., & Everard, R. (2015, July). *Stammering and the social model of disability: Implications for therapy*. Paper presented at the International Fluency Association 8th World Congress on Fluency Disorders, Lisbon, Portugal.

St. Louis, K. O. (Ed.). (2015). *Stuttering meets stereotype, stigma, and discrimination: An overview of attitude research*. Morgantown, WV: West Virginia University Press.

The Stuttering Foundation. (2005). *Adult stuttering therapy: Dr. Charles Van Riper* [DVD]. Memphis, TN: Author.

Trichon, M., & Tetnowski, J. (2011). Self-help conferences for people who stutter: A qualitative investigation. *Journal of Fluency Disorders, 36*(4), 290–295.

Venkatagiri, H. S. (2009). What do people who stutter want—fluency or freedom? *Journal of Speech, Language, and Hearing Research, 52*(2), 500–515.

Williams, D. E. (1957). A point of view about 'stuttering.' *Journal of Speech and Hearing Disorders, 22*, 390–397.

Yairi, E., & Seery, C. H. (2015). *Stuttering: Foundations and clinical applications* (2nd ed.). Boston, MA: Pearson Higher Education.

Yaruss, J. S., & Quesal, R. W. (2006). Overall Assessment of the Speaker's Experience of Stuttering (OASES): Documenting multiple outcomes in stuttering treatment. *Journal of Fluency Disorders, 31*(2), 90–115.

CHAPTER 4

A Perspective on Stuttering in the Social Context

James M. Mancinelli

INTRODUCTION

When two individuals encounter each other and begin a communicative interaction, that interaction is occurring within a specific social context. The verbal communication may be as simple as a basic greeting, an exchange of information, and then farewells. On the other hand, it may develop into a very complex conversational exchange, and that complexity is multidimensional as Hymes and other ethnographers have noted (Hymes, 1964, 1967). It is, however, crucial that we understand that this communicative event is embedded within a social context, and that makes all the difference for people who stutter (PWS). This chapter intends to show that for PWS, the social interaction becomes an object of evaluation and interpretation. PWS create a social history based on all of the communicative interactions they have experienced over time. This chapter will discuss a sociological framework for stuttering and describe its elements, relevance, and application to the assessment and treatment of those who stutter. Finally, many of the sociological terms introduced are new to the discipline of speech and language pathology and therefore a glossary of terms is provided in Appendix 4–A of this chapter.

THE SOCIOLOGICAL NATURE OF STUTTERING

Stuttering is a disorder that is more accurately explained by appealing to a multifactorial onset. (Smith & Kelly, 1997; Smith & Weber, 2017), and those factors continue to play a role in the communicative life of an adult who stutters. Furthermore, stuttering is also a stigmatizing disorder with a strong sociological component because it emerges within a social interaction (Boyle, 2013; Goffman, 1963; Krause, 1982; Lemert, 1970; Sheehan, 1953, 1970; Zhang & Kalinowski, 2012). There is reference to the sociological factors that contribute to disfluency in the literature (Zhang & Kalinowski, 2012) as well as a more direct discussion (Boyle, 2012; Lemert, 1970; Sheehan, 1970). Although environmental factors have been noted as etiologically relevant in the onset and persistence of stuttering (Smith & Weber, 2017), stuttering as a *social fact* about PWS during communicative interactions has been a largely overlooked dimension of the disorder (Acton & Hird, 2004; Butler, 2014; Goffman, 1963).

The Elements of a Sociological Framework

The sociological elements of stuttering cannot be underestimated. Stuttering is an emergent phenomenon, enmeshed within social interactions, and occurs at the intersection of the speaker, the listener, and the social context (Goffman, 1963). As a multifactorial disorder it emerges during the social interaction due to idiosyncratic variables (Acton & Hird, 2004; Lemert, 1970; Sheehan, 1970; Smith and Kelly, 1997). This gives stuttering a non-linear character in that a small change in one parameter (such as communication partner) can cause a large change in another (verbal fluency, tension). The most common historical models of stuttering were linear in that it was proposed that it grew from a simple form (sound repetitions) to a more complex form with increasing level of severity, secondary behaviors, and more aberrant speech disruptions. When stuttering is viewed within a sociological framework, however, its non-linearity becomes the defining character because the social interaction itself is a non-linear, dynamic, and variable phenomenon which has cognitive and emotional consequences for PWS.

The application of a sociological framework to stuttering has explanatory power and a history in the literature (Lemert, 1970; Sheehan, 1953, 1970). It includes the social context, the social identity of the communication partners, stigmatization and stereotyping, the type of talk, the evaluation and interpretation of the flow of the interactions, and disclosure/avoidance. The transactional and dyadic nature of verbal communication is influenced by the social context, culture, roles, and social relationships (DeFleur, Kearney, Plax, & DeFleur, 2005; Goffman, 1964). A description of stuttering that doesn't incorporate these factors in a systematic way leaves a gap in our complete understanding of the disorder. After all, the verbal fluency of a PWS, their primary focus during a communicative interaction, can be affected by those factors (Lemert, 1970).

Systematic investigations into the sociological nature of stuttering have been rare (Acton & Hird, 2004; Fraser & Scherer, 1982) and this is unfortunate. The interplay between the PWS, the listener, and the social context creates a communicative interaction, which is evaluated and interpreted during and after the interaction. The resulting interpretation can be framed very differently for each communicator (Blumer, 1969; Goffman, 1986). For example, the normally fluent speaker (NFS) can speak with a PWS while thinking about commonly held stereotypes about people who stutter, or simply accept the fact without preconceived notions. On the other hand, a PWS may frame the same interaction as a negative experience based on assumptions that he may have about the listener's general perceptions of PWS. Therefore, framing a communicative interaction for a PWS necessarily includes decisions about his social presentation and social identity during the interaction. This in turn necessarily includes a decision to try to conceal stuttering by using avoidance strategies, or *covering* (Goffman, 1963), in order to try to present himself as an NFS or to stutter freely and present a more authentic social self.

The Social Context

Every social interaction begins with a relationship between communication partners. In the case of those who are familiar with each other (e.g., friends, family members, colleagues), the expected course of the interaction is to prevent a disruption in that relationship (Goffman, 1967). For example, when interacting with a family member, the expectation is that the interaction will present no threats to the social relationship. Of course, a social interaction can take any direction and produce any number of scenarios, but the obligation of the interaction is to preserve the expected social presentation of each person. There are, however, many social encounters that occur daily between unfamiliar interactants who have no relationship until the end of the encounter when a new relationship has been defined by each person based on the evaluation and interpretation of that interaction. The thread that links each person during that interaction is the talk that occurs throughout it. One can see how this is complicated for PWS, because they must consider the *amount* and *type* of talk required by that particular social context. This can put a PWS at a distinct disadvantage due to the variability of his fluency, and the variability of the reactions of listeners. The communicative event occurring within that social interaction may contain powerful threats to the social identity of a PWS as he tries to present a social self that is expected by the other interactant, i.e., an NFS. Therefore the expected social relationship within that communicative event is disrupted as a result of the unexpected appearance of stuttering.

The social context within which verbal communication occurs contains not only the people, but also the amount and type of talk, context, culture, roles, and social relationships (DeFleur et al., 2005; Goffman, 1964; Lemert, 1970). The type of talk is referred to as *talk-in-interaction* within the sociological framework of stuttering.

Talk-in-Interaction

The primary situational threat for a PWS is referred to as *talk-in-interaction,* and examples of talk-in-interaction include conversations, interviews, reportage, depositions, or essentially any talk that involves two or more interactants (Goffman, 1963; Psathas, 1995; Sacks, Schegloff, & Jefferson, 1974; Schegloff, 1987; ten Have, 2007). Typically, a PWS finds himself within the context of a primary situational threat whenever he is in a communicative interaction involving one or more normally fluent speakers, and 98% to 99% of individuals are normally fluent speakers (Bloodstein & Bernstein Ratner, 2008; Ham, 1990). Variables within any form of talk-in-interaction (e.g., overlapping talk during a conversation, which for normally fluent speakers may be a naturally occurring element of any social interaction) can affect verbal fluency, comfort, anxiety, and communicative effectiveness during a social interaction for a PWS (Crocker et al., 1998). Within a sociological framework, the type of talk becomes a fully integrated element of the interaction and not a peripheral variable. The type of talk has the potential to affect the verbal fluency of the PWS and as a consequence his social identity within that interaction. Conversational analyses have shown that interactants respond to each other's talk in an ordered way, observing rules of turn taking and overlap and getting cues from pauses and gestures (Jefferson, 1989; Sacks et al., 1974; Schegloff et al., 1977; ten Have, 2007). However, it is not known whether the same conversational rules are adhered to in a communicative interaction between a PWS and NFS, since this has not been systematically investigated. Furthermore, every social interaction involves real-time evaluation and interpretation as the interactants are signaling to each other how the flow of the encounter is progressing with verbal and nonverbal signals (Blumer, 1969; ten Have, 2007). Thus, a rule-ordered conversational encounter not only includes the talk itself, but also the ongoing interpretations and evaluations of both parties. Furthermore, communicative interactions can have a range of values for PWS based on the social context and the type of talk, creating real threats to their speech fluency (Crocker et al., 1998; Goffman, 1963; Jones et al., 1984; Shelton, Alegre, & Son, 2010; Yang et al., 2007). Two possible threats are stereotyping and stigmatization of a PWS by his communicative partner.

Stereotyping and Stigmatization

The term *stigma* is defined as a "deeply discrediting" attribute or trait that marks an individual and reduces that person "from a whole and usual person to a tainted, discounted one" in the eyes of the other interactant (Goffman, 1963, p. 3). The individual who possesses an attribute that is devalued by society at large faces public stigma, negative stereotyping, prejudicial treatment, and discrimination (Boyle, 2012; Goffman, 1963). Internalization of these negative societal attitudes and reactions may result in social isolation and damaging psychosocial effects on the well-being of the PWS (Boyle, 2012). Stuttering meets the criteria of a stigmatizing attribute because of negative stereotypes about PWS and social stigma through interactions with others, which devalue the social identity of the stigmatized individual (Boyle, 2013; Goffman, 1963; Jones, Farina, Hastorf, Markus, Miller, & Scott, 1984).

The definition of stigma as a discrediting mark or attribute has remained stable since Goffman (1963) and its current conceptualization as a *dialectic, transactional process* between interactants in a social setting is now the prevailing characterization (Crocker et al., 1998; Jones et al., 1984; Shelton, Alegre, & Son, 2010; Yang et al., 2007). The stigmatizing stereotypes for PWS are rooted in the social interactions throughout their lives, which inform and color every ensuing communicative interaction. Stigmatization is dynamic in that it is refreshed and renewed with each encounter, as stereotypes are brought to mind for both parties.

There is a special relationship between a stigmatizing attribute and a negative stereotype (Goffman, 1963). Attributes of stuttering include the stereotypes of shyness, anxiousness, fearfulness, reticence, nervousness, tense demeanor, guardedness, sensitiveness, lack of intelligence, frustration, and introversion (Healey, 2010; Kalinowski, Stuart, & Armson, 1996; MacKinnon, Hall, & MacIntyre, 2007; Von Tiling, 2011; Woods & Williams, 1976). The negative stereotypes about a PWS develop out of the inferences that an NFS makes about a PWS during a communicative interaction, as well as the prevalent societal stereotypes. Some of these include characterizing the PWS as anxious, tense, or embarrassed and then applying those traits to the personalities of PWS in general (White & Collins, 1984). These stereotypes about PWS are stable across various social groups, such as teachers, lay people, and health care workers (Boyle, 2013). These stereotypes even exist in the media (e.g., *A Fish Called Wanda*, Porky Pig), lending support to societal thinking about PWS (Boyle, 2013). Boyle (2013) found that 40% of PWS concurred with the negative stereotypes associated with stuttering, reflecting an internalization of the public's view of stuttering, leading to self-stigmatization. Self-stigmatization, in turn, may have negative effects on social interaction by affecting the level of comfort, degree of anxiety, and cognitive effort on the part of PWS, as well as their verbal fluency.

The stigma of stuttering makes itself known as soon as a PWS begins to speak, making it a visible stigma. Other examples of visible, non-concealable stigmas include individuals with significant scarring from burns, a blind person, or a child with a craniofacial anomaly. Goffman considers these individuals to be *discredited*, meaning that they are instantly identifiable due to the visibility of their stigma (Goffman, 1963). Conversely, Goffman refers to an individual with a stigmatizing attribute that is concealable, but has the potential to be visible, as *discreditable* (Goffman, 1963). Although stuttering is referred to in the literature as a visible stigma (Boyle, 2013; Goffman, 1963; Van Riper, 1982), suggesting that a PWS is immediately discredited, its true nature can be more accurately defined as *fluid* or *dynamic* in relation to its visibility. For example, an NFS who is not familiar with his communicative partner as being a PWS is surprised when his anticipated identity as an NFS does not match his actual identity as a PWS (Goffman, 1963). The PWS begins the interaction in a concealed state until he begins to speak, at which time his stigma may become fully disclosed, and the tension, the discomfort, and the opportunities for judgment and stereotyping arise. On the other hand, for the NFS who knows that his communication partner is a PWS, there is no mismatch in identities, i.e., his stigmatizing attribute is known at the outset of the interaction, and this reduces the probability of negative reactions on the part of the NFS (Collins & Blood, 1990; Healey et al., 2007; Healey, 2010; Lee & Manning, 2010). From the perspective of a PWS, he is instantly fully disclosed as a PWS if he is stuttering freely during the communicative interaction; or he can choose to remain silent or utilize other avoidance strategies in an attempt to keep his stigma concealed from the listener. Therefore, it is apparent that a PWS has a choice in any communicative interaction. Speech-language pathologists prefer that the individual disclose his stuttering; however, a PWS who understands the social risks associated with self-disclosure, and hopes to preserve a social identity as a normally fluent speaker (NFS), may attempt to avoid stuttering. Conversely, it is possible that a PWS can pass as fluent as long as he remains concealed, and concealing his stuttering may be a natural response to avoid rejection or stereotyping (Bloodstein, 1995; Murphy, 1999; Sheehan, 1970; Van Riper, 1982). As a consequence, PWS can be in *either* state before or during a social interaction and can move from concealed to disclosed (in Goffman's terms *discreditable* to *discredited*, respectively) as their attempts to conceal their stuttering from others fail. This can cause feelings of great discomfort, tension, and anxiety during the interaction, as well as anger, guilt, shame, feelings of helplessness, feelings of suffering, and stigmatization as affective reactions to stuttering (Corcoran & Stewart, 1998; Daniels & Gabel, 2004; Murphy, 1999; Van Riper, 1982). This potential shift from one state of disclosure to another during the interaction is an example of the sociological variables impacting the communicative interaction.

When a stigmatized individual is interacting with a non-stigmatized individual, it is referred to as a *mixed situation* (Goffman, 1963). Mixed situations challenge both speakers due to the potential development of discomfort and tension. This happens for a few reasons. First, a disclosed PWS is not always certain that the other interactant will truly accept him, and this uncertainty can produce discomfort during the interaction. Second, the concealed PWS must *manage information* about his stigma, and this can be taxing and produce tension. This information includes deciding whether to remain concealed or to disclose during the social interaction, to lie or not to lie, to avoid words or specific sounds; to decide when it is best to disclose, with whom and how. As a consequence, a PWS begins to *partition* his life into what Goffman (1963) calls *forbidden*, *civil*, and *back* places, and PWS are very familiar with partitioning their social space. *Forbidden places/settings* are defined as places where exposure will result in expulsion from that particular social setting. This seems a bit extreme in relation to PWS and would most likely not occur in common social settings in contemporary American society, although it is possible; however, a PWS may consider certain careers or employment opportunities as forbidden places, e.g., air traffic controller, sales personnel. *Civil places/settings* are defined as those places where the stigmatized individual is accepted, although some discomfort lingers, and this is probably the norm in today's society. *Back places/settings* are defined as those where the stigmatized individual can be himself and stutter freely. Thus, PWS partition their social worlds based on the comfort and safety of the social context (Goffman, 1963; Panchakis, 2007; Ragins, 2008) and must decide on the information they will offer about their actual social identity (i.e., to stutter freely or to remain concealed in a social interaction). The majority of communicative interactions for a PWS are mixed situations and most likely in civil places and/or back places, suggesting that choosing to stutter freely in these situations comes with less negative consequences.

It is not surprising that a PWS would choose to avoid stuttering and thus make attempts to remain concealed during the communicative event in order to avoid the social stigma associated with the attribute of stuttering. It is also not surprising that after years of experiencing publicly held negative feelings and attitudes toward stuttering, PWS develop social selves built on the many negative social interactions they have experienced (Acton & Hird, 2004). Through these interactions with a PWS, communication partners also take a mental measure of the PWS, and they too construct a social identity for the PWS. The social identity of a PWS is thus interactionally defined and constructed by the interactants who build social facts about each other. These facts inform and are informed by the social encounter (Blumer, 1969; Goffman, 1963).

Social Identity

Identity is not a unitary construct. It comprises social identity, personal identity, and ego identity (Goffman, 1963). All three are pertinent to the study of individuals who stutter. *Social* identity is the one constructed through social interaction and it is this identity which will be an important element in this discussion; *personal* identity allows for the consideration of the individual's idiosyncratic way in managing stuttering during the interaction; and *ego* identity allows for the consideration of what a PWS feels about stuttering and its management. Every human being brings his/her psychological traits and characteristics into every social interaction, but the psychological traits and characteristics of each individual are not constructed anew with each social encounter. The *psychological* identity of a person is not formed or re-formed with every social interaction (Blumer, 1969). The social interaction, however, *is constructed* by the speakers as they evaluate their encounter (Blumer, 1969; Goffman, 1963).

As an individual moves through a myriad of social interactions during the day, he presents two identities (Goffman, 1963). The first is his *virtual identity* defined by two elements: the anticipated category of which he is a member and the attribute(s) of that particular category. For example, a man can be identified as a man (CATEGORY) by his physical appearance (ATTRIBUTE). The second identity is the individual's *actual identity* and is defined as the category and attribute(s) that he presents to the world. For example, the same man (CATEGORY) may also be deaf (ATTRIBUTE). A key element to the difference between these identities is that the virtual identity is *anticipated* by any other interactant and the actual identity is presented. If these two identities do not match, then there is an incongruity between them and the other interactant must adjust to this discrepancy by managing the information presented by this social presentation, e.g., communicating with a deaf individual and the decisions and challenges that it presents to a hearing person. The obvious application of this principle to a PWS is that the incongruity between the anticipated identity, as an NFS, and the actual identity, as a PWS, can lead to stereotyping and potential stigmatization. A PWS can "pass" until he stutters, when his stigmatizing attribute is visible immediately (Goffman, 1963, p. 48). Once the stigma of stuttering becomes visible during an interaction, there is an incongruity of social identity, possibly creating tension and discomfort for both parties (Goffman, 1963). Furthermore, as noted above, a listener's negative reactions to a stuttering event can serve to increase the disfluency (Bloodstein, 1995; Healey, 2010; Yovetich & Dolgoy, 2001) and reinforce any negative stereotypes about the self that a PWS may harbor (Boyle, 2013; Crocker, Major, & Steele, 1998; Van Riper, 1982).

Individuals have a social identity that affects how they interact in social settings, implying that the presentation of the self can and may differ from the private self (Goffman, 1963). This is certainly demonstrated in the daily life of a PWS, when the decision to stutter openly or attempt to conceal it is actually more of a decision about social identity. That is, in any form of talk with an NFS, a PWS who is attempting to conceal his stuttering makes that the focus of the interaction in order to present a social identity as a normally fluent speaker (Starkweather, 1987). Fluency is a desired outcome, but establishing and/or maintaining a social identity as an NFS is paramount, at least until he can integrate stuttering into his social identity through the process of self-acceptance, to present himself authentically in social contexts. A therapeutic technique that has commonly been viewed as a tool for facilitating self-acceptance in a PWS is self-disclosure, although it comes with social risks.

Disclosing the fact that one stutters during a communicative interaction places the PWS at risk for rejection, stereotyping, and stigmatization (Bloodstein, 1995; Cooper & Cooper, 1996; Goffman, 1963; Guitar, & Hoffman, 1979; Ham, 1990; Murphy, 1999; Ruscello, Lass, & Brown, 1988; Sheehan, 1970; Turnbaugh, St. Louis & Lass, 1981; Van Riper, 1982; Woods & Williams, 1976). Attempts to avoid stuttering and remain free of these negative social responses puts added pressure on a PWS and creates different risks, such as artificiality and convoluted discourse in order to avoid a particular feared sound or word which had been stuttered in the past. As a result, the communicative event can become disorienting and confusing for the listener, highlighting the aberrancy of the speech of the PWS and drawing the listener's attention to the signal itself and not the content. This is paradoxical and contrary to the purpose of PWS who wish to present themselves as NFS (Starkweather, 1987). Based on an encounter such as this, the listener thinks that the PWS is inarticulate, confirming a socially held stereotype about PWS. Therefore, the decision to stutter freely and thereby openly disclosing to the listener his actual identity may be freeing in one sense, yet self-sabotaging in another. The internal dissonance that this creates for the PWS can only diminish if his actual identity as a PWS is revealed.

The pressure of the decision to stutter freely, or attempt to conceal stuttering in order to avoid the stigma and stereotyping associated with it, is a constant for most PWS (Blumer, 1969; Boyle, 2012; Butler, 2014; Goffman, 1963). Furthermore, the listener becomes aware very quickly that his communication partner is a PWS and evaluates and interprets the interaction based on that fact—whereas for the PWS, managing his social identity now receives equal valence with his speech fluency and the content of the message. Managing the presentation of his social self as a PWS in order to avoid the stigmatizing views about a PWS becomes a primary focus (Goffman, 1959, 1963).

Evaluation and Interpretation of the Ongoing Interaction

Any social interaction begins with the individual evaluating the situation and commenting internally on its progress and flow, forming the basis of an interpretation of that interaction (Blumer, 1969). This is the foundational principle of symbolic interactionism. Symbolic interactionism closely examines the way the social identity of an individual develops through his interaction with the world, how that interaction is framed by each individual, and how it is interpreted and evaluated for meaning. Symbolic interactionism understands human interactions in this very distinctive and particular way, viewing a social interaction as interactants interpreting and evaluating each other's actions instead of merely reacting to them (Blumer, 1969; Goffman, 1963). Individuals respond and react to *situations* even though they may have encountered the same social contexts in the past, evaluating and interpreting them when they are encountered again (Blumer, 1969). People who stutter are aware of the reactions of their listeners (Bloodstein & Bernstein Ratner, 2008; Yovetich & Dolgoy, 2001) but it is the interpretation of those reactions by a PWS that affects the ongoing action of the communicative event. The positive or negative meaning of that interpretation is idiosyncratic and variable, but its impact can have immediate effects for the PWS, such as anxiety, fear, discomfort, and guilt. Because stuttering emerges during social interactions as a result of many variables and idiosyncratic factors (Smith & Kelly, 1997), understanding how interactions are constructed can shed light on how a PWS views and understands those interactions. This perspective can inform the study of disfluency, in that verbal communication becomes an organized social encounter comprising the evaluation of the encounter, the interpretation of that encounter, and social identity (Blumer, 1969; Goffman, 1964).

A PWS enters every communicative context with a history of these transactional experiences and their interpretations, coloring the interaction of the moment. Similarly, an NFS may also have had social interactions with a PWS that impact the current encounter. Each individual has built a *stuttering persona* out of those past experiences. Stuttering as a behavior is intimately linked to the *active relationship* between the speaker and the listener in a particular communicative context (Acton & Hird, 2004; Goffman, 1963; Lemert, 1970;).

Sociologically, every communicative interaction for a PWS is a new one, because stuttering is always intermittent. As noted above, for a PWS the communicative event includes a continual evaluation and interpretation of speech fluency as a measure of success or effectiveness, as well as the listener's reactions to it (Bloodstein & Bernstein Ratner, 2008; Starkweather, 1987;). Throughout his life, a heterogeneous history of these evaluations and interpretations is created (Butler, 2014; Goffman, 1963;). For a PWS the communicative event itself becomes an object of attention and evaluation—the context, the type of talk, the other interactant's response to his stuttering, and his success at not bringing attention to his speech. These internal evaluations over time lead to hierarchies of comfort and/or fear regarding communication events and all of their components. The same hierarchies can be used in treatment to desensitize a PWS to those social interactions and/or social contexts. A PWS views the communicative event as a true sociological object because it can be "indicated or referred to" by the speakers (Blumer, 1969, p. 11). As a consequence, the degree of fluency and the solidity of their social identity as an effective communicator are the parameters being evaluated. Both the PWS and the listener are now evaluating the communicative event as one shared object, but from two different perspectives (Bloodstein & Bernstein Ratner, 2008; Blumer, 1969; Cooper & Cooper, 1996; Goffman, 1963; Ham, 1990; `Turnbaugh, Guitar, & Hoffman, 1979; Woods & Williams, 1976; Yovetich & Dolgoy, 2001). Under these circumstances, the stigmatizing attribute of stuttering, now visible and interpretable, involuntarily generates disclosure. The role of self-disclosure in a social interaction is then a question worth pursuing.

State of Disclosure

Self-disclosure is considered the final step in the self-acceptance process for any stigmatized person (Goffman, 1963), yet self-disclosure can be extremely challenging for a PWS because of its possible consequences. A PWS has choices to make at the outset of a communicative interaction, regardless of social context: to stutter freely and openly, thereby disclosing his stigma; or to attempt to conceal and/or prevent stuttering by using avoidance strategies and thereby increasing the likelihood that he can present himself as an NFS. For some people who stutter, this is very possible, and these people can fall into the traditional *covert* group of people who stutter. This is not the case for all people who stutter due to the severity of their disfluency and their history of social interactions as a PWS. Disclosure is a constant feature in the lives of people who stutter because it makes them vulnerable to stereotyping and stigmatization during any social interaction. The decisions they make result in another episode in their social history of stuttering.

Self-disclosure is considered a process on a continuum that involves revealing personal information about oneself to another (Chelune, 1987; Derlega & Chaiken, 1977; Derlega, Metts, Petronio, & Margulis, 1993; Jourard, 1964; Ragins, 2008) and is commonly used by psychotherapists and counselors in treatment with individuals who are stigmatized due to physical, social, psychological, ethnic, and/or socioeconomic factors (Charmaz, 2010; Panchakis, 2007; Poindexter & Shippy, 2010; Ragins, 2008; Ryan, Kempner, & Emlen, 1980; Westbrook, Bauman, & Shinnar, 1992). Evidence from other stigmatized populations (e.g., people living with HIV/AIDS, sexual minorities, people of lower socioeconomic status, and people from ethnic backgrounds different from the majority) indicates that the benefits of self-disclosure are numerous. These include an increase in self-esteem, more positive self-evaluation, an increase in self-efficacy, and a reduction in the cognitive effort necessary to remain concealed in order to avoid public stigma (Derlega et al., 1993; Panchakis, 2007). Furthermore, the individual who self-discloses is supposed to experience a sense of relief, closer personal relationships, and reduced stress and to have the opportunity to affiliate with other people like him, something that is precluded if one remains concealed (Ragins, 2008). Self-disclosure also permits authenticity in that concealing an aspect of the self is no longer necessary (Ragins, 2008). The incongruity between the anticipated and actual identity of the individual is no longer present. Historically, speech-language pathologists have encouraged PWS to self-disclose because of those benefits. More specific to PWS, self-disclosure can be beneficial in reducing the stress and tension associated with a communicative interaction.

It is generally accepted that encouraging a PWS to self-disclose can increase self-acceptance by reducing feelings associated with stigmatization and negative attitudes toward stuttering, increasing comfort during the communicative encounter, and reducing the heightened sensitivity to his stuttering. He may stutter more freely, facilitating a feeling of authenticity and naturalness (Collins & Blood, 1990; Goffman, 1963; Guitar & Peters, 2013; Healey et al., 2007; Healey, 2010; Sheehan, 1970; Van Riper, 1982). Encouraging self-disclosure is a common therapeutic technique employed by most speech-language pathologists who work with people who stutter. Self-disclosure can take the form of a clear statement to the listener such as "I am a person who stutters" to simply stuttering freely without attempts to avoid disfluencies. There is anecdotal evidence that a PWS can use humor, sarcasm, self-deprecating comments, or be very direct as methods for disclosure (Van Riper, 1982). However, data on the benefits of self-disclosure from the perspective of PWS are rare. Mancinelli (2016) conducted a study examining self-disclosure from the perspective of 25 adults who stutter.

The results indicated that the participants rated the benefit of disclosing higher than they did not disclosing to their communication partner, based on the frequency distribution of the Likert response data; however, the findings of the paired *t*-tests revealed that whether or not the participants disclosed that they were PWS had no effect on their level of comfort, cognitive effort during the task, or level of anxiety. The results of the paired *t*-tests across participants for the dependent variables of total syllables spoken, total syllables stuttered, and total word count across conditions for all participants indicated that there was a non-significant difference as a result of disclosing or not disclosing that they were PWS at the outset of the experimental task, suggesting that state of disclosure had no effect. These findings are surprising in that disclosure is considered to be an ameliorating factor on tension, stress, and anxiety, with potential to increase verbal fluency for a PWS during a communicative event (Blood, Blood, Tellis, & Gabel, 2003; Collins & Blood, 1990; Healey, 2010; Healey, Gabel, Daniels, & Kawai, 2007; Lee & Manning, 2010; Manning, 2010; Manning, Burlison, & Thaxton, 1999; Rosenberg & Curtiss, 1954).

There is, however, evidence from the perspective of the listener that self-disclosure is helpful during a communication event. The studies on the listener's reactions to PWS who self-disclose are moderately substantial and describe benefits to the listener (Blood, Blood, Tellis, & Gabel, 2003; Collins & Blood, 1990; Healey, 2010; Healey et al., 2007; Lee & Manning, 2010; Manning, Burlison, & Thaxton, 1999; Rosenberg & Curtiss, 1954). For example, (a) listeners prefer speakers who self-disclose over those who do not (Collins & Blood, 1990; Healey, 2010; Healey et al., 2007; Lee & Manning, 2010); (b) listeners respond more favorably to speakers who self-disclose than to speakers who employ stuttering modification techniques (Healey, 2010; Lee & Manning, 2010; Manning et al., 1999); (c) listeners perceived speakers who self-disclose as more friendly (Healey et al., 2007); (d) disclosure is best done by the PWS at the outset of the communicative event (Healey et al., 2007) as opposed to waiting until the end of the interaction; and (e) listeners perceive self-disclosure more positively if the speaker's stuttering was more severe (Collins & Blood, 1990; Lee & Manning, 2010).

Even though increased verbal fluency is not a direct goal of self-disclosure, it can be a secondary effect due to a reduction in tension and fear during the communicative event. Removing the internal obstacles of fear, tension, and anticipatory struggle through self-disclosure may produce a concomitant increase in verbal fluency, as well as facilitating self-acceptance over time. Ultimately, the goal of any therapy with a PWS that includes self-disclosure is to reduce the negative feelings associated with stuttering and foster a more authentic social presentation of the self.

The Sociology of the Communicative Event in Stuttering

Stuttering is a dynamic, emergent phenomenon that rises up from a confluence of variables during a communicative interaction with another speaker (Smith & Kelly, 1997). This necessitates the need to create a framework for analyzing the sociological variables associated with the communicative event involving a PWS and another interactant. As discussed earlier, the sociological framework includes the social context, the stigmatization and stereotyping of the PWS, the type of talk in which the interactants are engaged, the evaluation and interpretation of the flow of the interaction by each person, and the social identity of each interactant (Figure 4–1). The state of disclosure is included as part of evaluation and interpretation because the decisions that are made in real time during the interaction regarding disclosure have effects on the eventual evaluation and interpretation of the communicative event.

Although there are standard components to any communicative event (Hymes, 1964, 1967), in the case of a PWS interacting with an NFS, the interaction must be viewed as fluid, changeable, non-linear, and under constant evaluation and interpretation for its adherence to the expected societal norms for dyadic communication by both parties. As non-linear and idiosyncratic phenomena, not all of the sociological elements have an equal valence for all people who stutter in all social interactions. For example, in some interactions, the type of talk may be a primary threat, whereas in another interaction it may be the social context itself. The level of self-acceptance is a major determinant. One can envision, for example, a PWS who has integrated stuttering into his personal and social identities as more comfortable and self-accepting. Conversely, a PWS who is covert or who still uses avoidance strategies in order to preserve his virtual identity as an NFS may feel variable effects during an interaction. Furthermore, his evaluation and interpretation of that communicative event will reflect those valences.

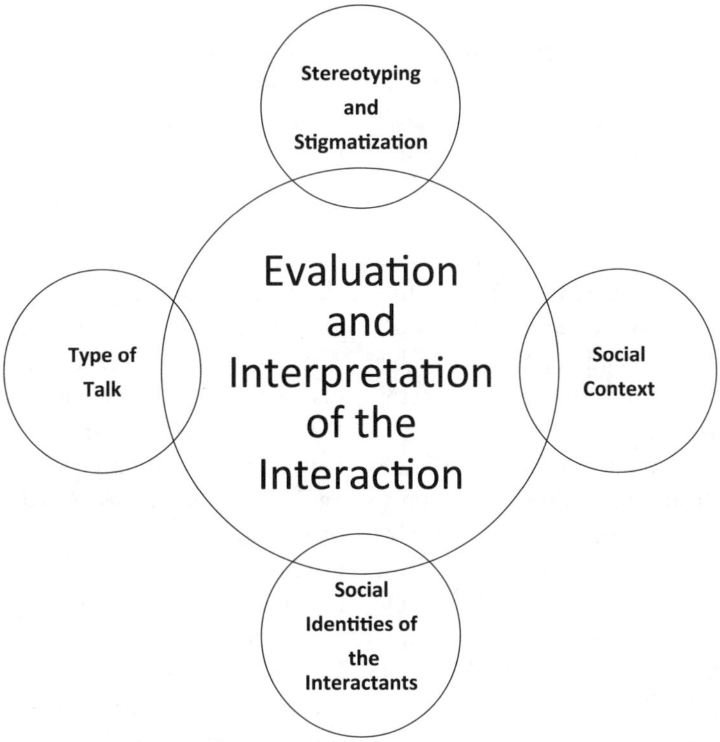

Figure 4–1. The communicative event within a sociological framework.

The evaluation and interpretation of the communicative event hold a central place in the model of the sociological framework. The graphic in Figure 4–1 emphasizes the relationships between the active elements of the framework during the communicative event. For a PWS, this process during a given communicative interaction includes an evaluation of his speech fluency as well as the listener's reactions to his speech. Essentially, a PWS attaches meaning and value to his speech by *evaluating* the degree of fluency and *interpreting* it as a measure of success or communicative effectiveness (Bloodstein & Bernstein Ratner, 2008; Starkweather, 1987). Every communicative interaction for a PWS is a new one, due to the inherent intermittency of stuttering (Butler, 2014; Goffman, 1963). Over time, this creates a heterogeneous history of evaluations and interpretations of those communicative events. Therefore, in the case of a PWS, the entire communicative event itself becomes an *object* of attention and evaluation (Blumer, 1969), and as an object it can be referred to and commented on. These internal evaluations lead to hierarchies of comfort and/or fear regarding communicative interactions. Clinicians are familiar with these hierarchies because they are sometimes used in treatment to desensitize a PWS to those types of social interactions or contexts. The communicative interaction can be assessed and parsed, with the degree of fluency and the solidity of his social identity as an effective communicator being the primary parameters evaluated.

During the interaction, both the PWS and the listener are evaluating the communicative event from two different perspectives (Bloodstein & Bernstein Ratner, 2008; Blumer, 1969; Cooper & Cooper, 1996; Goffman, 1963; Ham, 1990; Turnbaugh, Guitar, & Hoffman, 1979; Woods & Williams, 1976; Yovetich & Dolgoy, 2001). The PWS has now constructed a social identity for the listener through that communicative interaction while his social identity as a PWS is once again confirmed.

A PWS constructs a social identity from the communicative interactions that he experiences daily and how he frames those experiences (Blumer, 1969; Goffman, 1963, 1986). However, this is not a necessary process for normally fluent speakers. Historically, their social identity as an NFS is highly consistent during communicative events, with no incongruity between their anticipated identity and their actual identity (Goffman, 1963). Conversely, this is an interesting process for a PWS in that there is a *social history* related to stuttering in his life. In unfamiliar social contexts with unfamiliar communication partners, there will be an incongruity between the anticipated identity and the actual identity that emerges during that social interaction. Interestingly, that social history contains *inconsistent* social identities due to the intermittency of stuttering and partitioning of the social contexts. As an example, consider a PWS whose work context includes many people, all of whom know that he is a PWS. In the workplace, even though the type of talk, the interactants, and the social contexts may vary, his co-workers are aware that he is a PWS, so the pressure to present himself socially as an NFS is greatly reduced. This does not, however, necessarily eliminate any incongruity in social identity as a PWS due to the intermittency of stuttering. A communicative interaction on a day when his stuttering is worse may be framed by the PWS as ineffective, whereas for the NFS it may be framed simply as "he's having a bad day," with more focus placed on the content of the message, not the signal itself. In this example, variability leads both interactants to a reevaluation and reinterpretation of the interaction, because the PWS presented with less fluency. Outside of the workplace where the pressure to present a oneself as an NFS in order to reduce or eliminate stigmatization, a PWS relies on strategies for concealment, partitioning, or disclosing by stuttering freely, depending on how much he has integrated the stigma of stuttering into his personal identity (Goffman, 1963). Every social interaction is a new one and the sociological elements of an interaction drive the outcome for a PWS, especially in mixed situations.

A PWS typically finds himself in mixed situations, that is, in social contexts with normally fluent speakers. These situations may be threatening, neutral, or safe in reference to his comfort, anxiety, and cognitive effort. The decision to stutter freely or attempt to conceal his stuttering in order to avoid the stigma and stereotyping associated with it becomes paramount (Blumer, 1969; Boyle, 2012; Butler, 2014; Goffman, 1963). Therefore, the challenge in any communicative interaction is to decide whether to present his actual identity as a PWS or to attempt to conceal that identity by using avoidance strategies (Butler, 2014; Goffman, 1963). Should he confirm the social fact that he is a PWS, which may be apparent to the listener, by self-disclosing or should he attempt to preserve a false identity of an NFS at all costs—for example, by ending the interaction to reduce the opportunity for stuttering? This raises the issue of the value and short-term benefits of self-disclosure in the case of this readily visible stigma.

There is support from a sociological perspective that self-disclosure has a positive effect in that it is the last step on the path to self-acceptance for a stigmatized individual (Goffman, 1963). From the speech pathology perspective, self-disclosure does have positive effects on the communicative interaction between a PWS and an NFS (Healey et al., 2007; Manning, 2010). Therefore, it seems to make sense to foster self-disclosure in the PWS. It is commonly used therapeutically to reduce the reliance on avoidance strategies, to make the communicative event more comfortable and less stressful, and to make the listener more comfortable as well. It is important that we consider a very crucial factor regarding the visible stigma of stuttering: the speaker is immediately disclosed to the listener through his stuttering, and as a consequence, the role of voluntary self-disclosure in the short term is debatable. This requires closer examination.

I contend that self-disclosure is more likely to have optimal short-term benefits for the listener but optimal long-term benefits for the PWS. The reasoning is simple: At the outset of the communicative interaction in any social context, a PWS who manifests stuttering makes announcing it irrelevant. It is apparent to the listener that he is speaking with a PWS. There is evidence in the literature supporting the fact that listeners do appreciate when a PWS self-discloses at the outset of the communicative interaction (Collins & Blood, 1990; Healey et al., 2007; Healey, 2010; Lee & Manning, 2010). The listener will now evaluate and interpret this interaction based on the social fact that his communication partner is a PWS, which opens up the possibility for stereotyping and stigmatization. The PWS is now vulnerable to the evaluation and interpretation of the interaction by the NFS. If he states openly that he is a PWS, the discomfort and uncertainty felt by the listener regarding how to manage the interaction may be neutralized, allowing the listener to focus on the content of the message and not the signal itself. For the PWS, nothing has changed regarding speech fluency, but by disclosing to the listener, he can reduce the pressure imposed by the social context and his speech can be accepted for what it is. Self-disclosure at the outset of the interaction may help to reduce the stereotyping tendencies of unfamiliar communication partners, especially traits such as lack of confidence, shyness, and reticence to speak, even being inarticulate. It is the case, however, that every interaction is a new one for a PWS due to the variability and intermittency of stuttering. Therefore, the act of self-disclosure can potentially have either a positive or a negative value in a particular interaction based on the type of talk, the social context, the social identity of the other interactant, and the perceived evaluation by the listener. The short-term benefit is therefore variable for a PWS. The stigma of stuttering is immediately visible, and a PWS may not see the value in verbally self-disclosing to a communication partner because it is redundant. Therefore, this leaves him with the only remaining self-disclosure option, which is whether to stutter freely or to conceal it, and this may not be palatable for people who stutter. It may be that the true value of self-disclosure for a PWS comes in the *evaluation and interpretation* of the communication interaction once the stigma becomes visible. I believe that therapeutic effort must be put into self-acceptance, which fosters a reduction in anxiety and cognitive effort across social contexts, reflecting on how a PWS evaluates and interprets his communicative interactions.

CLINICAL IMPLICATIONS

The Affective, Behavioral, and Cognitive Aspects of Stuttering

It is a commonly held principle that clinicians must address the affective (A), behavioral (B), and cognitive (C) aspects of stuttering in therapy. As a dynamic, multifactorial disorder, the affective, behavioral, and cognitive aspects emerge idiosyncratically in varying proportions, though consistently, in people who stutter. Addressing the ABCs of stuttering certainly allows the clinician to obtain a multidimensional impression of how a PWS feels about, thinks about, and responds to his stuttering. This therapeutic approach is consistent with the understanding that stuttering is an emergent phenomenon and is more than a disruption of the rhythm of speech, more than a summation of types of disfluencies. As inclusive as this is, it does not account for the sociological framework within which stuttering occurs in a well-defined way, leaving a critical gap in a clinician's potential plan. Therefore, I suggest that we raise the etiological and therapeutic profile of the social context by adding it to the ABCs.

Incorporating the Sociological Framework into Therapeutic Planning

The sociological framework of stuttering includes the social context of the communicative interaction, the evaluation and interpretation of the interaction by both interactants, the social identities of the interactants, stereotyping and stigmatization, and the type of talk. I encourage my clients who stutter to journal daily about their communicative interactions throughout the day. This will reveal if they are partitioning the interactions (e.g., avoiding perceived unsafe spaces) or restricting their interactions to familiars or to a certain type of talk. They can reflect on their decisions about disclosure and how they choose to do so and reflect on their levels of comfort, anxiety, and cognitive effort across social contexts. The following are recommendations and suggestions based on the aspects of the framework. They have not yet been tested in a systematic way.

The Social Context

It is necessary that we have a very clear sense of the social contexts which are the most challenging for a particular individual. Historically, speech-language pathologists have asked clients to formulate a hierarchy which reflects their least fluent to their most fluent scenarios. We can augment this hierarchy by asking the client to include social contexts, certain people, types of talk, listeners in a specific role, etc. It may be more helpful to have a client formulate one hierarchy of strictly social contexts within which he finds himself least/most fluent, then create one for people, roles, and types of talk (telephone, teaching, public speaking, etc.). An example of a general treatment goal addressing the social context could be the following:

> *The client will create a hierarchy for types of social interactions, people, roles, and types of talk ranking each list from the easiest to the most challenging.*

The specificity of these hierarchies can be used as a foundation for treatment plans which can help the client to precisely address these sociological elements of the communicative event. The multidimensional social history that results from these hierarchies will aid treatment efficacy and relevance for the client. For example, once the client has created the hierarchies for each of the elements noted above, the clinician and the client can then choose which category is of primary importance. If the client feels that it is the type of social interaction that has the most negative effects on the communicative interaction, then the treatment would start desensitizing the client to the interactions on the hierarchy. This is not new; however, what is new is the fact that when a clinician looks at the hierarchical arrangement in total, a more inclusive picture of the client as a verbal communicator emerges. That is, engaging with a sales clerk in a store with a line behind him is the most challenging social interaction; or speaking with a physician over the phone about medical issues is more challenging than speaking with a physician in person. Yet, speaking with a family member over the phone is not challenging at all, indicating that for this client stuttering emerges more when the type of talk interacts with the social role of the other speaker. This can then be addressed from the cognitive, behavioral, and affective perspectives for this client. The overarching point is that for a PWS, it is not simply the talk, or the person, or the social situation, but the interplay of all variables that affect verbal fluency and their evaluation and interpretation of a particular communicative interaction.

Type of Talk

The type of talk has historically been an area of focus in the treatment of people who stutter. For example, if a client informs the clinician that telephone conversations and public speaking are difficult for him, the clinician can then institute a desensitization program focusing on those types of talk. Type of talk, however, includes the rules for engaging in that talk. Conversational analyses show that there are measurable components to conversational speech between two or more interactants that can inform a clinician's treatment plan. This requires observing and assessing the client engaging in conversational talk, and optimally in varied social contexts, perhaps during the intake interview process and in a telephone conversation. The outcome of such an observation is valuable because it provides a real-time, objective measure of the client's ability to comply with conversational rules. Typically, two individuals in a dyadic communicative interaction overlap each other's talk and understand the role of pausing (for a comprehensive description of conversational analysis, see Psathas, 1995; Sacks et al., 1974; Schegloff, 1968, 1987; Schegloff, Jefferson, & Sacks, 1977; ten Have, 2007). Does a PWS follow the rules of conversation? If so, does that adherence have any effect on verbal fluency, delivery of content, comfort, cognitive effort (planning) and/or tension? Conversely, if the rules of conversation are not followed, how does that inform our treatment plan for the client? A goal in the treatment plan to address those findings could play an important role in the movement toward self-acceptance. That is, if the client can be reassured that he is adhering to the commonly used rules of conversation, then the opportunities for deeper insights into his communicative effectiveness increase. A client will need training in the rules of conversation and how to identify them in a dyadic communicative event and that is a crucial first step. Subsequent to that training, a treatment goal addressing the type of talk and adherence to the rules of conversation could be the following:

> *The client will engage in a conversational interaction with two unfamiliar students and will assess his adherence to the rules of conversation during video review with the clinician.*

Stereotyping and Stigmatization

Boyle (2013) has developed a very efficient and focused method for assessing stigmatization in PWS, the *Self-Stigma of Stuttering Scale* (4S), with a flexibility that is valuable to both researchers and clinicians. All of the items, which are in the form of statements, reflect commonly held stereotypes and attributes associated with PWS. This scale asks the client to indicate what he believes other people in the general public think about people who stutter (14 statements in 3 sections) and what he believes about people who stutter (19 statements in 3 sections). It is a 1 to 5 Likert scale, where 1 = strongly disagree, and 5 = strongly agree. The 4S takes between 5 and 7 minutes to complete and it yields an overall stigma score. However, the clinician can also examine the client's responses to each of the 6 sections.

Stereotyping and stigmatization are a social fact for PWS. They can be subjected to it during every interaction. Using the 4S, clinicians now have a means for assessing it objectively. The results from the 4S can be used to address a client's belief system about his stuttering and this can be very fruitful toward the goal of self-acceptance. Results from the 4S can facilitate insights into how the PWS thinks about the listener and the role that those thoughts and perceptions play in his construction of communicative interactions. Two examples of treatment goals using the findings from the 4S and addressing the stereotyping and stigmatization could be the following:

> *The client will journal about his responses to statements on the Self-Stigma of Stuttering Scale (4S) that reflect a sense of self-stigmatization and be prepared to discuss his journal entry at the next therapy session.*

> *The client will journal about how he believes his sense of self-stigmatization affects his communicative interactions with other speakers.*

Social Identity

The sociological framework of the communicative interaction includes the construction of a social identity for interactants engaged in a communicative event. In the case of the PWS, the construction of a social identity involves the potential for stereotyping and stigmatization by the other interactant, especially if the PWS and the other interactant are not familiar with each other. The listener reaction, the response to that reaction by the PWS, and the ensuing evaluation and interpretation are all elements used to construct the social identities of each person during that interaction. The listener may become a "patient listener" in the evaluation of the PWS; and the PWS may remain inarticulate and nervous in the evaluation of the listener. In order to formulate a comprehensive treatment plan, the clinician should gain insight into the processes and criteria his/her client uses to evaluate the social identity of the client's communication partner and how that affects the construction of the client's own identity during that interaction. Is the clinician's construction of the social identity of the listener based on observable behaviors occurring within that interaction? Does the clinician base the construction of the listener's social identity on his/her own socio-communicative history of stuttering and measure it against the observations of the current interaction? The answer is probably "yes" to both. However, *integrating* the sociological framework into the therapy plan in a systematic way broadens and deepens the clinician's communicative profile of the client, especially when combined with the affective, behavioral, and cognitive aspects of treatment. The long-term goal would be to facilitate a stable social identity for the PWS so that, despite the intermittency and the variability of his disfluency, as well as the non-linearity of social interactions, the PWS remains authentically himself. An example of a treatment goal addressing social identity could be:

> *The client will make journal entries reflecting on his perceptions of his communicative partners during a social interaction and his internalized reactions to those perceptions.*

This could be implemented by having the client reflect in his journal how he is perceiving his communication partners, using his hierarchy of partners, as a guide. He can then reflect on how that perception affected his own identity within that interaction. For example, did he feel as though he presented himself as a reticent speaker because all of his answers were very clipped to avoid stuttering? Did he do this because his communication partner was high on his list of difficult communication partners? Did that social identity have an effect on the communicative interaction as a whole? Is it typical for him to adopt the "reticent speaker" identity with listeners like this? How can he construct another identity in similar interactions in the future?

Social identity is a foundational concept in the study and treatment of stigmatized individuals regardless of their stigmatizing attribute. People who stutter may prefer to live authentically and helping them do so requires addressing the issue of social identity. The value of self-help groups cannot be underestimated in this regard (see Chapter 10 in this book for a discussion of self-help groups)

Evaluation and Interpretation

The importance of this aspect of the framework cannot be overstated and as a consequence, assessing this process for each client and then incorporating those findings into the treatment plan is imperative. The variability, intermittency, and dynamism of stuttering are tied to its emergent character. Stuttering emerges within the social interaction when a certain set of variables arise. Those same variables may have been present in a similar interaction earlier but with different effects on fluency. Therefore, the new interaction is *necessarily* evaluated differently, and this in turn will generate new affective and cognitive interpretations. Clinicians need to be aware of the processes of evaluation and interpretation that their client uses in order to provide a treatment plan that addresses those processes. For example, some clients may evaluate each interaction in a dichotomous manner, that is, either "good" or "bad" and their interpretation of the interaction is based on that evaluation. For other clients, that dichotomy does not apply and communicative interactions are evaluated based on level of comfort, or level of cognitive effort, and not on verbal fluency. Incorporating these features of a client's disfluency into the treatment plan can have a significant effect on the movement toward self-acceptance across social contexts. I view this element of the sociological framework to be an ongoing focus of therapy. An example of a treatment goal addressing the evaluation and interpretation processes could be:

> *The client will evaluate and interpret the parameters of fluency, comfort, cognitive effort, and tension during the review of a communicative interaction with a normally fluent speaker.*

Even though this goal can be an ongoing one in a client's treatment plan, the clinician can vary the focus—for example, on social context, interactants, and/or type of talk. For example, the clinician may propose that the client journal about communicative interactions addressing the goal above. Pertinent questions could be, "How did you evaluate your interaction with the school principal from the fluency, comfort, and cognitive effort perspectives? Which parameter was more difficult to evaluate? Do you know why that is?" Follow-up questions could be, "How did you interpret your evaluation? Was it realistic? What affected your interpretation? Is it possible to interpret this evaluation in another way?" Again, the purpose is to obtain a three-dimensional view of the client as a speaker in a social context, and not simply "a speaker."

CONCLUSION

Social interaction is an integral part of the human condition. Throughout the day, we are engaged with each other as we teach, learn, hold conversations, and even deceive. These interactions necessarily involve predictions, interpretations, and evaluations by the interactants (Hari, Henriksson, Malilnen, & Parkkonen, 2015), and each one of those elements creates a social history for a PWS and impacts all interactions subsequently. In this chapter the sociological framework of stuttering was presented so that clinicians can add a pragmatic dimension to their understanding of the disorder and to formulate assessment protocols and treatment plans that can offer insights and assistance in the daily lives of people who stutter. There is value in systematically investigating the daily lives of people with communication disorders by using ethnographic principles (Kovarsky & Crago, 1990–1991). From a research perspective, the sociological framework of stuttering opens up the possibility of developing an ethnography of stuttering which could provide a glimpse into the everyday lives of PWS. For example, using the journal entries of PWS who are asked to reflect on the elements of the sociological framework can offer insights about differences and similarities between the communicative lives of PWS and NFS. These data could be gathered from many sources over a specified period of time and then analyzed qualitatively for themes and meaning.

The *Overall Assessment of the Speaker's Experience of Stuttering* (OASES) (Yaruss & Quesal, 2006) was certainly an important step in the right direction and is an invaluable tool for evaluating the psychosocial aspects of stuttering. This is also true of the 4S (Boyle, 2013) because it provides a formal and objective measure of stereotyping and stigmatization in people who stutter. I propose that we must refine our description, assessment, and treatment of stuttering by bringing the sociological elements into sharper focus. After all, stuttering emerges during a social interaction and any analysis of the phenomenon is incomplete without consideration of the sociological framework to the communicative event. The assessment and treatment discussion above should be viewed as a starting point. More importantly, clinicians now have a framework within which to develop socially relevant goals, and researchers a platform from which to launch further investigations that examine the communicative lives of PWS.

The lives of people who stutter are complicated by the decisions they must make as they enter and exit social interactions. Observing, recording, and analyzing those interactions, the "daily rounds" of their lives (Goffman, 1963), can certainly improve our understanding of stuttering as well as inform our treatment planning.

REFERENCES

Acton, C., & Hird, M. J. (2004). Toward a sociology of stammering. *Sociology, 38*(3), 495–513.

Blood, I. M., Blood, G. W., Tellis, G. M., & Gabel, R. M. (2003). A preliminary study of self-esteem, stigma, and disclosure in adolescents who stutter. *Journal of Fluency Disorders, 28*(2), 143–159.

Bloodstein, O. (1995). *A handbook on stuttering.* Clifton Park, NY: Delmar Cengage Learning.

Bloodstein, O., & Ratner, N. B. (2008). *A handbook on stuttering.* Clifton Park, NY: Delmar Cengage Learning.

Blumer, H. (1969). *Symbolic interactionism: Perspective and method.* Englewood Cliffs, NJ: Prentice-Hall.

Boyle, M. P. (2012). *Self-stigma of stuttering: Implications for self-esteem, self-efficacy, and life satisfaction* (Unpublished doctoral dissertation).

Boyle, M. P. (2013). Assessment of stigma associated with stuttering: Development and evaluation of the Self-Stigma of Stuttering Scale (4S). *Journal of Speech, Language, and Hearing Research, 56*(5), 1517–1529.

Butler, C. (2014). Wanted—straight talkers: Stammering and aesthetic labour. *Work, Employment and Society, 28*(5), 718–734.

Charmaz, K. (2010). Disclosing illness and disability in the workplace. *Journal of International Education in Business, 3*(½), 6–19.

Chelune, G. J. (1987). A neuropsychological perspective of interpersonal communication. In J. H. Berg & V. J. Derlega (Eds.), *Self-disclosure: Theory, research, and therapy* (pp. 9–34). New York, NY: Plenum Press.

Collins, C. R., & Blood, G. W. (1990). Acknowledgment and severity of stuttering as factors influencing nonstutterers' perceptions of stutterers. *Journal of Speech and Hearing Disorders, 55*(1), 75–81.

Cooper, E. B., & Cooper, C. S. (1996). Clinician attitudes toward stuttering: Two decades of change. *Journal of Fluency Disorders, 21*, 119–135.

Corcoran, J. A., & Stewart, M. (1998). Stories of stuttering. *Journal of Fluency Disorders, 23*(4), 247–264.

Crocker, J., Major, B., & Steele, C. (1998). Social stigma. In D. Gilbert, S. Fiske, & G. Lindzey (Eds.), *The handbook of social psychology* (pp. 89–107). New York, NY; Boston, MA: McGraw-Hill.

Daniels, D. E., & Gabel, R. M. (2004). The impact of stuttering on identity construction. *Top Language Disorders, 24*(3), 200–215.

DeFleur, M. H., Kearney, P., Plax, T. G., & DeFleur, M. L. (2005). *Fundamentals of human communication: Social science in everyday life.* New York, NY: McGraw-Hill.

Derlega, V. J., & Chaiken, A. L. (1977). Privacy and self-disclosure in social relationships. *Journal of Social Issues, 33*(3), 105.

Derlega, V. L., Metts, S., Petronio, S., & Margulis, S. T. (1993). *Self-disclosure.* Newbury Park, CA: Sage.

Fraser, C., & Scherer, K. R. (1982). *Advances in the social psychology of language.* Cambridge, UK: Cambridge University Press.

Goffman, E. (1959). *The presentation of the self in everyday life.* New York, NY: Random House.

Goffman, E. (1963). *Stigma; notes on the management of spoiled identity.* Englewood Cliffs, NJ: Prentice-Hall.

Goffman, E. (1964). The neglected situation. *American Anthropologist, 66*(6), 133–136.

Goffman, E. (1967). *Interaction ritual: Essays on face-to-face behavior.* New York, NY: Pantheon.

Goffman, E. (1986). *Frame analysis: An essay on the organization of experience.* Boston, MA: Northeastern University Press.

Guitar, B., & Peters, T. J. (2013). *Stuttering: An integration of contemporary therapies*. Memphis, TN: The Stuttering Foundation of America.

Ham, Ham R. (1990). What is stuttering: Variations and stereotypes. *Journal of Fluency Disorders, 15*(5–6), 259–273.

Hari, R., Henriksson, L., Malinen, S., & Parkkonen, L. (2015). Centrality of social interaction in human brain function. *Neuron, 88*.

Healey, E. C. (2010). What the literature tells us about listeners' reactions to stuttering: Implications for the clinical management of stuttering. *Seminars in Speech and Language, 31*(4), 227–235.

Healey, E. C., Gabel, R. M., Daniels, D. E., & Kawai, N. (2007). The effects of self-disclosure and non-self-disclosure of stuttering on listeners' perceptions of a person who stutters. *Journal of Fluency Disorders, 32*(1), 51–69.

Hymes, D. (1964). Introduction: Toward ethnographies of communication. *American Anthropologist, New Series, 66*(6, Part 2), 1–34.

Hymes, D. (1967). Models of the interaction of language and the social setting. *Journal of Social Issues, 23*(2), 8–28.

Jefferson, G. (1989). Preliminary notes on a possible metric which provides for a "standard maximum" silence of approximately one second in conversation. In D. Roger & P. Bull (Eds.), *Conversation: An interdisciplinary perspective* (pp. 166–196). Philadelphia, PA: Multilingual Matters.

Jones, E. E., Farina, A., Hastorf, A. H., Markus, H., Miller, D. T., & Scott, R. A. (1984). *Social stigma: The psychology of marked relationships*. New York, NY: W. H. Freeman.

Jourard, S. M. (1964). *The transparent self: Self-disclosure and well-being*. Princeton, NJ: Van Nostrand.

Kalinowski, J., Stuart, A., & Armson, J. (1996). Perceptions of stutterers and nonstutterers during speaking and nonspeaking situations. *American Journal of Speech-Language Pathology, 5*(2), 61–67.

Kovarsky, D., & Crago, M. (1990–1991). Toward the ethnography of communication disorders. *National Student Speech Language Hearing Association Journal, 18*, 44–55.

Krause, R. (1982). A social psychological approach to the study of stuttering. In C. Fraser & K. Scherer (Eds.), *Advances in the social psychology of language* (pp. 77–122). Cambridge, UK: Cambridge University Press.

Lee, K., & Manning, W. H. (2010). Listener responses according to stuttering self-acknowledgment and modification. *Journal of Fluency Disorders, 35*(2), 110–122.

Lemert, E. M. (1970). Sociological perspectives. In J. Sheehan (Ed.), *Stuttering: Research and therapy* (pp. 172–187). New York, NY: Harper & Row.

MacKinnon, S. P., Hall, S., & MacIntyre, P. D. (2007). Origins of the stuttering stereotype: Stereotype formation through anchoring–adjustment. *Journal of Fluency Disorders, 32*(4), 297–309.

Mancinelli, J. M. (2016). *The effects of self-disclosure on the communicative interaction between a person who stutters and a normally fluent speaker* (Doctoral dissertation). Retrieved from Proquest Dissertations & Theses. (Publication number 10241459)

Manning, W. (2010). *Clinical decision making in fluency disorders*. Clifton Park, NY: Delmar Cengage Learning.

Manning, W. H., Burlison, A. E., & Thaxton, D. (1999). Listener response to stuttering modification techniques. *Journal of Fluency Disorders, 24*, 267–280.

Mitchell, S. D. (2009). *Unsimple truths: Science, complexity, and policy*. Chicago, IL: University of Chicago Press.

Murphy, B. (1999). A preliminary look at shame, guilt, and stuttering. In N. B. Sacks & E. V. Healey (Eds.), *Stuttering research and practice: Bridging the gap* (pp. 131–143). Mahwah, NJ: Erlbaum.

Panchankis, J. E. (2007). The psychological implications of concealing a stigma: A cognitive- affective behavioral model. *Psychological Bulletin, 133*(2), 328–345.

Poindexter, C. C., & Shippy, R. A. (2010). HIV diagnosis disclosure: stigma management and stigma resistance. *Journal of Gerontological Social Work, 53*, 366–381.

Psathas, G. (1995). *Conversation analysis: The study of talk-in-interaction*. Thousand Oaks, CA: Sage.

Ragins, B. R. (2008). Disclosure disconnects: Antecedents and consequences of disclosing invisible stigmas across life domains. *Academy of Management Review, 33*(1), 194–215.
Rosenberg, S., & Curtiss, J. (1954). The effect of stuttering on the behavior of the listener. *Journal of Abnormal Psychology, 49*(3), 255.
Ruscello, D. M., Lass, N. J., & Brown, J. (1988). College students' perceptions of stutterers. *NSSLHA Journal, 16*, 115–120.
Ryan, R., Kempner, K., & Emlen, A. C. (1980). The stigma of epilepsy as a self-concept. *Epilepsia, 21*(4), 433–444.
Sacks, H., Schegloff, E. A., & Jefferson, G. (1974). A simplest systematics for the organization of turn-taking for conversation. *Language, 50*(4), 696–735.
Schegloff, E. A. (1968). Sequencing in conversational openings. *American Anthropologist, 70*(6), 1075–1095.
Schegloff, E. A. (1987). Analyzing single episodes of interaction: An exercise in conversation analysis. *Social Psychology Quarterly, 50*(2), 101–114.
Schegloff, E. A., Jefferson, G., & Sacks, H. (1977). The preference for self-correction in the organization of repair in conversation. *Language, 53*(2), 361–382.
Sheehan, J. G. (1953). Theory and treatment of stuttering as an approach-avoidance conflict. *Journal of Psychology, 36*(1), 27–49.
Sheehan, J. G. (1970). *Stuttering: Research and therapy.* New York, NY: Harper & Row.
Shelton, J. N., Alegre, J. M., & Son, D. (2010). Social stigma and disadvantage: Current themes and future prospects. *Journal of Social Issues, 66*(3), 618.
Smith, A., & Kelly, E. (1997). Stuttering: A dynamic multifactorial model. In R. Curlee & G. Siegel (Eds.), *Nature and treatment of stuttering: New directions* (2nd ed., pp. 204–217). Needham Heights, MA: Allyn & Bacon.
Smith A., & Weber, C. (2017). How stuttering develops: The multifactorial dynamic pathways theory. *Journal of Speech, Language, and Hearing Research, 60*, 2483–2505.
St. Louis, K. O., & Lass, N. J. (1981). A survey of communicative disorders students' attitudes toward stuttering. *Journal of Fluency Disorders, 6*(1), 49–79.
Starkweather, C. W. (1987). *Fluency and stuttering.* Englewood Cliffs, NJ: Prentice-Hall.
ten Have, P. (2007). *Doing conversation analysis.* London, UK: Sage.
Turnbaugh, K. R., Guitar, B. E., & Hoffman, P. R. (1979). Speech clinicians' attribution of personality traits as a function of stuttering severity. *Journal of Speech and Hearing Research, 22*(1), 37–45.
Van Riper, C. (1982). *The nature of stuttering.* Englewood Cliffs, NJ: Prentice-Hall.
Von Tiling, J. (2011). Listener perceptions of stuttering, prolonged speech, and verbal avoidance behaviors. *Journal of Communication Disorders, 44*(2), 161–172.
Westbrook, L. E., Bauman, L. J., & Shinnar, S. (1992). Applying stigma theory to epilepsy: A test of a conceptual model. *Journal of Pediatric Psychology, 17*(5), 633–649.
White, P. A., & Collins, S. R. C. (1984). Stereotype formation by inference: A possible explanation for the "stutterer" stereotype. *Journal of Speech and Hearing Research, 27*(4), 567–570.
Woods, C. L., & Williams, D. E. (1976). Traits attributed to stuttering and normally fluent males. *Journal of Speech and Hearing Research, 19*(2), 267–278.
Yang, L. H., Kleinman, A., Link, B. G., Phelan, J. C., Lee, S., & Good, B. (2007). Culture and stigma: Adding moral experience to stigma theory. *Social Science & Medicine, 64*(7), 1524–1535.
Yaruss, J. S., & Quesal, R. W. (2006). Overall assessment of the speaker's experience of stuttering (OASES): Documenting multiple outcomes in stuttering treatment. *Journal of Fluency Disorders, 31*(2), 90–115.
Yovetich, W. S., & Dolgoy, S. (2001). The impact of listeners' facial expressions on the perceptions of speakers who stutter. *Journal of Speech-Language Pathology and Audiology/Revue d'Orthophonie Et d'Audiologie, 25*(3), 145–151.
Zhang, J., & Kalinowski, J. (2012). Culture and listeners' gaze responses to stuttering. *International Journal of Language & Communication Disorders / Royal College of Speech & Language Therapists, 47*(4), 388.

APPENDIX 4–A

Glossary of Terms Pertinent to the Sociology of Stuttering

actual identity	This is the identity of an individual that one experiences during a social, e.g., a PWS.	Goffman (1963)
covering	The methods used by stigmatized persons to prevent disclosing their stigma. A PWS uses word avoidance or even silence.	Goffman (1963)
disclosing	When stigmatized persons openly display their stigma in social settings.	Goffman (1963)
discreditable	This refers to the undisclosed state of a stigmatized person. That is, there is the potential for the stigma to be discovered.	Goffman (1963)
discredited	This refers to the *disclosed state* of a stigmatized person. The stigma is publicly known or acknowledged.	Goffman (1963)
ego identity	This identity allows for the consideration of what individuals feel about their stigma and its management during an interaction.	Goffman (1963)
emergent phenomenon	Any real-world phenomenon that results from a confluence of factors interacting with each other, implying complexity. Stuttering as a phenomenon demonstrates this concept.	Mitchell (2009)
managing information	This refers to the process of divulging information about oneself, how much to divulge, what to divulge, and/or when to divulge it during a social interaction.	Goffman (1963)
partitioning	This describes the process whereby a stigmatized person separates his daily reality into three distinct settings: 1. *Forbidden places* are those places where exposing the stigma will cause expulsion from that situation. 2. *Civil places* are those places where he is accepted as a stigmatized person, although some may feel uncomfortable.	Goffman (1963)

partitioning *continued*	3. *Back places* are those places where the stigmatized individual can safely and comfortably be himself.	
social identity	The identity constructed through social interaction. It allows for the consideration of stigma in the daily life of a PWS.	Goffman (1963)
talk-in-interaction	This term refers to the object of study in conversational analysis (CA) and developed out of Goffman's theories on social interaction. It is meant to capture the concept that the talk in a social interaction provides information about how the interaction is organized and its features. It refers to forms of talk such as conversation, interviews, courtroom proceedings, depositions, and reportage. It is the talk of everyday life.	Sacks et al. (1974); Schegloff (1987); Jefferson (1989); Psathas (1995); ten Have (2007)
virtual identity	This is the identity of an individual that one anticipates/expects in a social interaction, e.g., a fluent speaker.	Goffman (1963)

CHAPTER 5

The Impact of Perfectionism on Stuttering

Barbara J. Amster and Evelyn R. Klein

INTRODUCTION

The purpose of this chapter is to explore the clinical implications of perfectionism and its possible impact on stuttering. We begin with a scenario:

Bobby is the second of two boys in the Smith family. Bobby, like his older brother Johnny, started to stutter at age 4. But unlike his older brother, Bobby's stuttering did not go away and now at age 7, Mrs. Smith is concerned because Bobby is stuttering "severely." Mrs. Smith comments that she and her husband reacted to the stuttering in both boys in the same manner, trying not to draw attention to it. This worked for Johnny but not for Bobby. Mrs. Smith describes the two boys as very different from each other. Johnny is very easygoing, not easily upset, but Bobby was described as being very hard on himself, often berating himself if his homework or schoolwork was not flawless. Could Bobby's perfectionistic personality style make it more likely for his stuttering to become chronic?

Some people feel that striving for perfection is admirable, but actually having the expectation that everything should be perfect can lead to feelings of inadequacy and frustration. Errors and mistakes are a natural part of being human. You probably know people who have the tendency to be perfectionistic, who are often self-critical if their unattainable standards are not met. Many people have this tendency. Some of them are people who stutter (PWS) and some are not. As clinicians who have treated many people who stutter over the years and have come to know our clients well, we have found that many of our adult clients who stutter were very self-critical, not only about their speech but also about their appearance, job performance, and relationships. Several of our pediatric clients who stutter often became very upset when their coloring went outside the lines or their stack of blocks wasn't perfectly aligned. Could these clients also be perfectionists? Could it be that a tendency toward perfectionism has some connection to stuttering?

An intriguing aspect of stuttering is that many young children go through a period of disfluency, but most recover. Estimates of recovery vary but are as high as 80% (Yairi & Ambrose, 1992). Yet for some people, stuttering persists and becomes chronic. Chronic or persistent stuttering has been related to an interaction of environmental and constitutional factors (Shapiro, 2011). Theorists have investigated predictive factors for recovery and persistence (Yairi, Ambrose, Paden, &

Throneburg, 1996). Various factors—age at onset, duration of the disorder, family history of persistent or recovered stuttering, and scores on language/nonverbal measures—appear to have some predictive value (Yairi et al., 1996). For instance, children who begin to stutter at an earlier age are more likely to recover, as are those who have been disfluent less than 15 months post onset. Children who have concomitant language impairments are less likely to remit and those with a family history of stuttering are at greater risk, but if the history indicates that family members recovered, that would be a better prognostic indicator. Nevertheless, the search for vulnerabilities for chronic stuttering continues, including environment (Starkweather & Gottwald, 1990), speech-motor system (Kleinow & Smith, 2000), temperamental characteristics (Anderson, Pellowski, Conture, & Kelly, 2003), personality (Manning & Beck 2013), and social anxiety (Messenger, Onslow, Packman, & Menzies, 2004). Could it be that individuals who show a cognitive style that heightens their awareness of speech difficulties set unrealistic goals for performance, which leads to rumination and worry, making them more vulnerable to the biophysical predisposition to stutter? Perhaps being perfectionistic is another vulnerability making stuttering more likely to persist?

CONCEPTUALIZATION OF PERFECTIONISM

The definition and conceptualization of perfectionism varies among investigators (Flett & Hewitt, 2002; Frost, Marten, Lahart, & Rosenblake, 1990). In early explanations, perfectionism was viewed as a maladaptive, unidimensional personality orientation based on cognitive factors in the form of illogical beliefs, attitudes, and thoughts (Burns, 1980a, 1983; Flett & Hewitt, 2002). Perfectionistic individuals were described as living with unrealistic personal standards, leading to feelings of incompetence and low self-esteem (Burns, 1980a, 1980b). Hamachek (1978) suggested that the definition of perfectionism should distinguish between normal and neurotic perfectionism. Normal perfectionism involves the functional pursuit of excellence, whereas neurotic perfectionism includes self-denigration as a result of standards that are impossible to meet (Hamachek, 1978). In this view, neurotic perfectionists are overly concerned about making mistakes and doubt their abilities. Hamachek's use of the term "neurotic perfectionism" is similar to later conceptions of maladaptive perfectionism.

Perfectionism has also been conceptualized as a more complex multidimensional construct including intrapersonal and interpersonal aspects (Flett & Hewitt, 2002). One characteristic of perfectionism that is frequently noted in the literature is the tendency to be less tolerant of mistakes and more self-critical (Burns, 1980a; Frost et al., 1990). This characteristic of perfectionism is noted in both unidimensional and multidimensional constructs. Frost, Turcotte, Heimberg, Mattia, Holt, and Hope (1995) in an experiment involving the Stroop Color Naming Task (1935) reported that people who have high levels of concern over mistakes react more negatively to making mistakes and are more likely to conceal their mistakes from others. Flett, Hewitt, Blankstein, and Gray (1998) reported that individuals who focus on failure and mistakes can be described as perfectionistic and this may lead to anxiety and depression. DiBartolo, Li, Averett, Skotheim, Smith, Raney, and McMillen (2007) describe the more negative aspects of perfectionism as maladaptive cognitive styles. They found that the negative and maladaptive evaluative concerns in perfectionism put an individual at risk for psychological distress. Flett and Hewitt (2006) take issue with the theory that there are positive and negative types of perfectionism, indicating that positive aspects of perfectionism are often confused with conscientiousness. They also state that "negative perfectionism involves avoidance tendencies because of a concern about making mistakes" (p. 480). Negative perfectionism may relate to stuttering as PWS tend to avoid speaking situations and social interactions. Similarly, avoidance is considered a key factor in stuttering (Bloodstein & Bernstein Ratner, 2008; Shapiro, 2011; Starkweather, 1987; Van Riper, 1982).

Another conceptualization of perfectionism considers perfectionism to be divided into three dimensions (Hewitt & Flett, 1990; Stoeber & Carr, 2015). *Self-oriented perfectionists* are very self-critical if they believe they have not met their *own* expectations. *Other-oriented perfectionists* believe it is important for *others* to strive to be perfect. They are very critical of others who don't meet their expectations. *Socially prescribed perfectionists* strive for perfection because they believe *others expect* them to be perfect and that they will be judged poorly by those who are highly critical of them.

Stoeber and Carr (2015) studied 388 university student volunteers and found that individuals with high self-oriented perfectionism tended to be highly reactive to positive and negative stimuli. This type of perfectionism was positively correlated with avoidance and fear. Other-oriented perfectionism predicted less negative affect and those with higher levels tended to be highly defensive when feeling threatened. These individuals were less sensitive and generally experienced less negative affect compared with those lower in other-oriented perfectionism. Those with socially prescribed perfectionism were found to be more maladaptive. Their perfectionism was negatively correlated with goal-driven persistence and affective well-being. Additionally, Wyatt and Gilbert (1998) investigated perfectionism, social rank, and status in 113 undergraduate psychology students (who did not stutter) and found that socially prescribed perfectionism was significantly positively correlated with measures of shame, submissiveness, and defeat. Self-oriented perfectionists saw themselves as more inferior to others. According to Schlenker and Leary (1985), perfectionistic individuals tend to be socially tense and may have difficulty initiating socially affiliated behaviors.

Hewitt, Habke, Lee-Baggley, Sherry, and Flett (2008) studied perfectionistic self-presentation (PSP), which they describe as a deleterious interpersonal style involving promoting a public image of perfection and avoiding displays or self-disclosures of any perceived imperfections. They found that perfectionistic individuals who had elevated PSP scores, particularly those who hid their imperfections, responded to social interaction in ways that intensified emotional distress. This may be pertinent to PWS who often avoid social interactions in order to hide their perceived imperfect speech.

Dunkley, Zuroff, and Blankstein (2003) offer a different construct for perfectionism. They divide perfectionism into two dimensions that they call *personal standards* (PS) and *self-criticism* (SC). PS includes the setting and striving for high standards for oneself, whereas SC involves harsh self-criticism and concern about criticism from others. Furthermore, individuals with SC have been shown to show symptoms of depression and anxiety (Dunkley, Blankstein, Masheb, & Grilo, 2006).

Tangney (2002) discusses the importance of what she calls the "self-conscious emotions," which are shame, guilt, embarrassment, and pride for perfectionists. She states: "perfectionists are apt to be especially familiar with the self-conscious emotions because they focus so much energy on self-evaluation." Tangney (2002, p. 199). These self-conscious emotions, especially shame, are often experienced by PWS (Murphy, 1999).

Because of the varied conceptualizations of perfectionism, there is also some controversy about measuring it. The *Burns Perfectionism Scale* (Burns, 1980a) is a unidimensional measure focusing on the more maladaptive features of perfectionism. The Burns scale is "heavily weighted on personal standard setting and concern over mistakes" (Frost et al., 1990, p. 451). Concern over mistakes appears to be a significant characteristic of perfectionistic individuals (Frost et al., 1990).

A more multidimensional conceptualization led to two separate measures of perfectionism with the same name, the *Multi-Dimensional Perfectionism Scale* (MPS) (Flett & Hewitt, 2002; Frost et al., 1990; Hewitt & Flett, 1990, 1991). The Hewitt and Flett (1991) MPS differentiated three perfectionism dimensions: other-oriented, self-oriented, and socially prescribed perfectionism, previously described in this chapter. The Frost et al. (1990) MPS distinguished six dimensions: concern over mistakes, personal standards, parental expectations, parental criticism, doubts about actions, and organization. Based on a different multidimensional conceptualization, Slaney, Rice, and Ashby (2002) developed the *Almost Perfect Scales* (APS), which categorizes perfectionists into adaptive and maladaptive groupings. Hill, Huelsman, Furr, Kibler, Vicente, and Kennedy (2004) noted that the choice of a preferred perfectionism instrument is debatable and suggested that a single measure capturing the constructs from both MPS scales would be useful for researchers. They proposed a new multidimensional measure, the *Perfectionism Inventory* (Hill et al., 2004), which uses eight constructs they believe to be fundamental to perfectionism: concern over mistakes; high standards for others; need for approval; organization; perceived parental pressure; planfulness; rumination; and striving for excellence. In 2010, Kim developed a self-report scale to capture both positive and negative consequences of perfectionism, which was found to be a reliable and valid measure in a follow-up study by Stoeber, Hoyle, and Last (2013).

Shafran, Cooper, and Fairburn (2002) suggested that multidimensional perfectionism scales are not clinically relevant because it is the more maladaptive aspects of perfectionism that require intervention. They suggest using a unidimensional model. They also suggest that avoidance of tasks is a maintaining factor of clinical perfectionism. Furthermore, Shafran and Mansell (2001) noted that it is the negative aspects of perfectionism that are associated with psychopathology, deserve intervention, and can interfere with treatment. The unidimensional model, with its emphasis on concern over making mistakes, might actually be more relevant to use in evaluating perfectionism in people who stutter. These different measures of perfectionism could indicate that perfectionism as a construct has a variety of interpretations depending on the views of researchers who study it.

The Development of Perfectionism

Frost et al. (1990) note that most theorists working in the area of perfectionism describe perfectionists as individuals who place importance on their parents' expectations and evaluations of them. They were brought up in environments in which love was conditional and to experience love they had to meet increasing levels of perfection in performance.

In their review article, Morris and Lomax (2014) indicate that there is strong evidence that supports the role of parent behavior in the development of perfectionism in children. Controlling parents tended to predict more maladaptive perfectionism. Flett, Hewitt, Oliver, and Macdonald (2002) looked at the role of the familial environment on the development of perfectionism and found that anxious parents encourage perfectionism in their children through focusing on mistakes and the negative outcomes that come from making mistakes. Further, they discuss various factors contributing to the development of perfectionism, including specific characteristics of the child such as temperament. They posit that perfectionists have temperaments characterized by "high levels of emotionality, including high fearfulness, along with high levels of persistence" (p. 111). This is similar to the findings of temperament in children who stutter discussed later in this chapter. Perfectionistic traits may run in families and an investigation of the genetics of perfectionism appears warranted but has been presently overlooked.

Children who grow up in environments with conditional positive approval may develop a sense of self that is defined by performance standards. Performance appraisals and fear of making mistakes and possibly failing are key features in perfectionism as described by Frost et al. (1990). Individuals concerned with meeting standards imposed by others have been found to fear negative evaluations by others (Hewitt & Flett, 1991).

Mitchell, Broeren, Newhall, and Hudson (2013) investigated the impact of perfectionistic child-rearing behaviors which were experimentally manipulated in a copying task in clinically anxious and non-anxious children. Perfectionistic child-rearing practices were described as focusing on imperfection and mistakes in children. They found that all of the children showed an increase in self-oriented perfectionism when they randomly received high perfectionistic rearing behaviors. In contrast, children who received non-perfectionistic child-rearing practices improved significantly in task accuracy performance. Therefore, children performed better when parents did not react in a perfectionistic manner.

Stuttering and Perfectionism

A link between stuttering and perfectionism has been investigated (Amster, 1995; Amster & Klein, 2008, 2007, 2005; Brocklehurst, Drake, & Corley 2015). Perfectionism has been mentioned in the stuttering literature as a temperamental factor to explain how stuttering develops or is maintained (Riley & Riley, 2000). As discussed above, perfectionism, like stuttering, is challenging to operationally define (Flett & Hewitt, 2002; Perkins, 1990). A frequently noted feature of perfectionism is the tendency to be less tolerant of perceived mistakes and more self-critical (Burns, 1980a; Frost et al., 1990).

Few experimental studies have explored whether PWS are perfectionistic. In one study, Amster (1995) surveyed 47 PWS and 22 matched controls using the Burns Perfectionism Scale in both its original format (Burns, 1980a) and an adapted format in which subjects answered the questions on the Burns Scale as they thought they would have responded as a child of about 4 or 5 years of age. Amster (1995) noted that the PWS were more perfectionistic and viewed themselves to have been more perfectionistic as children than people who did not stutter. Amster and Klein (2008) used the Burns Perfectionism Scale with 8 PWS and had similar results. All participants at baseline scored in the perfectionistic range on the Burns Perfectionism Scale (Burns, 1980a) and on an adaptation of the Burns Perfectionism Scale (Amster, 1995). All participants considered themselves to have been perfectionistic as children, with childhood recollections of perfectionism remaining stable from baseline to completion of treatment (using a combination of Cognitive Behavioral Therapy and Stuttering Modification [CBT-SM]) and 15 weeks after treatment ended at follow-up. However, self-ratings of current adult level of perfectionism showed a different profile as perfectionism significantly decreased across CBT-SM treatment. PWS reduced their perfectionistic tendencies with CBT-SM and continued to show reductions 15 weeks after treatment ended. Amster and Klein (2005) conjectured that people who stutter are concerned about their speech errors and view them as mistakes leading to negative emotional reactions. Because of this, people who stutter may try to hide their stuttering, leading to escape and avoidance behaviors. Avoidance behaviors are often thought to be key features of chronic stuttering (Bloodstein & Bernstein Ratner, 2008; Shapiro, 2011; Starkweather, 1987; Van Riper, 1982). Perfectionism, especially concern over making mistakes, may lead to heightened awareness and concern about speech errors, and the resulting distress may lead to avoidance. Consequently, perfectionism could be a personal characteristic related to the development and maintenance of chronic stuttering.

Brocklehurst, Drake, and Corley (2015) used a different perfectionism scale, the Frost Multidimensional Perfectionism Scale (FMPS; Frost et al., 1990) on 81 PWS and 81 matched controls in an online survey. They found that the PWS were not abnormally perfectionistic when looking at the total perfectionism score. However, being a PWS was associated with higher scores on the Concern about Mistakes–Doubts about Actions subscale but slightly lower scores on the Personal Standards subscale. These individuals also perceived their stuttering to be more severe. Further, Brocklehurst et al. (2015) indicated that this outcome supported the findings of Amster (1995) and Amster and Klein (2007, 2008).

If PWS are more concerned about making mistakes, they might be more distressed about their perceived speech errors, thereby more intense in their reactions to disfluency. In efforts to gain control of their speech, PWS may expend increased levels of energy, resulting in tension, effort, and struggle, the types of behaviors thought to make stuttering persist (Starkweather, 1987).

The authors of this chapter believe that having the personal characteristic of perfectionism can be a catalyst for the development and maintenance of chronic stuttering.

Potential Neurophysiological Connections with Perfectionism and Concern About Mistakes

McGirr and Turecki (2009) found that perfectionism is associated with increased sympathetic nervous system indicators and cortisol responses which can affect a number of physiological systems in the body. Similarly, Wirtz, Elsenbruch, Emini, Rudisuli, Groessbauer, and Ehlert (2007) found that perfectionism was associated with increased cortisol production in men in response to stress. They used the German version of the Frost Multidimensional Perfectionism Scale and found that for their 50 middle-aged male subjects during a public speaking task, high scores in the subtest Concern over Mistakes and Doubts significantly predicted the cortisol response, indicating that this aspect of perfectionism affects the neuroendocrine stress response.

Hewitt et al. (2008) analyzed physiological data of individuals who showed perfectionistic self-presentation and found that they had higher levels of heart rate when discussing past mistakes.

Heightened concern about mistakes appears to be a central feature of maladaptive perfectionism. Amster and Klein (2008) and Brocklehurst, Drake, Corley (2015) noted that PWS showed increased concern about making mistakes. Interestingly, Arnstein, Lakey, Compton, and Kleinow (2011), in a study of neural correlates of speech monitoring, found that these responses (error-related negativity [ERN] and the error positivity [Pe]) were both higher in PWS than in matched controls. In fact, ERN was higher whether or not the PWS actually made an error. Their results support theories that stuttering occurs from overmonitoring of the speech plan. This overmonitoring of the speech plan could be underlying neurophysiological support for the increased concern about mistakes found in both the Amster and Klein (2008) and Brocklehurst,

Drake, and Corley (2015) studies. It would be interesting to see whether their subjects also scored high on concern about mistakes on one of the perfectionism scales. One of the authors of this study, Jennifer Kleinow, is contributing a chapter to this book that further explores the neural emotional underpinnings of stuttering (see Chapter 2).

PERSONALITY, SOCIAL ANXIETY, AND STUTTERING

Messenger, Onslow, Packman, and Menzies (2004) used the *Fear of Negative Evaluation* (FNE) Scale and the *Endler Multidimensional Anxiety Scale–Trait* with 34 stuttering and 34 control participants. They found that those who stutter expected negative social evaluations, whereas controls did not. The findings produced a large effect size. Further, their results indicated that as a group, PWS have anxiety mostly restricted to the social domain. They postulated that social anxiety mediates stuttering in daily speaking exchanges affecting severity because of the relationship among anxiety, respiration, and speaking. Stuttering may also lead to social anxiety. Social anxiety can also be influenced by heightened awareness and worry about what you are going to say, how you are going to say it, and how people will evaluate you.

This is further reflected by Manning and Beck (2013), who investigated individuals' hypersensitivity to potential criticism and fear of social evaluation as personality characteristics in people who stutter. They scored participants on the *Assessment of DSM-IV Personality Disorders, ADP-IV* and found that 45 of the 50 adult participants in treatment for developmental stuttering did not show personality disorders. Only 5 participants were identified with a personality disorder. These findings were in contrast to those of Iverach et al. (2010), who found that 64% of 93 adult participants who stutter had a personality disorder (using the *Five Factor Inventory* by Costa & McCrae, 1992). Their higher neuroticism factor was interpreted to reflect interpersonal difficulties directly related to stuttering. The contrasting findings in these two studies could be due to differences in participants and the personality measurement scales used. Manning and Beck (2013) believe that a likely consequence of stuttering is excessive anxiety related to concern and fear of social evaluation. They concluded that future research should focus on "how emotional processes either facilitate or diminish healthy functioning among people who stutter" (p. 16).

It could be that these individuals have heightened awareness of mistakes and are overly concerned with the evaluations of themselves and others. These are factors associated with perfectionistic thinking which also leads to feelings of increased anxiety.

Temperament, Emotional Reactivity, and Perfectionism

Although the connection between perfectionism and stuttering has not been widely investigated, researchers have explored temperament and personality characteristics and their association with persistent stuttering. For example, Anderson et al. (2003) found that preschool-age children who stutter were more likely than their matched controls to have temperamental characteristics of hypervigilance, slowness to adapt to change, and irregularity in biological functions. They suggested that these characteristics might differentiate those who persist in stuttering from those who recover. Guitar (2003) examined the temperamental trait of reactivity, defined as the intensity of reaction by measuring the startle response in 14 adults who stutter and 14 matched controls. This study provided some evidence that

PWS may have more reactive temperaments than people who do not stutter. According to Anderson et al. (2003), a more highly reactive individual would tend to react strongly to disappointment or perceived failure. A reactive temperament may predispose an individual to experience feelings of disappointment with perceived speech errors. Amster and Klein (2005) speculated that individuals with more reactive temperaments might also be perfectionistic, as they would likely show undue concern over perceived mistakes. Eggers, De Nil, and Van den Bergh (2010) gave the *Children's Behavior Questionnaire* to 116 children who stutter (CWS) and matched controls and found that the children who stutter performed differently on temperamental factors of *Negative Affectivity* and *Effortful Control*, further supporting that CWS differ from typically developing children in temperamental characteristics. In contrast, Alm (2014), in a review article, did not find that there was evidence for increased risk for persistent stuttering in children with emotionally reactive temperaments.

Relating temperament to perfectionism, Kobori, Yamagata, and Kijima (2005) based a study on the Flett et al. (2002) transactional model of perfectionism. This model divides perfectionism into the three types previously discussed: self-oriented (a strong motivation for self-perfection), other-oriented (a strong motivation for others to be perfect), and socially prescribed (perceptions of unrealistically high standards imposed by others to be perfect). They administered the *Multidimensional Perfectionism Scale* (MPS) (Hewitt & Flett, 1991) and the *Temperament and Character Inventory* (Cloninger, Svrakic, & Przybeck, 1993) to 428 Japanese undergraduate students. Self-oriented perfectionism was associated with the temperamental characteristics of low novelty seeking (preference for sameness), high reward dependence (a need for feedback), and high persistence (ability to stay with a task to completion). These temperamental traits are similar to those mentioned by Anderson et al. (2003). The children who stutter in this study were more likely to be withdrawn in new situations, to display more intense reactions to disappointment or failure, and to show greater persistence with an activity.

Ed Conture and colleagues have investigated emotional reactivity and emotional regulation in preschool children who stutter in several studies (Arnold, Conture, Key, & Walden, 2011; Karrass, Waldren, Conture, Graham, Arnold, Hatfield, & Schwenk, 2006). Emotional reactivity can be defined as automatic and forceful reactions to an external *emotional* stimulus, and emotional regulation can be used to describe an individual's ability to manage and respond to an *emotional* experience. These studies have revealed greater emotional reactivity experienced by preschool children who stutter compared with controls, and relative lack of ability to flexibly control attention and regulate their emotions as well as fluent speech. We, the authors of this chapter, speculate that children who are more emotionally reactive and have difficulty with emotional regulation are also perfectionistic.

Modifiability of Perfectionism

An important consideration about maladaptive perfectionism is that while its effects can be detrimental (Blatt, 1995; Flett et al., 1998), it can be modified with appropriate treatment. Ferguson and Rodway (1994) used Cognitive Behavioral Therapy (CBT) with individuals who were perfectionistic and found that CBT may be effective in treating perfectionism and associated problems, which they measured using the *Burns Perfectionism Scale*. In a series of experiments involving automatic perfectionistic thoughts, Flett et al. (1998) reported that perfectionistic thoughts increase distress and that cognitive-behavioral interventions may be particularly useful in reducing their frequency. Perfectionism has been associated with a variety of clinical disorders, including depression, eating disorders, anxiety disorders, and social phobias (Shafran & Mansell, 2001), and cognitive restructuring appears to be an effective treatment.

DiBartolo, Frost, Dixon, and Almodovar (2001) investigated a brief cognitive restructuring intervention on perfectionists' responses to a public speaking task. Using the Frost et al. (1990) MPS, they identified perfectionistic subjects who scored high and low in the subtest Concern over Mistakes. Subjects with elevated scores in Concern over Mistakes were significantly more troubled by thoughts of negative speech-related outcomes. Also, the brief cognitive restructuring intervention was more successful for subjects with a high score on the MPS subtest Concern over Mistakes, and these subjects reported feeling significantly better able to cope than they had prior to the intervention. In addition, they reported decreased anxiety ratings about the speaking task. These results provide promising support for the benefits of cognitive restructuring when PWS show perfectionistic tendencies. See Chapter 6 in this book for a further discussion on the use of Cognitive Behavioral Therapy for PWS.

The *Cool Kids Program* (Mitchell, Newall, Broeren, & Hudson, 2013), is a manualized CBT treatment that has been investigated with 67 children (by Lyneham, Abbott, Wignall, & Rapee, 2003). It was found to reduce anxiety in children (6–13 years of age). Using self-report questionnaires at baseline, post-treatment, and at 6-month follow-up, results indicated that self-oriented perfectionism (SOP) and self-prescribed perfectionism (SPP) decreased immediately following treatment. However, only maternal ratings of children's SOP predicted improvement in child ratings of anxiety at 6-month follow-up time. Although this treatment was not focused on CWS, it did identify perfectionism as a trait that includes concern over mistakes associated with increased expectations and criticism from parents. Higher SOP in children predicted greater anxiety reduction when CBT was used. Stuttering has been linked with perfectionism (Amster & Klein, 2008; Klein & Amster, 2004) and anxiety (Alm, 2014; Manning & Beck, 2013).

We, the authors of this chapter, are not saying that maladaptive perfectionism causes stuttering, but we speculate that having this trait may be a precipitating and perpetuating factor making stuttering more likely to persist. Maladaptive perfectionism may be a potentially important personality characteristic to consider when applying Smith and Weber's (2017) Multifactorial Dynamic Pathways Theory of stuttering development. We consider perfectionism to be a cognitive style. When the necessary predisposing biophysical factors are present, this cognitive style affects the cognitive, emotional, and social factors, in turn causing PWS to struggle in an attempt to control their speech or avoid speaking in an effort to elude the negative feelings of lack of control and the potential negative reactions from others. These types of behaviors can make stuttering more severe and persistent. We believe that any behavioral treatment of stuttering such as stuttering modification or fluency shaping could greatly benefit from some cognitive restructuring techniques such as CBT, which can change the perfectionistic cognitive pattern, thereby reducing the emotional and social consequences. We are not suggesting this to alter fluency, but believe that it could improve PWS' quality of life by making PWS less hard on themselves. We further encourage the use of a perfectionism scale such as the Burns Scale or the Multidimensional Perfectionism Scales in any diagnostic assessment of stuttering, as they may give valuable information for clients who show this cognitive style. A version of the Burns Scale can be found in Table 5–1, and an adaptation of the Burns

Table 5–1. Burns Perfectionism Scale

This inventory lists a number of attitudes or beliefs that people sometimes hold. Decide how much you agree with each statement according to the following code:

+2 = I agree very much
+1 = I agree somewhat
0 = I feel neutral about this
–1 = I disagree slightly
–2 = I disagree strongly

Fill in the blank preceding each statement with the number that best describes **how you think most of the time**. Be sure to choose only one answer for each attitude. There is no "right" or "wrong," so try to respond according to the way you usually feel and behave.

_______ **1. If I don't set the highest standards for myself, I am likely to end up a second-rate person.**

_______ **2. People will probably think less of me if I make a mistake.**

_______ **3. If I cannot do something really well, there is little point in doing it at all.**

_______ **4. I should be upset if I make a mistake.**

_______ **5. If I try hard enough, I should be able to excel at anything I attempt.**

_______ **6. It is shameful for me to display weaknesses or foolish behavior.**

_______ **7. I shouldn't have to repeat the same mistake many times.**

_______ **8. An average performance is bound to be unsatisfying to me.**

_______ **9. Failing at something important means I'm less of a person.**

_______ **10. If I scold myself for failing to live up to my expectations, it will help me to do better.**

Scoring: Add up scores on all items noting that plus and minus numbers cancel each other out. The higher the score, the more perfectionistic the mindset.

A score of minus 20 = a non-perfectionistic mindset
A score of plus 20 = a high degree of perfectionism

Source: Reprinted with permission from David D. Burns. Burns, D. D. (1980, November). The perfectionist's script for self-defeat. *Psychology Today*, 34–52.

Scale to examine a retrospective view of perfectionistic traits during childhood can be found in Table 5–2; a version of the Frost Multidimensional Perfectionism Scale can be found on the web at http://www.bbc.co.uk/science/humanbody/mind/surveys/perfectionism/

When using the Burns Scale, a higher score up to a score of +20 indicates a more perfectionistic mindset, whereas a lower score, as low as –20, indicates a non-perfectionistic mindset.

In therapy, we try to show our clients how imperfect "normal" speech actually always is. We have them monitor the speech disruptions of others including family members. We especially like to have them monitor those who are usually considered great speakers, such as news commentators or politicians. We want our clients to notice when these speakers display typical disfluencies such as pauses, fillers, and reformulations. Our clients are often amazed when their attention is drawn to the "speaking

Table 5–2. Amster Adaptation of the Burns Perfectionism Scale

This inventory lists a number of attitudes or beliefs that people sometimes hold. Decide how much you agree with each statement according to the following code:

+2 = I agree very much
+1 = I agree somewhat
0 = I feel neutral about this
–1 = I disagree slightly
–2 = I disagree strongly

Fill in the blank preceding each statement with the number that best describes **as you think you might have felt as a child of about age four or five**. Be sure to choose only one answer for each attitude. There is no "right" or "wrong" answer.

_______ **1. If I don't set the highest standards for myself, I am likely to end up a second-rate person.**

_______ **2. People will probably think less of me if I make a mistake.**

_______ **3. If I cannot do something really well, there is little point in doing it at all.**

_______ **4. I should be upset if I make a mistake.**

_______ **5. If I try hard enough, I should be able to excel at anything I attempt.**

_______ **6. It is shameful for me to display weaknesses or foolish behavior.**

_______ **7. I shouldn't have to repeat the same mistake many times.**

_______ **8. An average performance is bound to be unsatisfying to me.**

_______ **9. Failing at something important means I'm less of a person.**

_______ **10. If I scold myself for failing to live up to my expectations, it will help me to do better.**

Scoring: Add up scores on all items noting that plus and minus numbers cancel each other out. The higher the score, the more perfectionistic the mindset.

A score of minus 20 = a non-perfectionistic mindset
A score of plus 20 = a high degree of perfectionism

Source: Adapted from Burns, D. D. (1980, November). The perfectionist's script for self-defeat. *Psychology Today*, 34–52.

mistakes" of others, although these disfluencies are different than stuttering.

For preschool children, drawing less negative attention to disfluency may in turn help to reduce their heightened concern over what they perceive as a mistake in speaking. There are successful preschool treatments for stuttering (for example, the Lidcombe Program, Demands and Capacities, Parent-Child Interaction Therapy). Although these treatments differ in their approach, their outcomes are positive (Guitar, Kazenski, Howard, Cousins, Fader, & Haskell, 2015; Millard, Nicholas, & Cook 2008; Starkweather & Gottwald,1990). We hypothesize that one of the ingredients that leads to success is that the parents are involved and guided in the child's treatment in a constructive manner. This may diminish the parents' sense of helplessness, worry, and anxiety, leading to less perfectionist parental child-rearing behaviors such as unintentionally harsh criticism of the child's speech errors.

Perhaps the tendency for perfectionism to develop can be diminished by reducing the parents' outward display of anxiety and critical comments.

In addition to traditional preschool stuttering intervention, we also encourage parents to relax their expectations of perfection throughout the day, including during play or art activities. We encourage fun and potentially messy activities such as finger-painting or knocking down block towers. We find ourselves using the term "No big deal" when the children show any distress and model this type of attitude with the parents. In line with Ashby, Kottman, and Martin (2004), we promote safe risk taking and mistake making. We recommend that parents monitor and reduce their own verbalizations to their children about what worries them. We believe that encouraging more relaxed parenting could buffer the development of maladaptive perfectionism. This sentiment is echoed by Doreen Lenz Holte in discussing the eventually successful treatment of her son. "We learned that Eli, like many kids who stutter, had perfectionistic tendencies – and we needed to create an environment that tolerated and encouraged messiness, emotive expression, and some bad manners" (Holte, 2011, p. 47).

Traditional behavioral treatment may in fact foster perfectionistic tendencies in both children and adults because an emphasis on fluency may encourage the unattainable goal of using "speech tools" at all times. When disfluency inevitably happens, the individual berates him/herself and may use struggle and tension to try to get back to a more fluent state.

Preliminary studies (Amster & Klein, 2008; Brocklehurst et al., 2015) suggest that individuals who exhibit chronic stuttering appear to have perfectionistic tendencies. Individuals who show high levels of maladaptive perfectionism may experience more therapeutic success when given treatment that addresses this tendency, such as Cognitive Behavioral Therapy. See Chapter 6 in this text for information on application of CBT for PWS.

The possibility that maladaptive perfectionistic tendencies are an ingredient that increases an individual's distress about stuttering, regardless of stuttering severity, is worthy of further consideration.

REFERENCES

Alm, P. A. (2014). Stuttering in relation to anxiety, temperament and personality: Review and analysis with focus on causality. *Journal of Fluency Disorders, 40*, 5–21.

Amster, B. J. (1995). Perfectionism and stuttering. In C. Starkweather & H. Peters (Eds.), *Stuttering: Proceedings of First World Congress on Fluency Disorders* (Vol. II, pp. 540–543). Nijmegen, Netherlands: Nijmegen University Press.

Amster, B. J., & Klein, E. R. (2005, November). *A preliminary study of perfectionism and stuttering: Follow-up to treatment.* Paper presented at the meeting of the American Speech-Language-Hearing Association, San Diego, CA.

Amster, B. J., & Klein, E. R. (2008). Perfectionism in people who stutter: Preliminary findings using a modified cognitive-behavioral treatment approach. *Behavioural and Cognitive Psychotherapy, 36*, 35–40.

Amster, B. J., & Klein, E. R. (2007). The role of perfectionism in stuttering: A follow-up study. In J. Au-Yeung & M. M. Leahy (Eds.), *Research, treatment, and self-help in fluency disorders: New horizons—proceedings of the Fifth World Congress on Fluency Disorders* (pp. 361–367). Dublin, Ireland: International Fluency Association.

Anderson, J. D., Pellowski, M. W., Conture, E. G., & Kelly, E. M. (2003). Temperamental characteristics of young children who stutter. *Journal of Speech, Language, and Hearing Research, 46*, 1221–1233.

Arnold, H. S., Conture, E. G., Key, A. P. F., & Walden, T. (2011). Emotional reactivity, regulation and childhood stuttering: A behavioral and electrophysiological study. *Journal of Communication Disorders, 44*, 276–293.

Arnstein, D., Lakey, B., Compton, R. J., & Kleinow, J. (2011). Preverbal error-monitoring in stutterers and fluent speakers. *Brain and Language, 116*, 105–115.

Ashby, J. S., Kottman, T., & Martin, J. L. (2004). Play therapy with young perfectionists. *International Journal of Play Therapy, 13*, 35–55.

Blatt, S. J. (1995). The destructiveness of perfectionism: Implications for the treatment of depression. *American Psychologist, 50*, 1003–1020.

Bloodstein, O., & Bernstein Ratner, N. (2008). *A handbook on stuttering* (6th ed.). Clifton Park, NY: Thomson Delmar Learning.

Brocklehurst, P. H., Drake, E., & Corley, M. (2015). Perfectionism and stuttering: Findings of an online survey. *Journal of fluency Disorders, 44*, 46–62.

Burns, D. (1980a, November). The perfectionist's script for self-defeat. *Psychology Today*, 34–52.

Burns, D. (1980b). *Feeling good: The new mood therapy.* New York, NY: William Morrow.

Burns, D. (1983). The spouse who is a perfectionist. *Medical Aspects of Human Sexuality, 17*, 219–230.

Cloninger, C. R., Svrakic, D. M., & Przybeck, T. R. (1993). A psychobiological model of temperament and character. *Archives of General Psychiatry, 50*, 975–990.

Costa, P. T., & McCrae, R. R. (1992). *Revised NEO Personality Inventory (NEO-PI-R) and NEO Five-Factor Inventory (FFI): Professional Manual.* Lutz, FL: Psychological Assessment Resources.

DiBartolo, P. M., Frost, R. O., Dixon, A., & Almodovar, S. (2001). Can cognitive restructuring reduce the disruption associated with perfectionistic concerns? *Behavior Therapy, 32*, 167–184.

DiBartolo, P. M., Li, C. Y., Averett, S., Skotheim, S., Smith, L. M., Raney, C., & McMillen, C. (2007). The relationship of perfectionism to judgmental bias and psychopathology. *Cognitive Therapy Research, 31*, 573–587.

Dunkley, D. M., Blankstein, K. R., Masheb, R. M., & Grilo, C. M. (2006). Personal standards and evaluative concerns dimensions of "clinical" perfectionism: A reply to Shafran et al. (2002, 2003) and Hewitt et al. (2003). *Behaviour Research and Therapy, 44*, 63–84.

Dunkley, D. M., Zuroff, D. C., & Blankstein, K. R. (2003). Self-critical perfectionism and daily affect: Dispositional and situational influences on stress and coping. *Journal of Personality and Social Psychology, 84*, 234–252.

Eggers, K., De Nil, L. F., & Van den Bergh, B. R. H. (2010). Temperament dimensions in stuttering and typically developing children. *Journal of Fluency Disorders, 35*, 355–372.

Ferguson, K. L., & Rodway, M. R. (1994). Cognitive behavioral treatment of perfectionism: Initial evaluation studies. *Research for Social Work Practices, 4*, 283–308.

Flett, G. L., & Hewitt P. L. (2002). Perfectionism and maladjustment: An overview of theoretical, definitional, and treatment issues. In G. L. Flett & P. L. Hewitt (Eds.), *Perfectionism: Theory, research, and treatment* (pp. 5–31). Washington, DC: American Psychological Association.

Flett, G. L., & Hewitt, P. L. (2006). Positive versus negative Perfectionism in psychopathology: A comment on Slade and Owens's Dual Process Model. *Behavior Modification, 30*, 472–495.

Flett, G. L., Hewitt, P. L., Blankstein, K. R., & Gray, L. (1998). Psychological distress and the frequency of perfectionistic thinking. *Journal of Personality and Social Psychology, 75*, 1363–1381.

Flett, G. L., Hewitt, P. L., Oliver, J. M., & Macdonald, S. (2002). Perfectionism in children and their parents: A developmental analysis. In G. L. Flett & P. L. Hewitt (Eds.), *Perfectionism: Theory, research, and treatment* (pp. 89–132). Washington, DC: American Psychological Association.

Frost, R. O., Marten, P., Lahart, C., & Rosenblake, R. (1990). The dimensions of perfectionism. *Cognitive Therapy and Research, 14*, 449–468.

Frost, R. O., Turcotte, T. A., Heimberg, R. G., Mattia, J. I., Holt, C. S., & Hope, D. A. (1995). Reactions to mistakes among subjects high and low in perfectionistic concern over mistakes. *Cognitive Therapy and Research, 19*, 195–205.

Guitar, B. (2003). Acoustic startle responses and temperament in individuals who stutter. *Journal of Speech, Language, and Hearing Research, 46*, 233–240.

Guitar, B., Kazenski, D., Howard, A., Cousins, S., F., Fader E., & Haskell, P. (2015). Predicting treatment time and long-term outcome of the Lidcombe Program: A replication and reanalysis. *American Journal of Speech-Language Pathology, 24*, 533–544.

Hamachek, D. E. (1978). Psychodynamics of normal and neurotic perfectionism. *Psychology, 15*, 27–33.

Hewitt, P. L., & Flett, G. L. (1990). Perfectionism and depression: A multidimensional analysis. *Journal of Social Behavior and Personality, 5*, 423–438.

Hewitt, P. L., & Flett, G. L. (1991). Perfectionism in the self and social contexts: Conceptualization, assessment, and association with psychopathology. *Journal of Personality and Social Psychology, 60*, 456–470.

Hewitt, P. L., Habke, A. M., Lee-Baggley, D. L., Sherry, S. B., & Flett, G. L. (2008). The impact of perfectionistic self-presentation on the cognitive, affective, and physiological experience of a clinical interview. *Psychiatry, 71*, 93–122.

Hill, R. W., Huelsman, T. J., Furr, M. R., Kibler, J., Vicente, B. B., & Kennedy, C. A. (2004). A new measure of perfectionism: The perfectionism inventory. *Journal of Personality Assessment, 82*, 80–91.

Holte, D. L. (2011). *Voice unearthed: Hope, help, and a wake-up call for the parents of children who stutter.* n.p.: Author.

Iverach, L., O'Brian, S., Jones, M., Block, S., Lincoln, M., Harrison, E., . . . Onslow, M. (2010). The five factor model of personality applied to adults who stutter. *Journal of Communication Disorders, 43*, 120–132.

Karrass, J., Waldren, T. A., Conture, E. G., Graham, C. G., Arnold, H. S., Hatfield, K. N., & Schwenk, K. A. (2006). Relation of emotional reactivity and regulation to childhood stuttering. *Journal of Communication Disorders, 39*, 402–423.

Kim, J. M. (2010). *The conceptualization and assessment of the perceived consequences of perfectionism* (Thesis). Department of Psychology, University of Michigan. Retrieved from http://hdl.handle.net/2027.42/77633

Kleinow, J., & Smith, A. (2000). Influences of length and syntactic complexity on the speech motor stability of the fluent speech of adults who stutter. *Journal of Speech, Language, and Hearing Research, 43*, 548–559.

Kobori, O., Yamagata, S., & Kijima, N. (2005). The relationship of temperament to multidimensional perfectionism. *Personality and Individual Differences, 38*, 203–211.

Lyneham, H. J., Abbott, M. J., Wignall, A., & Rapee, R. M. (2003). *The Cool Kids family program.* Sydney, Australia: Macquarie University Anxiety Research Unit (MUARU).

Manning, W., & Beck, J. G. (2013). Personality dysfunction in adults who stutter: Another look. *Journal of Fluency Disorders, 38*, 184–192.

McGirr, A., & Turecki, G. (2009). Self-critical perfectionism is associated with increases in sympathetic indicators in a controlled laboratory stress paradigm. *Psychosomatic Medicine, 7*, 589–590.

Messenger, M., Onslow, M., Packman, A., & Menzies, R. (2004). Social anxiety in stuttering: Measuring negative social expectancies. *Journal of Fluency Disorders, 29*, 201–212.

Mitchell, J. H., Broeren, S., Newhall, C., & Hudson, J. L. (2013). An experimental manipulation of maternal perfectionistic anxious rearing behaviors with anxious and non-anxious children. *Journal of Experimental Child Psychology, 116*, 1–18.

Mitchell, J. H., Newall, C., Broeren, S., & Hudson, J. L. (2013). The role of perfectionism in cognitive behavior therapy outcomes for clinically anxious children. *Behaviour Research and Therapy, 51*, 547–554.

Millard, S. K., Nicholas, A., & Cook, F. M. (2008). Is Parent–Child Interaction Therapy effective in reducing stuttering? *Journal of Speech, Language, and Hearing Research, 51*, 636–650.

Morris, L., & Lomax, C. (2014). Review: Assessment, development, and treatment of childhood perfectionism: A systematic review. *Child and Adolescent Mental Health, 19*, 225–227.

Murphy, W. (1999). A preliminary look at shame, guilt, and stuttering. In N. Bernstein Ratner & E. C. Healey (Eds.), *Stuttering research and practice: Bridging the gap* (pp. 131–144). Mahwah, NJ: Erlbaum.

Perkins, W. H. (1990). What is stuttering? *Journal of Speech and Hearing Disorders, 55*, 370–382.

Riley, G., & Riley, J. (2000). A revised component model for diagnosing and treating children who stutter. *Contemporary Issues in Communication Science and Disorders, 27*, 188–199.

Schlenker, B. R., & Leary, M. R. (1985). Social anxiety and communication about the self. *Journal of Language and Social Psychology, 4*, 171–192.

Shafran, R., Cooper, Z., & Fairburn, C. G. (2002). Clinical perfectionism: A cognitive-behavioral analysis. *Behaviour Research and Therapy, 40*, 773–791.

Shafran, R., & Mansell, W. (2001). Perfectionism and psychopathology: A review of research and treatment. *Clinical Psychology Review, 21*, 879–906.

Shapiro, D. A. (2011). *Stuttering intervention: A collaborative journey to fluency freedom* (2nd ed.). Austin, TX: Pro-Ed.

Slaney, R. B., Rice, K. G., & Ashby, J. S. (2002). A programmatic approach to measuring perfectionism: The almost perfect scales. In G. L. Flett & P. L. Hewitt (Eds.), *Perfectionism: Theory, research, and treatment* (pp. 63–88). Washington, DC: American Psychological Association.

Smith, A., & Weber, C. (2017). How stuttering develops: The multifactorial dynamic pathways theory. *Journal of Speech, Language, and Hearing Research, 60*, 2483–2505.

Starkweather, C. W. (1987). *Fluency and stuttering.* Englewood Cliffs, NJ: Prentice-Hall.

Starkweather, C. W., & Gottwald, S. R. (1990). The demands and capacities model II: Clinical applications. *Journal of Fluency Disorders, 15*, 143–157.

Stoeber, J., & Carr, P. J. (2015). Perfectionism, personality, and affective experiences: New insights from revised Reinforcement Sensitivity Theory. *Personality and Individual Differences, 86*, 354–359.

Stoeber, J., Hoyle A., & Last, F. (2013). The consequences of perfectionism scale: Factorial structure and relationships with perfectionism, performance perfectionism, affect, and depressive symptoms. *Measurement and Evaluation in Counseling and Development, 46*, 178–191.

Stroop, J. R. (1935). Studies of interference in serial verbal reactions. *Journal of Experimental Psychology, 18*, 643–662.

Tangney, J. P. (2002). Perfectionism and the self-conscious emotions: Shame, guilt, embarrassment, and pride. In G. L. Flett & P. L. Hewitt (Eds.), *Perfectionism: Theory, research, and treatment* (pp. 199–215). Washington, DC: American Psychological Association.

Wirtz, P. H., Elsenbruch, S., Emini, L., Rudisuli, K., Groessbauer, S., & Ehlert, U. (2007). Perfectionism and the cortisol response to psychosocial stress in men. *Psychosomatic Medicine, 69*, 249–255.

Wyatt, R., & Gilbert, P. (1998). Dimensions of perfectionism: A study exploring their relationship with perceived social rank and status. *Personality and Individual Differences, 24*, 71–79.

Yairi, E., & Ambrose, N. (1992). A longitudinal study of stuttering in children: A preliminary report. *Journal of Speech and Hearing Research, 35*, 755–760.

Yairi, E., Ambrose, N., Paden, E. P., & Throneburg, R. N. (1996). Predictive factors of persistence and recovery: Pathways of childhood stuttering. *Journal of Communication Disorders, 29*, 51–77.

Van Riper, C. (1982). *The nature of stuttering.* Englewood Cliffs, NJ: Prentice-Hall.

CHAPTER 6

Cognitive Behavioral Therapy (CBT) for People Who Stutter

Evelyn R. Klein and Barbara J. Amster

INTRODUCTION

Several years ago we were treating a group of adults who stutter and what was interesting about this group was that everyone had been through years of treatment for stuttering but no one had been exposed to anything other than techniques to work directly on their speech. They were surprised to learn that the first part of our treatment approach was going to focus on their thoughts just prior to, during, and after stuttering events. The prospect of this therapeutic model intrigued them. We taught the group about automatic thoughts that are often fleeting but penetrate our minds in a way that can leave us in distress. Group members recalled situations in which they felt upset about their speech. The idea began to hit home when our clients started reminiscing about specific circumstances. John recalled a time he was upset for days when a 4-year-old child presumably hung up the phone on him when he stuttered while asking to speak to the child's mother. John later learned that the phone call had been dropped because of poor reception and that the child's mother actually wanted to speak with him. His assumptions about what happened were inaccurate and his distress was needlessly self-imposed. These types of cognitive distortions can play havoc on one's emotional sense of well-being, whether one stutters or not. Fortunately, Cognitive Behavioral Therapy (CBT) can be useful in changing these self-defeating thoughts. It has been applied successfully to treat depression, anxiety, eating disorders, perfectionism, obsessive-compulsive disorders, phobias, posttraumatic stress disorder, chronic medical conditions, and many more (Beck, 2011).

CBT is a treatment that has been used with people who stutter (PWS). CBT can be an effective adjunct to typical therapeutic interventions for PWS that focus on reducing stuttering and increasing fluent speech. For individuals whose stuttering is chronic, recovery from stuttering often involves more than changing speech output. As Bill Murphy (1999), a speech-language pathologist (SLP) and a person who stutters, stated in his chapter on shame, guilt, and stuttering, PWS will have limited success speaking if they focus on only speech motor work. He believed that a person's emotional system impacts stuttering in a big way. We agree.

The two emotions Murphy expressed are quite interesting (Murphy, 1999; Van Riper, 1982). PWS often experience shame and guilt related to negative self-evaluation. Shame involves emotional pain related to feelings of being dishonorable or worthless as an individual. Shame creates a feeling of being exposed and embarrassed as a person. The distress people feel can be so painful that it can make them want to avoid encounters. It can also provoke a sense of anger toward others, who they feel shame them. Guilt is slightly different from shame in that it relates to feelings of remorse for specific offensive actions that the person has done. To simplify, shame can be thought of as an internal state or sense of feeling flawed, whereas guilt tends to be more often associated with doing something wrong and feeling badly about it. While guilt is not pleasant, its side effects are not as damaging to a person as the consequences of shame. These emotions can run very deep. One woman with whom we worked told us that she wouldn't speak to her newborn son during the first years of his life because she was afraid that her stuttering would influence the way he would learn to speak and that he would eventually stutter. To her, that would have been the worst thing she could do to her baby! When asked how she communicated with him, she said she took care of his basic needs such as diapering, feeding, bathing, and holding him but decided it best not to speak to him. Speaking to the baby became her husband's responsibility. She deprived both herself and her child of the enjoyment of talking because of her strong sense of shame and guilt about stuttering. The sense of shame and guilt related to stuttering can rob the person who stutters of worthwhile encounters and joy.

This chapter explores the role of CBT in working with PWS. We begin with the foundations of CBT and discuss the cyclic nature of emotions related to an individual's personal world, automatic thoughts, feelings, and behaviors. We discuss the evolution of CBT along with its inspiring history, research, and use in the treatment of PWS. We also share a guide for using our educational CBT approach with PWS.

A word of caution is needed for SLPs when treating clients who present with any serious mental health concerns. Referral to appropriate mental health professionals such as clinical psychologists, psychiatrists, social workers, and others with appropriate licensure is in order when a client presents with serious depression, anxiety disorder, suicidal ideation, or other concerning mental health needs beyond our scope of practice. The American Psychological Association (APA.org) is a good resource for locating psychologists and gaining additional information about mental health issues.

COGNITIVE BEHAVIORAL THERAPY (CBT): THE IMPORTANT UNDERPINNINGS OF HOW THOUGHTS AFFECT BEHAVIOR

It can be a challenge to think about your own thoughts. Working with CBT in treating PWS requires identification, exploration, and modification of one's thoughts. All of us have thoughts throughout the day as we interact with a variety of people in various situations. Based on our experiences at any given moment, automatic and unplanned thoughts enter our minds. If thoughts are negative, they can result in unpleasant emotions.

Thoughts can arise from feelings rooted in core beliefs. Core beliefs are personal ideas about yourself, other people, the world, and the future. They develop over time but start in childhood. They are dependent on one's personality and predisposition and are influenced by genetics and environmental experiences. Core beliefs can have a negative slant and appear during times of distress. When they are more negative, they tend to relate to three broad realms: *helplessness* (having to do with feelings of incompetence, weakness, vulnerability), *unlovability* (having to do with feelings of being different, undesirable, defective, not good enough), or *worthlessness* (having to do with feeling immoral, dangerous, toxic, unacceptable) (Beck, 2005). Negative interpretations can become overly emphasized in a person's mind, especially when they are replayed. Core beliefs about what is important and what matters in life develop over time and reflect personal experiences and ongoing interactions within our relationships, both close ones and casual encounters. Any one of us is susceptible to negative emotions. CBT is intended to help people change their views, change the way they allow things to disturb them, and replace them with more positive interpretations.

The goal of CBT is to become better able to control one's thoughts so that life experiences become less distressing. The idea behind CBT is to challenge and modify those beliefs you have about yourself and others that may be inaccurate and damaging. We want to feel good about our lives but sometimes life's situations are unpleasant and influence our thoughts and emotions. How we deal with our emotions is crucial to life's satisfaction. This is also true for PWS (totaling approximately 60 million people in the world; Helgadóttir, 2010), as they navigate many encounters where speech may be challenging. PWS may have experienced situations over time that have affected their thoughts, emotions, physical sensations, and actions. Such experiences can certainly affect our sense of self-acceptance and fulfillment. Treatment plans incorporating CBT can help. Beck's 10 basic principles of CBT (Beck, 2011) can be incorporated into treatment plans for PWS by SLPs who learn the tenets of this approach. Table 6–1 provides an overview of these principles.

Although the 10 principles apply to treatment in general, therapy is individualized and based upon the person's goals. Nevertheless, beliefs about self-worth often permeate treatment. Eloquently noted by Beck (1976) in Fry's chapter (2013), "cognitions, in the form of negative automatic thoughts, appraisals, images, assumptions and beliefs, are linked to and help to explain individuals' affective, somatic and behavioural responses to events" (p. 303). Beck's focus reflects the role that thoughts and behaviors play in creating unhelpful and self-perpetuating negative beliefs.

Beck (2014) found that clients benefited substantially by identifying their core beliefs, not a simple task. For PWS, Sheehan (2006) referred to this as the *giant in chains* complex in his book on effective counseling in stuttering therapy. PWS may think that if they didn't stutter, they would accomplish more in life and life would be better. In this situation, the PWS has overly attributed stuttering as the cause of problems in his or her life. That type of core belief requires an adjustment. Therapists can work on helping clients identify and reevaluate their beliefs. With highly critical people, role-plays, imagery, and psychodramas have been successful in changing beliefs. The intent is to change dysfunctional beliefs and thoughts to improve perceptions and relationships. Of great importance in the process is the need to: (1) assess and share information about the client's progress, (2) work from an informed agenda, (3) provide collaborative homework, and (4) ask the client for feedback along the way. Beck believes that future challenges include incorporating sound CBT principles and strategies through continuing education at the graduate level for health and mental health practitioners. This can include SLPs who work with individuals who have communication needs such as PWS.

In contrast to other psychotherapies, CBT relies on a problem-oriented application. Therapists seek solutions to current situations instead of dwelling on the past. The foundation is based on coping so that individuals can live a better life with less discomfort. Homework between sessions is an integral part of the treatment, and the patients hopefully learn to care for themselves more successfully. This

Table 6–1. Basic Principles of CBT for People Who Stutter

Principle 1	CBT is based on the formulation of patients' problems and an individual conceptualization of each patient in cognitive terms. The therapist identifies current thinking that contributes to the patients' feelings and problem behaviors.
Principle 2	CBT requires a sound therapeutic alliance. Therapist actively listens with warmth and empathy. Feedback is solicited from the patient at the end of the session.
Principle 3	CBT emphasizes collaboration and active participation. Therapy is teamwork. Patient decides problems to discuss and identifies distorted thinking.
Principle 4	CBT is goal oriented and problem focused. The therapist guides the patient to examine problems and set specific goals.
Principle 5	CBT emphasizes the present. The therapist helps the patient examine current problems based on dysfunctional thinking. The therapist helps patients set goals and identify thoughts and beliefs and teaches patients to do this on their own.
Principle 6	CBT is educative and aims to teach the patient to be his or her own therapist with an emphasis on relapse prevention.
Principle 7	CBT aims to be time limited. The amount of sessions varies depending on the patient's individual needs.
Principle 8	CBT sessions are structured: introduction, mood check, review of week, setting the session agenda, reviewing and discussing homework, setting new homework (automatic thought record), and eliciting feedback.
Principle 9	CBT teaches patients to identify, evaluate, and respond to their dysfunctional thoughts and beliefs. Therapists help patients to have more realistic perspectives and to feel better emotionally by *guided discovery* using questions and *behavioral experiments* to test their thinking.
Principle 10	CBT uses a variety of techniques to modify thinking, mood, and behavior. Therapeutic techniques relate to the therapist's skills and the patient's needs.

Source: Adapted from Beck (2011).

short-term treatment helps people gain better problem-solving strategies as they use an automatic thought record (ATR) and relaxation exercises in individual and group therapy situations. See Appendix 6–A for a sample ATR.

The ATR is a tool to help people analyze and question their thoughts in situations that create unpleasant emotional reactions. For example, if a PWS thinks people will laugh at him or her when speaking, he or she may stop talking, limit speech, or feel badly when stuttering. Using the ATR, the therapist can gather details about the situation or event that caused distress and then help the PWS by answering some of the following questions (Beck, 2011):

1. What evidence is there to prove the distressing thought is true (or false)?
2. What would you tell friends to help them if they had the same experience or thought?
3. What does the thought do for you, how does it make you feel?

4. Is it possible that you are worrying unnecessarily, especially if you have little control over the situation?
5. What would be the worst thing that could happen if the thought were true?
6. How would your life be different if you didn't believe the thought?
7. Would it be beneficial to extinguish the thought?

Ultimately, the thought is to be replaced with a more representative thought that is less anxiety provoking. Keeping a diary of thoughts and responses helps the person process and change those unhelpful and distressing thoughts. CBT encourages individuals to face their fearful thoughts and reduce them. It can be beneficial to face one's fears and realize that although unpleasant, they don't need to affect daily life.

When people enter social situations, they have pre-conceived notions about their ensuing encounters. These notions, when negative, can activate assumptions of potential danger leading to the use of self-imposed safety behaviors such as avoidance. Ironically, SLPs may even recommend safety behaviors in treatment. In an online survey with 169 SLPs who were asked to identify strategies to help their PWS clients manage anxiety, 92% recommended rehearsing speech prior to talking, 81% recommended seeking safe speaking partners in threatening social situations, 57% recommended clients avoid difficult words, and 51% suggested reducing unnecessary talking (Helgadóttir, Menzies, Onslow, Packman, & O'Brian, 2014). In other words, they may actually be teaching clients safety behaviors that have been found to maintain fears and encourage avoidance, the exact strategies that make stuttering more debilitating. In contrast, therapeutic techniques such as CBT can help PWS approach social situations in a more functional manner.

Figure 6–1, adapted from Clark (2000) and Clark and Wells (1995) by Helgadóttir (2010), helps explain the impact of negative early learning experiences, such as bullying, on the interpretation of social situations.

Clark (2005) identified three assumptions to explain how social anxiety is maintained when people enter a social situation. Socially anxious individuals process information based upon: (1) extremely high standards for social performance; (2) conditional beliefs about consequences of performing in certain ways; and (3) unconditional beliefs about oneself. This model relates to PWS as they have a higher chance of having social anxiety compared with

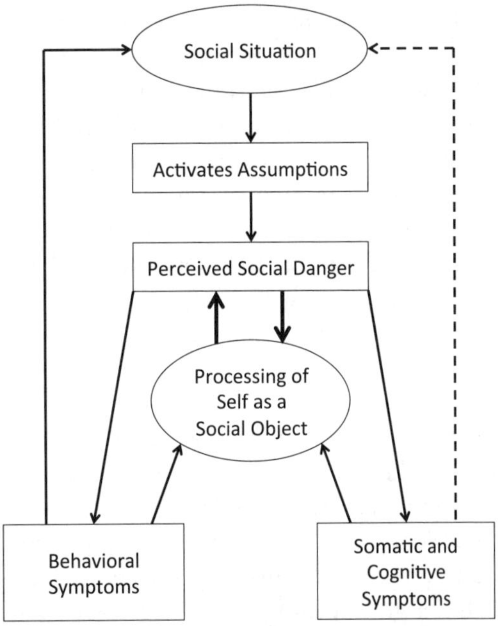

Figure 6–1. A model explaining processes that can occur when negative learning experiences influence social situations. *Source*: Reprinted with permission from Clark, D. M., & Wells, A. (1995). A cognitive model of social phobia. In R. G. Heimberg, M. R. Liebowitz, D. A. Hope, & F. R. Schneier (Eds.), *Social phobia: Diagnosis, assessment, and treatment* (pp. 69–93). New York, NY: Guilford Publications. © Guilford Publications, 1995.

matched controls (Iverach et al., 2009). They tend to predict how they will be viewed during speaking situations where they feel they will stutter with tension. To cope, they may completely avoid the situation, switch to use "safer" words, or decide not to speak during the situation. Negative self-talk can heighten negative beliefs and further perpetuate difficulties (Fry, Botterill, & Pring, 2009).

People who experience maladaptive perfectionism, related to setting goals that are often unattainable and then feel dissatisfied with their performance, may be more susceptible to negative self-talk. Hirsch and Hayward (1998) reflect on the *feeling like a failure* phenomenon. In their study about an adult who suffered with perfectionism, anxiety, and depression, progress was made only after he began to challenge his flaws and mistakes. CBT was an effective treatment method for reducing perfectionism in that case. For PWS, similar feelings may be true even though much of their speaking time may be fluent.

Social perfectionism can further perpetuate negative perceptions of oneself. Social perfectionism (discussed in http://stutteringjack.com/cognitive-behaviour-therapy-cbt-a-treatment-for-stuttering-or-not/) relates to worry about what others think. People who experience social perfectionism have deep concerns over making mistakes, including stuttering, and this can lead to self-prescribed safety behaviors such as avoidance. Such behaviors add to anxiety and make speech more stressful. The goal in CBT is to reduce worry about what other people think. Using CBT, the PWS is encouraged to make mistakes and stutter on purpose while reducing frustration, thoughts of failure, and other self-defeating thoughts. CBT has been found to be an effective tool in managing maladaptive perfectionism. Chapter 5 in this book discusses the role of perfectionism in stuttering.

Brundage, Winters, and Beilby (2017) investigated the need for psychosocial support for PWS, specifically related to the fear of negative evaluations. Their study investigated judgment bias in social situations. This study compared PWS with those who did not stutter, exhibiting various levels of heightened anxiety related to their perception of social threats. All study participants reported the absence of generalized anxiety disorder, psychiatric disorder, or any communication disorder with the exception of stuttering. Using the measure *Fear of Negative Evaluation* (FNE; Watson & Friend, 1969), PWS were placed into one of two groups, those who had high FNE scores (top 25% of distribution) and those with low FNE scores. The investigators found that the PWS group with high FNE scores perceived significantly greater social threat for mildly negative social situations compared with PWS with lower FNE scores, as well as people who did not stutter. Thus, PWS with high FNE scores appear to overestimate that a negative event will occur and exaggerate the possible consequences even for less threatening situations. Extrapolating from these findings, it appears that SLPs should consider working with clients on "affective, behavioral, and cognitive reactions to communicative situations when providing treatment" (Brundage, Winters, & Beilby, 2017, p. 9). As the authors of this chapter, we believe that CBT can help reduce negative judgment bias by modifying preconceived notions.

Efficacy of CBT

CBT was developed to help people identify and examine their core beliefs in an effort to change self-defeating thoughts. The underlying premise is that thoughts affect emotions and emotions affect one's sense of well-being. One of the first randomized controlled studies using CBT was conducted with depressed patients. It validated CBT as an effective treatment and found it to be as effective as antidepressant medication (Beck, Rush, Shaw, & Emery, 1979). This groundbreaking finding led the way for additional studies. CBT became a treatment of choice as a way to help patients respond more appropriately and modify their negative thinking. As noted above, there are 10 basic principles that underlie treatment for individuals who receive this therapy (see Table 6–1).

In recent years, CBT has expanded to include treatment for more varied populations and disorders (Beck, 2014). Combined with a greater interest in technology for effective treatment delivery, there are more intervention modalities being used with evidence-based outcomes. More than 1,000 randomized controlled studies and meta-analyses show efficacy for CBT. CBT has even been used effectively for test anxiety, relationship issues, and procrastination, to name a few. It is used with children and adults of all ages, including athletes, the homeless, those with chronic pain, tinnitus, and many more. There are more than 100 computer-based treatment programs using CBT and they are helping reduce anxiety, depression, insomnia, headache, pain, and more.

According to reviews of 106 meta-analytic studies on the efficacy of CBT (Hofmann, Asnaani, Vonk, Sawyer, & Fang, 2012), with a myriad of mental health problems, 11 studies compared rates of response between CBT and other treatments. CBT was found to have the highest therapeutic response rates in 7 of the 11 reviews. Thus, CBT has a strong evidence base. What makes this treatment approach worthwhile is that it addresses the faulty beliefs one has about oneself, others, interactions, current relationships, and future aspirations. Maladaptive automatic thoughts can perpetuate emotional distress. Therefore, the target of treatment is to challenge one's distressing automatic thoughts and modify them. For those who undergo CBT, gains are often made even after therapy ends, with a positive effect on social skills. The evidence for CBT has been impressive and it has been recommended as a first-line intervention.

CBT AND STUTTERING

While Hofmann et al. (2012) investigated CBT with a variety of mental health disorders, McDonald (2012) investigated literature on CBT specific to stuttering. He found six articles, including two that were randomized clinical trials (RCTs). McDonald found that CBT was not consistently effective in reducing stuttering's frequency or severity but showed positive alterations in stuttering-related thoughts and attitudes. Blomgren (2010) discussed the negative feelings and attitudes PWS develop due to embarrassment and anxiety when speaking, and Craig, Hancock, Tran, and Craig (2003) noted that PWS have anxiety levels that are higher than the general population. Higher anxiety often results in more difficulties, both emotionally and physically (Menzies, Onslow, Packman, & O'Brian, 2009). RCTs provide us with evidence-based research to compare individuals who receive CBT with those who don't.

In 2008, Menzies et al. investigated the effects of CBT on anxiety and stuttering. Thirty adults were randomly assigned to the experimental or control groups with the experimental CBT group receiving 10 weeks of CBT therapy followed by 14 hours of speech therapy. Social anxiety was measured. Those who met criteria for social phobia when the study began no longer met diagnostic criteria after CBT therapy. However, CBT did not change percent of syllables stuttered to any greater degree than speech restructuring alone. The authors speculated that by reducing anxieties about stuttering, the PWS can stutter more freely and not feel embarrassed or anxious about it, thereby feeling more relaxed speaking as a PWS.

In another study, by Moleski and Tosi (1976), 20 adults who stutter were randomized to receive a form of CBT (rational-emotive therapy) or systematic desensitization, with in vivo tasks, or to a control group. The tasks involved making phone calls to acquaintances and engaging in spontaneous discussions with strangers or not engaging in those in vivo exposures. Results of a battery of psychological and fluency measures indicated that CBT had better outcomes and reduced stuttering and lowered anxiety and negative attitudes about speaking than systematic desensitization or no treatment.

John Farroway, a PWS, who received treatments that helped him practically eliminate his stuttering, learned about CBT in his early seventies. Although he rarely stuttered, he was still avoiding situations, substituting words, and rarely speaking to more than one person at a time. Farroway (2014) decided to take part in a CBT treatment and found that it had a positive effect on how he thought and behaved. He began to control his *thinking errors* that entered his mind with little awareness. He described his thinking errors as: expectations that the worst would happen (catastrophizing), that he knew what others were thinking (mindreading), that he predicted what was going to happen (fortune-telling), and that he saw situations in only one way (all or nothing thinking). Through therapy he learned to challenge those thoughts and beliefs. By rescripting situations he found greater control and more positive outcomes.

Emotions and Automatic Thoughts in CBT for PWS

Over the past 40 years, CBT has been used for PWS with varying success. Burns and Brady (1978) realized early on that effective treatment for PWS should include cognitive therapy to reduce embarrassment, anxiety, and tension in feared situations. They focused on attitude restructuring to address maladaptive attitudes that included fear of rejection, self-blame, defeatism, and a sense of inferiority. Craig and Tran (2006) supported CBT as a treatment approach for adults who stutter. While studies have realized the value of CBT for PWS, many of those studies lacked control or comparison groups and long-term follow-up data (Menzies et al., 2009). In the Menzies et al. (2008) CBT study, four components of CBT were thought to be worthwhile procedures to decrease fear and anxiety. These included: exposure, behavioral experiments, cognitive restructuring, and attentional training.

According to Menzies et al. (2009), the following four CBT treatment strategies have been found beneficial for PWS, helping them to reduce their automatic negative thoughts. The first procedure, *exposure* (a common practice in behavior therapy), involved PWS being exposed to individualized situations based on a personal fear hierarchy (typically 10 to 15 situations). They had to remain in each situation until their anxieties began to lessen. This helped them accurately perceive the reality of speaking situations, knowing they could reduce their anxiety and consequent avoidance. *Behavioral experiments* included working directly on fears and anticipated negative judgments from others, along with voluntary stuttering and reality checks to help clients analyze situations more appropriately. Third, *cognitive restructuring* was instituted to help reduce automatic negative thoughts, especially dealing with perceived criticism. PWS learned to challenge their irrational thoughts using reframes in daily situations with scales such as the *Unhelpful Thoughts and Beliefs about Stuttering* (UTBAS) scale consisting of 66 statements related to stuttering (St. Clare et al., 2009). For each item, PWS would work on changing their thoughts and perceptions (cognitive restructuring) by: (1) identifying evidence for or against the thought; (2) reacting to a friend with the same thought; (3) identifying the purpose for worrying about the thought; (4) identifying what the thought does or does not do for you; and (5) contemplating the worst outcome if the thought came true. *Attentional training* was also incorporated as PWS learned to focus on meditative breathing and a thought mantra using the word "relax" twice daily for a total of 10 minutes.

CBT treatment has been adapted to many people with a variety of clinical needs, including PWS. Fry (2013) depicted a cognitive model that portrays the vicious cycle of stuttering. It begins with a negative automatic thought driven by a belief that the PWS thinks that stuttering and its negative interpretation will happen again. That creates an emotional response of fear and trepidation which causes physiological tension. The person's behavioral responses vary but generally lead to increased tension and more stuttering. CBT can be beneficial in breaking this vicious cycle.

The following excerpt from Williams' (1980) course on stuttering depicts a sense of what some PWS can experience, further supporting the need for cognitive-behavioral treatments.

> *As the moment to speak approaches, his fear rises sharply. His mouth feels dry, his palms and underarms are sweaty, his heart pounds, his breathing is rapid and shallow. He feels trapped and panic-stricken. Then the instant arrives when he must speak. He tries to retain some degree of composure as he frantically casts about to find some way of getting out the feared words. He instantly and automatically goes into his repertoire of coping behaviors as he struggles desperately for fluency. He may hold his breath and try to squeeze out the words with sheer force, he may shut his eyes tightly, clench his fists, jerk or twist his head around, contort his face in grotesque grimaces. He knows he is making a horrible spectacle of himself but he feels out of control. He may utter weird croaking or gasping sounds as his speech mechanism seems to have gone berserk. He may feel as though he is blanking out, almost fainting, out of contact with reality. Then, finally, he manages to complete the utterance, mangled and distorted though it has been. He feels exhausted, worn-out for the moment. Worse, he feels shamed and degraded. He may attempt a show of bravado, of casualness, but he wonders what his listeners think of him for his weird behavior. He has made a complete fool of himself, and he wishes he could disappear. He is relieved to have gotten out the words, but he feels horribly embarrassed. He may then utter the remaining words quite fluently, hoping that somehow they will cancel out his failure and convince the listeners that somehow he is still human. But he can't convince himself of this, and he knows that the same thing will happen again many times in the future. His confidence and self-esteem are near zero.* (http://www.mnsu.edu/comdis/kuster/jdwilliamslibrary/williamscourse.html)

Williams' depiction of stuttering is intense. With such emotions, PWS anticipate their next speaking experience and attempt to form safety behaviors such as avoidance. Gordon Blood (1995) supported this notion when he wrote a seminal article about behavioral-cognitive therapy for treating PWS. Counseling and attitude change were the focus of his treatment. He found that positive attitude change was related to reductions in disfluencies when used with biofeedback. He agreed with Cooper (1993), who noted that stuttering is a *chronic perseverative syndrome* with a sense of uncertainty relating to loss of control during speech. According to Blood's treatment study, therapeutic changes need to occur not only in speaking, but also in feeling and thinking. His treatment incorporated work on reducing negative emotions, fears, and avoidance.

To reduce negative emotions and fears, the PWS is taught to recount situations and automatic thoughts and to reflect on the meaning of the automatic thought and accompanying emotions. How those thoughts influenced the person's behaviors are worked through in therapy. The intent is to analyze and modify unproductive and distressing core beliefs. This approach is valuable when treating people with social anxiety and stuttering. Anxiety can worsen stuttering and lead to greater avoidance behaviors. It is estimated that about 50% of PWS are affected by social anxiety (Menzies et al., 2009), which further influences peer relationships, bullying, and fears of being judged negatively.

It makes sense that SLPs who are educated in applying CBT incorporate CBT for chronic stuttering. We feel strongly that applications of CBT for PWS should be taught in a counseling or fluency course during graduate school. There are also continuing education workshops and DVDs that offer training in this area. For more information, see http://www.stutteringhelp.org or https://www.beckinstitute.org/get-training/

Negatively charged thoughts can make a person feel bad. These thoughts are often automatic and enter the mind without warning. They may involve thoughts about: *how we think we were treated, what we think others think about us, what we think we should have done differently, what we think is wrong, and what we think needs to change.* Extensive analysis of the speaking moment and erroneous cognitions are familiar to many PWS. Perceived negative listener evaluation is a common thought of PWS, leading to social anxiety related to speaking (Craig, Blumgart, & Tran, 2009). CBT can be beneficial in helping people identify their cognitive distortions and contemplate alternatives to feel better. Figure 6–2 provides a cognitive conceptualization by Judith Beck (2011). Using this model, PWS can process relevant information related to their core beliefs along with conditional assumptions and coping strategies. The job of the therapist is then to help people who stutter realize how their thoughts, and what they say to themselves, can be detrimental. The next step is to work on applying compensatory strategies to anxiety-producing situations.

Considerations in Applying CBT with PWS

An important question when considering a treatment approach such as CBT for PWS is, *What factors influence stuttering severity?* Psychological characteristics that closely impact stuttering are necessary to identify, as they may influence an individual's treatment. A regression analysis (Manning & Beck, 2013) was conducted with 50 adults who were receiving treatment for stuttering. The regression analysis included trait anxiety, social anxiety, depression, and personality features as measured on the subscales of the *Overall Assessment of the Speaker's Experience of Stuttering* (OASES; Yaruss & Quesal, 2008) and percent syllables stuttered as measured by the *Stuttering Severity Instrument* (Riley, 1994). Results indicated that social anxiety and trait anxiety were significant predictors associated with stuttering severity. In contrast, depression or personality dysfunction was not significantly related to stuttering severity. This research supports the commonly held notion that speaking itself elicits heightened verbal communication anxiety for PWS and is related to stuttering severity.

Anxiety is thought to be a psychological concomitant of stuttering (Ingham, 1984) and is therefore often studied. Whether anxiety precedes stuttering or is a result of experiences as a PWS has been debated and is usually considered to be an outcome of the experiences as a PWS over time (Menzies et al., 2008). Ezrati-Vinacour and Levin (2004) conducted a study comparing 47 adults who stuttered with 47 adults who did not stutter. The PWS had greater trait anxiety (ongoing, long-lasting anxiety, a personal characteristic)

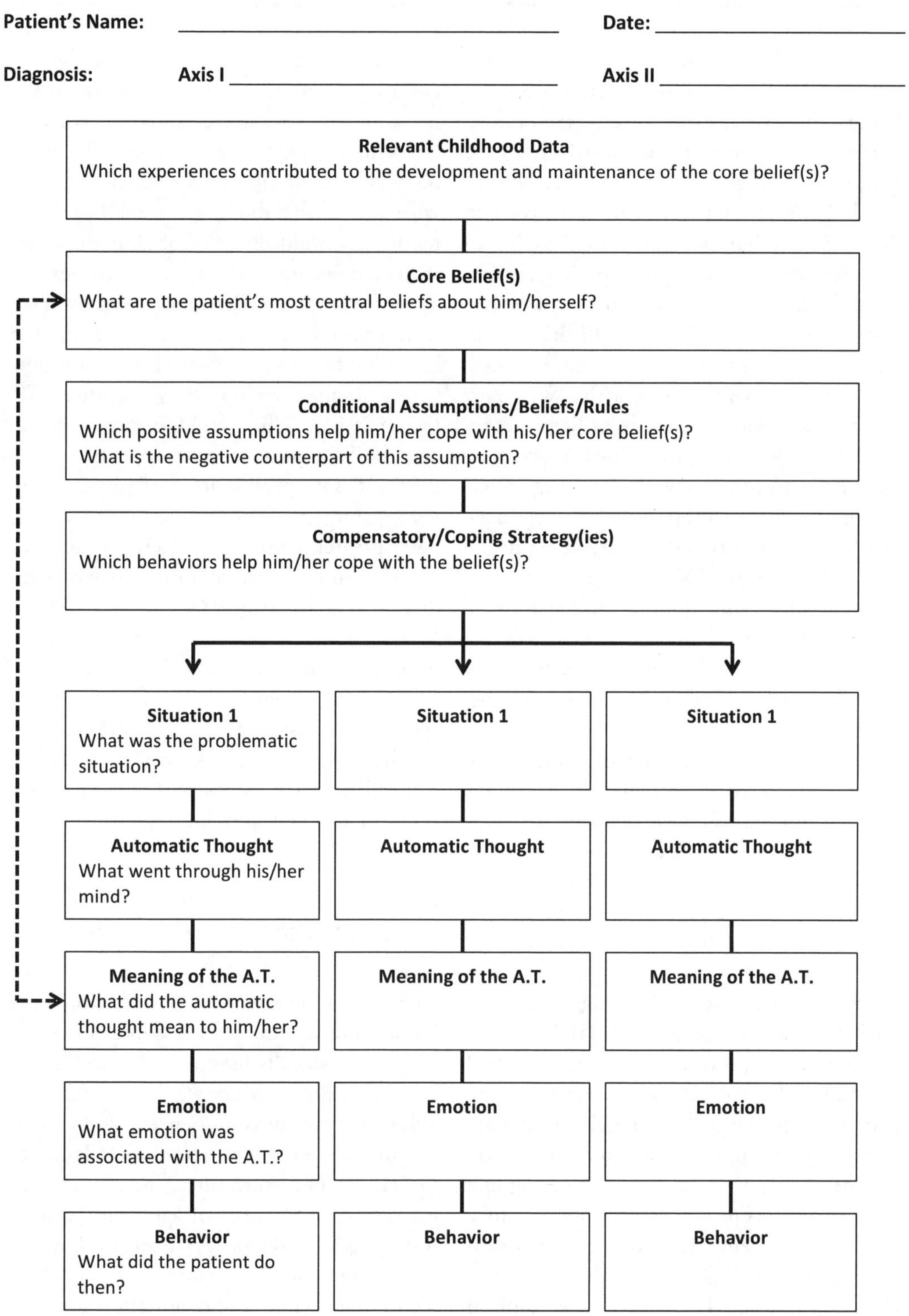

Patient's Name:
Date:
Diagnosis:
Axis I
Axis II
Relevant Childhood Data
Which experiences contributed to the development and maintenance of the core belief(s)?
Core Belief(s)
What are the patient's most central beliefs about him/herself?
Conditional Assumptions/Beliefs/Rules
Which positive assumptions help him/her cope with his/her core belief(s)?
What is the negative counterpart of this assumption?
Compensatory/Coping Strategy(ies)
Which behaviors help him/her cope with the belief(s)?
Situation 1
What was the problematic situation?
Situation 1
Situation 1
Automatic Thought
What went through his/her mind?
Automatic Thought
Automatic Thought
Meaning of the A.T.
What did the automatic thought mean to him/her?
Meaning of the A.T.
Meaning of the A.T.
Emotion
What emotion was associated with the A.T.?
Emotion
Emotion
Behavior
What did the patient do then?
Behavior
Behavior

Figure 6–2. Cognitive conceptualization diagram. *Source*: Reprinted with permission from *Cognitive behavior therapy worksheet packet*. Copyright 2011 by Judith S. Beck. Bala Cynwyd, PA: Beck Institute for Cognitive Behavior Therapy. © J Beck, 2011.

compared with controls in an experimental task. In addition, the more severe PWS were found to have greater state anxiety (temporary, unpleasant emotional arousal related to experiences) to social communication. The authors concluded that anxiety is a personality trait that often develops over time in PWS.

Negatively perceived experiences can promote anxiety in PWS, or anyone for that matter. Iverach, Menzies, O'Brian, and Onslow (2011) investigated anxiety in social situations involving speech with PWS. The researchers reviewed a decade of literature to see if there were changes in clinical practice in the treatment of anxiety in stuttering. They determined that there appears to be a connection between anxiety and concern about negative evaluations for PWS. Increased anxiety, fear of negative evaluation, and anticipation of social harm such as bullying often arise in the teenage years in PWS. They believe that it is imperative that mental health issues including anxiety be treated.

Alm (2014) agrees that thinking about oneself and what others may be thinking (social cognition) can have deleterious effects on speech. PWS may be concerned about the risk of stuttering, its potential consequences, and how to act for best results. This type of social cognition calls upon the medial prefrontal cortex (mPFC), usually active during rest when a person is not thinking about goal-directed activities (Fox et al., 2005). However, we know that propositional speech is goal directed and therefore social cognition may compete with the goal for speech and impact both language and speech motor processes. In other words, thinking about stuttering in a way that makes one more socially anxious may interfere with talking. This, in part, may explain why talking when alone or with a pet, away from potential social evaluation, may result in less stuttering for the person who stutters.

Another characteristic that has attracted investigation in PWS is temperament. Temperament can be defined as a person's innate, enduring disposition. Alm (2014) found that preschoolers who stutter showed no differences in shyness (a temperamental characteristic) and social anxiety when compared with peers who did not stutter but had a tendency toward the traits of inattention and hyperactivity-impulsivity. Alm believes that hyperactivity-impulsivity may be a prognostic indicator for chronic stuttering in children.

Shyness or psychological problems don't appear to affect relationships in young CWS (Alm, 2014). When children are preschool age, their social functioning appears to be no different from peers who don't stutter. However, young children who are sensitive may have greater emotional reactivity and feel greater muscle tension compared with children who do not stutter (Karrass et al., 2006). Investigators indicate that emotional sensitivity usually begins between 7 and 12 years of age, with greater vulnerability during the teenage years (De Nil & Brutten, 1991). As teens, children often want to keep their stuttering secret (Erickson & Block, 2013) and that may result in avoiding speaking.

Cognitive Restructuring and Treating Children Who Stutter

The current dynamic view of stuttering is that it is a neurodevelopmental disorder stemming from "an atypically functioning speech motor system" (Smith & Weber, 2016, p. 292). This vulnerable system is influenced by linguistic, cognitive, social, and emotional demands. Developmental stuttering generally emerges between 2 and 5 years of age and is variable during early childhood, occurring in about 5% of children, with approximately 75% to 80% recovering regardless of treatment (Blomgren, 2013; Smith & Weber, 2017, 2016).

Stuttering can be discouraging for even young children. Although sometimes difficult for young children to describe, they often feel frustrated and embarrassed as they become more aware of their disfluent speech and how it differs from others who can speak without struggling. Research indicates that preschool children are aware of their own stuttering and can be negatively affected by it (Vanryckeghem, Brutten, & Hernandez, 2005).

Working with parents is integral to supporting children who stutter (CWS). It can be especially beneficial when components of CBT are integrated into treatment. One comprehensive treatment that helps modify communicative interactions and attitudes about stuttering in families with young children is described by Yaruss, Coleman, and Hammer (2006) in their *family-focused treatment approach*. "The treatment involves several related components, including: (a) parent-focused strategies designed to help parents modify their communication behaviors and reduce their concerns about stuttering, and (b) child-focused strategies designed to help children modify their communication behaviors and develop healthy, appropriate communication attitudes" (p. 119). This approach helps parents learn about stuttering and modify communicative interactions to develop healthier thoughts about stuttering. Treatment involves six to eight 45-minute weekly appointments and includes education/counseling, communication modifications, and review/reassessment. Parents learn about reducing stress and speaking demands through the use of charting to analyze stuttering events and their children's reactions to them. Parents also learn to reduce time pressures, use slower, relaxed speech, and rephrase speech. Parents and children learn to speak in a more open way so that interpersonal stressors can be diminished and more positive attitudes can emerge.

In treating adolescents and adults who stutter, CBT is more direct and helps modify beliefs about how they think others perceive them. With an older group of children, the aim is to reduce anxiety about communication and avoidance. The goal is to change negative thoughts through discussions, anxiety management, and systematic desensitization procedures (Blomgren, 2013). Research by Blomgren, Roy, Callister, and Merrill (2005) found that CBT reduced anxiety about communication and avoidance in PWS regardless of whether there was a decrease in stuttering frequency. Although stuttering may have decreased minimally, the person who stuttered felt better in terms of self-acceptance.

Murphy, Yaruss, and Quesal (2007) discussed enhancing treatment for school-age children who stutter. Their work centered on reducing children's feelings of perceived negative reactions through desensitization and cognitive restructuring. Treatment included cognitive restructuring and self-acceptance with a 9-year-old boy. Treatment was effective in helping him reduce negative reactions, which were severe at times. As pointed out, many clinicians appear to be uncomfortable working with children on their negative reactions to stuttering and they prefer to work directly with fluency enhancing techniques (Cooper & Cooper, 1996). Murphy, Yaruss, and Quesal (2007) borrowed from the field of cognitive psychology and used CBT to help the boy identify that stuttering bothered him and that peers' comments made him upset. The child conveyed how he wanted to cry and how he was worried that others thought he was dumb. By using tenets of CBT, the goal was to help him reduce the emotional effects of teasing or bullying.

The approach by Murphy, Yaruss, and Quesal (2007) is intended to change attitudes and reactions. The first step requires learning about stuttering, specifically key facts about the disorder. With this foundation in place, the boy learned about others who stutter so that he didn't feel so alone. In conjunction with this, a stuttering pen pal was provided so that he had someone with whom he could correspond. (Similar connections can be made through http://www.westutter.org; the National Stuttering Association, NSAKids; or http://www.friendswhostutter.org) This increased the child's willingness to talk about stuttering and to stutter openly. Group interactions were another important component. The boy worked on examining his moments of stuttering and reducing physical tension, which helped him obtain better awareness and a greater sense of control. Additional strategies included pseudo-stuttering games to become more desensitized about the discomforts he felt related to stuttering. As he learned more about stuttering, he became better able to represent it in concrete ways such as bursting water balloons to playfully represent breaking out of a strong stuttering block. Negative thoughts were continually explored to help monitor and modify his reactions. The boy also drew pictures to express his feelings about stuttering in a concrete way to further desensitize his disfluencies. It was often beneficial to engage in pseudo-stuttering both inside the therapy room and out in public so that both the therapist and the child could observe other people's reactions to their stuttering and then follow up with a survey about what listeners really know about stuttering.

Positive self-talk is also an important part of CBT. Children are taught to challenge their negative thoughts and talk back to them. Self-statements that include thoughts such as "people will think I am stupid when I stutter" are changed to acknowledge that "I am not stupid and that stuttering is just something I do at times when I speak" (Murphy, Yaruss, & Quesal, 2007). The goal is to increase one's tolerance of stuttering. In the case review by Murphy, Yaruss, and Quesal (2007), the 9-year-old boy said he taught his friends about stuttering and they didn't think he was weird. He was then willing to use his learned stuttering modifications in more situations. The result was decreased stuttering, less negative thoughts about stuttering, greater communication success, and most importantly, self-acceptance.

CBT helps children learn that being a good communicator does not require being fluent. Treatment includes addressing beliefs and feelings about speech as the SLP gradually helps the child experience situations using a systematic and controlled fear hierarchy. The goal is to "deawfulize" (Murphy, 1989) stuttering and reduce the anxiety and anguish children feel over what they think others are thinking about their stuttering.

CWS usually want their stuttering to stop and don't want others to notice it. Another aspect of cognitive restructuring in stuttering treatment is purposeful self-disclosure to let others know that you stutter. Self-disclosing is suggested to reduce fear and avoidance. In our experience working with children who stutter, especially those approaching the teenage years, self-disclosure is something they don't want to do. In fact, they say others know they stutter and if they don't know it, that's fine. We have noticed some of our young clients becoming anxious and fidgety when the topic of self-disclosure is approached. If children are not ready or willing to self-disclose, even to someone they proclaim doesn't matter to them, don't push it. More time and work on thoughts and beliefs are needed. As children mature, they often become more concerned about peer acceptance and more aware of self-esteem issues. They want to fit in. Therefore, it is vital that the SLP address the least fearful activities first in CBT while systematically increasing more feared and challenging thoughts. This is typically used in creating a fear hierarchy to help children identify and change their cognitive distortions. Use of an ATR is not only useful for adults, but also helpful for children who are mature enough to process events and associated feelings. See Appendix 6–A for a sample of an ATR along with directions for use.

The emotional impact of stuttering on CWS can be significant. Kelman and Wheeler (2015), from the Michael Palin Centre in London, integrated CBT into their treatment for CWS and discussed its implementation. They found it to be a useful tool but recognize the need to make a referral for psychological support services when children are experiencing substantial anxiety or depression. Their cognitive model with children includes the following: (1) identifying emotions and cognitions; (2) forming links between emotions, cognitions, and behaviors; (3) improving therapeutic response through creative activities; (4) reframing cognitions to consider alternative explanations for events through self-talk and problem solving; (5) developing coping strategies within and beyond the clinic; (6) using CBT in a collaborative approach to expand confidence and tackle challenges; and (7) involving the child's social network to demonstrate how other people's responses can influence the child's progress. Kelman and Wheeler (2015) encourage the use of CBT for CWS due to evidence that CWS often experience negative peer reactions and social exclusion (Langevin, Packman, & Onslow, 2009).

As pointed out by Smith and Weber (2016), no single approach fits all children. They support the notion that treatment strategies need to be based on a multidimensional profile that is tailored to the child's linguistic, phonological, and/or heightened emotional reactivity or negative affect.

Treatment Studies Using CBT for PWS

Reddy, Sharma, and Shivashankar (2010), in their case series study using aspects of CBT with five adolescents and adults who stuttered, found the treatment to be partially effective in reducing dysfunctional thoughts, decreasing anxiety, as well as reducing stuttering. All five participants noted an improvement in quality of life following the treatment protocol, which included relaxation, mindfulness meditation, deep breathing and speech techniques. The second phase included cognitive restructuring, assertiveness training, and problem-solving techniques. Follow-up was not assessed, so the contribution of CBT among the other approaches couldn't be verified.

Menzies et al. (2008) were specifically interested in how CBT would impact stuttering and anxiety. The participants, 30 adults with chronic stuttering, were randomly assigned to either the experimental group (speech restructuring with CBT; $n = 15$) or the control group (speech restructuring only; $n = 15$). Prior to the study, each participant received a multi-axial psychiatric interview and a battery of tests. Sixty percent of the participants were initially diagnosed with social phobia (an anxiety disorder). In addition, percent syllables stuttered was calculated during 10 minutes of speaking in the clinic. All segments included video recordings and two 10-minute recorded phone calls with clinic strangers. Their CBT program involved 10 sessions for a total of 15 hours, prior to speech restructuring. Graded in vivo exposures were used in the sessions to reduce anxiety when speaking. The participants were taught to identify their automatic thoughts that contributed to their anxieties about speaking and confront those situations. The speech restructuring treatment included: (1) 14 hours per participant using a standardized version of prolonged and slow speech with a low level of speech naturalness, and (2) a group therapy day comprising stutter-free speech in the clinic combined with 4 individual sessions. Maintenance sessions were also offered to help control stuttering. Data were collected before, during, and after treatment, and again at one-year follow-up. The findings were interesting. The control group that received speech restructuring without CBT showed no improvement in social phobia symptoms at the one-year follow-up. However, those 15 adults in the experimental group who received speech restructuring with CBT (who also displayed 33% more fears on the hierarchy at baseline than those in the control group) had greater improvements and did not show signs of previous social phobia at the one-year follow-up mark. Although the CBT group did not improve significantly in speech fluency, they said they felt better and showed significantly less avoidance behaviors than before treatment. While CBT did not significantly reduce stuttering, it did have a big impact on participants' abilities to participate and interact socially. The authors speculated that CBT was effective in reducing the need for PWS to control their stuttering via speech restructuring.

Menzies et al. (2009), in their tutorial on how SLPs can incorporate CBT into treatment, recommend educating SLPs about decreasing anxiety while increasing communicative interactions. They also support working on quality of life issues to make therapeutic gains longer lasting. Based on their findings, Menzies et al. (2009) believe that if a PWS experiences anxiety, traditional speech therapy has a poor long-term response. In fact, two-thirds of adults who stutter did not preserve fluent speech with behavioral treatment alone (Martin, 1981). Research has shown that adding the cognitive component to treatment is worthwhile (Amster & Klein, 2008; Klein & Amster, 2004; Menzies et al., 2008).

Menzies et al. (2009) encourage SLPs to incorporate components of *exposure, behavioral experiments, cognitive restructuring*, and *attentional training* into their treatment for PWS. Exposure is often used in treating anxiety. The PWS is gradually exposed to situations that create anxiety and then confronts the event without escaping it. Using this strategy, anxiety typically begins to decline. With PWS, the clinician helps the client create a fear hierarchy to gradually work on exposures that are threatening. The fear hierarchies generally include 10 to 15 situations, with the most common ones being talking on the phone, talking to people of authority, meeting people initially, meeting less familiar friends, and making group presentations. The PWS also contemplates and reflects on expectations and then compares those with how the situations actually turned out. The basic fear is usually about how stuttering will produce negative evaluations for the PWS. In their tutorial, Menzies et al. (2009) also include behavioral experiments where the PWS stutters voluntarily and with greater severity than usual so that past negative predictions can be modified. Through these activities, unhelpful thoughts are analyzed and new, more accurate predictions are made. Cognitive restructuring helps the PWS challenge detrimental beliefs and modify irrational, critical thoughts. The UTBAS scale provides a list of 66 unhelpful, intrusive thoughts and beliefs people may have about stuttering. A new brief version, the UTBAS-6, can be found at http://jslhr.pubs.asha.org/epdf.aspx?doi=10.1044/2016_JSLHR-S-15-0167 (Iverach et al., 2016). The goal is for PWS to challenge their thoughts, providing evidence both for and against them. A thought that serves no purpose or does not advance one's functioning is discarded. PWS are taught to contemplate the real impact of others' behaviors during their social interactions. If someone laughs at or antagonizes the PWS, that doesn't prevent the PWS from accomplishing what was needed. The fourth part of the CBT work involves attentional training. Here, mindfulness is used to minimize intrusive thoughts. The PWS is taught to attend to other thoughts than the ones that are threat related. Practice focuses on breathing, counting, a mantra, and other distractors.

Koç (2010) also identified CBT as an effective treatment approach for treating stuttering. He began with the assumption that irrational thoughts fuel stuttering. In his research with three adolescents who stuttered between 13 and 19 years of age without ever receiving stuttering treatment, he instituted cognitive restructuring. The clients identified their thoughts and feelings and discussed their behaviors related to stuttering. They learned to detect, accept, and deal with their thoughts and feelings about stuttering. They considered excessive generalizations about stuttering, analyzed their destructive thoughts and inferences, and realized when they were engaging in cognitive distortions such as all-or-nothing thinking. They also examined their stuttering in detail. Through cognitive reorganization and behavioral therapy, they modified their thoughts, reflected more accurately on their distortions, and additionally decreased speech disfluencies.

Although not specifically about using CBT, Boyle (2011) discussed the importance of changing one's relationship with one's thoughts. He refers to PWS as experiencing increased negativity related to their emotional reactivity and negative thoughts about stuttering. Clients must learn that thoughts don't always represent truth and therefore don't need to be acted upon. Changing one's thoughts using imagery (as in a movie scene) can be helpful in changing a mental script. It is important to teach the client to let thoughts come and go, to view them as mental events not facts, and to reduce the overwhelming nature of thoughts by writing them down and thinking about them over time. The goal is to help clients think about how thoughts are created and if they realistically fit with current situations. Over time the client will think less negatively.

THE EDUCATIONAL MODEL OF CBT FOR PWS

Klein and Amster (2004) and Amster and Klein (2008) developed an *Educational CBT Model with PWS*, which is based on the CBT model used in clinical psychology. We adapted the model for SLPs who may not be formally trained in cognitive behavioral techniques. The first author of this chapter is both a licensed psychologist and certified/licensed SLP who has been trained in CBT. Although SLPs have training in case conceptualization and rapport building, they may be less familiar with selection and timing of CBT strategies. We believe our Educational CBT Model is beneficial for both SLPs and their clients with techniques that are easily applied.

The Educational CBT Model begins by teaching PWS about core beliefs and automatic thoughts. Throughout the day people experience fleeting thoughts based on their interactions and activities. Emotions flow through the mind, often without much concentrated thought, nevertheless impacting how we feel. Deep-seated beliefs and assumptions that people have about themselves, others, and the world must be identified, analyzed, and challenged if they are to change. In this educational model, PWS learn about those thoughts and how they are developed over time, accumulating with one's experiences. They tend to go unrecognized but affect the way we perceive reality and interact with others. Such core beliefs affect our relationships, child-rearing practices, financial decisions, performance at work, and certainly self-esteem, to name a few. They impact people's automatic thoughts throughout the day. Klein and Amster (2004) have the PWS identify, contemplate, and challenge their beliefs and thoughts about themselves and their stuttering.

Using the Educational CBT Model, PWS work with certified SLPs. After an initial evaluation, the SLPs review the results and together with the PWS develop three primary goals for the course of therapy. Initial goals for PWS tend to be broad and include statements such as: "I want to stop stuttering," "I want to feel that I'm OK," "I don't want people to look down on me." We work on helping our clients identify more immediate and direct goals, such as, "I want to talk with my co-workers at lunch" and "I want to answer the phone when someone calls." Goals become less focused on fluency and more focused on the tasks and feeling more comfortable speaking. Our clients like this direction, as the focus is more realistically obtainable.

During the initial training with the Educational CBT Model we introduce eight common cognitive distortions to make it easier for the clients to learn them for analyzing their thoughts. There are many lists of cognitive distortions (Freeman, Pretzer, Fleming, & Simon, 1990; Joyce-Beaulieu & Sulkowski, 2015), but we chose eight that were thought to be most relevant to PWS. These include: *All or Nothing Thinking; Not Seeing the Whole Picture; Taking It Personally; Focusing on the Negative; Mindreading; Fortune-Telling; Catastrophizing;* and *Should've, Could've, Would've.* Individual sessions focus on learning about automatic thoughts and cognitive distortions. For explanations of these cognitive distortions, see Appendix 6–B in this chapter. After each cognitive distortion is introduced, the PWS identifies situations where they recall having those thoughts. Using an ATR (see Appendix 6–A), it is easier for the PWS to identify distressing situations, accompanying automatic thoughts related to those situations, emotions that are felt during those times, and their newly recognized cognitive distortion(s) to challenge them. PWS work to identify positive, negative, and neutral responses concerning their specific situations, in both individual and group therapy. For instance, one group discussed John's situation. You may recall at the beginning of this chapter, he was the man who thought a 4-year-old child hung up the phone on him because he stuttered. Three thoughts were identified. The negative thought was *my stuttering was so bad a child even hung up on me and I won't try to call again.* The positive thought was *the phone reception was poor and the call was dropped, so I'll call again.* A neutral thought was *the child answered the phone and because the call was not for her, she hung up. I'll try another time and maybe someone else will answer the phone.* These variations helped the PWS look for different possibilities in his own situation. Throughout the program, the ATR is used. During the individual sessions, each client becomes better able to think about encounters during the week and modify his/her thoughts about them.

Group work is particularly important for PWS. During the first session, we introduce a video (*I Think They Think . . .* , Rapee, 2006) on social anxiety and social phobia about adults who don't stutter but who find it very difficult to speak to others in unfamiliar social settings. The group members discuss similarities and differences among themselves and the people in the video. They are also given blank 3 × 5 cards to write down their core beliefs about speaking, interactions, work, family, and other activities of their daily life. Group members each write their thoughts anonymously, and the cards, which get collected, are read aloud by the SLP. This activity can be very meaningful. Group members discuss everyone's beliefs without knowing who said which one. It gives PWS an opportunity to think about other people's perspectives, providing different interpretations for the same situation. For example, one client wrote, "Valued adults who progress at work can speak effectively to groups of people." Group members discussed the concept of what makes someone a valued person, how such thoughts originate, and how they come to be believed. Group members challenge the truth behind the thought, giving examples and relating diverse experiences. Group members learn from each other.

The Educational CBT Model teaches eight automatic distortions (see Appendix 6–B), one at a time, to the group of PWS. Each cognitive distortion in Appendix 6–B is reviewed and people share their personal experiences. As awareness grows, participants engage in thoughtful discussions about how core beliefs impact their automatic thoughts and how these influence their lives. Specific situations lead to important group work and new insights about how beliefs produce thoughts, perceptions, and consequent feelings. Individuals in the group often express many new insights with profound changes in their interpretations of others' behaviors and their own feelings.

As part of the process, we as group leaders are active participants in the group and share our own core beliefs and cognitive distortions. Participants have frequently said they greatly appreciate that we are open about sharing our own experiences and thoughts. We encourage SLPs to do that as well. Sharing one's own challenges and how to change them using CBT can make a positive impact. Clients have commented on feeling less alienated and more self-accepting.

Stuttering modification techniques are instituted during the last three weeks of this six-week treatment. These groups are usually eager to review physical areas of tension throughout their bodies, how various speech sounds are produced, and to practice stuttering modification techniques, including cancellations, pull-outs, and preparatory sets.

At the start of treatment, people often express feelings of panic, the tightness in their chests and mouths. They worry that they will forget to breathe and maybe lose control. Words such as "petrified, scared, stiff, and afraid" are used to describe sensations. Throughout the program, people who stutter lessen their avoidances and begin to take risks and talk in previously avoided situations. For instance, one client decided to chat at the lunch table with coworkers and another started to talk in the car pool with colleagues, all after many years of avoidance. The need to be accepted by others, to reduce worry about what others are thinking, and to release negative self-evaluation diminishes. These individuals realize that *mindreading* and *fortune-telling* are inaccurate and unhelpful. Our clients learn to challenge their automatic thoughts and distortions that have caused them anguish.

After treatment ends, we follow up with our clients, initially at 3 months and periodically after that. Our clients frequently report that the treatment model changed their lives for the better. They learn to reevaluate their automatic thoughts and assumptions and reframe encounters to lead more positive and productive lives despite whether or not they stutter.

Evidence for this Educational CBT Model was obtained with eight adult clients who were seen over a period of six weeks. Prior to the treatment sessions, each PWS received a battery of tests, including: a comprehensive case history, *Stuttering Severity Instrument* (Riley, 1994); the *Burns Perfectionism Scale* (Burns, 1980) with an adaptation of the Burns Scale to reflect on perfectionistic tendencies during childhood; *Liebowitz Social Anxiety Scale* (Sajatovic & Ramirez, 2001); *Locus of Control of Behavior* (Manning, 2001); and the *Modified Erikson Scale of Communication Attitudes* (Erikson, 1991). For the PWS, treatment included six 45-minute individual sessions and six 90-minute group sessions. The first three weeks were devoted solely to CBT. During the second three weeks, stuttering modification techniques were added.

Investigation of the Educational CBT Model (Amster & Klein, 2008; Klein & Amster, 2004) revealed statistically significant results: (1) reductions in syllables stuttered (from a mean of 7.32, SD = 6.6, to 2.72, SD = 3.1; $p = .01$), (2) reductions in negative communication attitudes as measured by the Erikson Scale of Communication Attitudes (from a mean of 19.00, SD = 3.5, to 12.38, SD = 5.0; $p = .004$), (3) reductions in anxiety as measured by the Liebowitz Anxiety Scale (from a mean of 56.25, SD = 23.9, to 32.13,

SD = 14.3; p = .02) and reductions in perfectionism as measured by the Burns Perfectionism Scale (from a mean of 9.75, SD = 5.1, to −2.38, SD = 8.1; p = .035), at follow-up. This program approach, geared toward SLPs working with PWS, had a very positive influence on our clients.

We are not suggesting that CBT is the cure for fluency disorders or that it will reduce stuttering. Rather, we are suggesting that CBT is a method to help modify thoughts that can lead to avoidance and shame. CBT can help PWS approach situations with greater self-acceptance and less concern about what others are thinking. This can make speaking less effortful and more enjoyable.

REFERENCES

Alm, P. A. (2014). Stuttering in relation to anxiety, temperament and personality: Review and analysis with focus on causality. *Journal of Fluency Disorders, 40*, 5–21.

Amster, B. J., & Klein, E. R. (2008). Perfectionism in people who stutter: Preliminary findings using a modified cognitive-behavioral treatment approach. *Behavioural and Cognitive Psychotherapy, 36*, 35–40.

Beck, A. T. (1976). *Cognitive therapy and the emotional disorders.* New York, NY: International Universities Press.

Beck, A. T. (1996). *The Beck Depression Inventory–II.* San Antonio, TX: The Psychological Corporation.

Beck, A. T. (2005). The current state of cognitive therapy: 40-year retrospective. *Archives of General Psychiatry, 62*, 953–959.

Beck, A. T., Epstein, N., Brown, G., & Steer, R. A. (1988). An inventory for measuring clinical anxiety: Psychometric properties. *Journal of Consulting and Clinical Psychology, 56*, 893–897.

Beck, A. T., Rush, A. J., Shaw, B. F., & Emery, G. (1979). *Cognitive therapy of depression.* New York, NY: Guilford.

Beck, J. S. (2011). *Cognitive behavior therapy: Basics and beyond* (2nd ed.). New York, NY: Guilford.

Beck, J. S. (2014). Recent developments in cognitive behavior therapy. *The Pennsylvania Psychologist, 74*, 16–17.

Blomgren, M. (2010). Stuttering treatment for adults: An update on contemporary approaches. *Seminars in Speech and Language, 31*, 272–282.

Blomgren, M. (2013). Behavioral treatment for children and adults who stutter: A review. *Psychology Research and Behavior Management, 6*, 9–19.

Blomgren, M., Roy, N., Callister, T., & Merrill, R. M. (2005). Intensive stuttering modification therapy: A multidimensional assessment of treatment outcomes. *Journal of Speech, Language, and Hearing Research, 48*, 509–523.

Blood, G. (1995). A behavioral-cognitive therapy program for adults who stutter: Computers and counseling. *Journal of Communication Disorders, 28*, 165–180.

Boyle, M. (2011). Mindfulness training in stuttering therapy: A tutorial for speech-language pathologists. *Journal of Fluency Disorders, 36*, 122–129.

Brundage, S. B., Winters, K. L., & Beilby, J. M. (2017). Fear of negative evaluation, trait anxiety, and judgement bias in adults who stutter. *American Journal of Speech-Language Pathology, 26*, 496–510.

Burns, D. (1980, November). The perfectionist's script for self-defeat. *Psychology Today*, 34–52.

Burns, D., & Brady, J. P. (1978). Stuttering and speech disorders. *Symposium on Behavior Therapy in Psychiatry.* Psychiatric Clinics of North America.

Clark, D. M. (2000). Cognitive behaviour therapy for anxiety disorders. In M. G. Gelder, Lopez-Ibor, & N. N. Andreason (Eds.), *New Oxford textbook of psychiatry.* Oxford, UK: Oxford University Press.

Clark, D. M. (2005). A cognitive perspective on social phobia. In W. R. Crozier & L. E. Alden (Eds.), *The essential handbook of social anxiety for clinicians* (pp. 193–218). Chichester, UK: John Wiley & Sons.

Clark, D. M., & Wells, A. (1995). A cognitive model of social phobia. In R. G. Heimberg, M. R. Liebowitz, D. A. Hope, & F. R. Schneier

(Eds.), *Social phobia: Diagnosis, assessment, and treatment* (pp. 69–93). New York, NY: Guilford.

Cooper, E. B. (1993). Second opinion. Chronic perseverative stuttering syndrome: A harmful or helpful construct. *American Journal of Speech-Language Pathology, 2*, 11–15.

Cooper, E. B., & Cooper, C. S. (1996). Clinician attitude towards stuttering: Two decades of change. *Journal of Fluency Disorders, 21*, 119–135.

Craig, A., Blumgart, E., & Tran, Y. (2009). The impact of stuttering on the quality of life in adults who stutter. *Journal of Fluency Disorder, 24*, 61–71.

Craig, A., Hancock, K., Tran, Y., & Craig, M. (2003). Anxiety levels in people who stutter: A randomized population study. *Journal of Speech, Language, and Hearing Research, 46*, 1197–1206.

Craig, A., & Tran, Y. (2006). Fear of speaking: Chronic anxiety and stuttering. *Advances in Psychiatric Treatment, 12*, 6.

De Nil, L. F., & Brutten, G. J. (1991). Speech-associated attitudes of stuttering and nonstuttering children. *Journal of Speech and Hearing Research, 34*, 242–252.

Erikson, R. L. (1991). Assessing communication attitudes among stutterers. *Journal of Speech and Hearing Research, 12*, 711–724.

Erickson, S., & Block, S. (2013). The social and communication impact of stuttering on adolescents and their families. *Journal of Fluency Disorders, 38*, 311–324.

Ezrati-Vinacour, R., & Levin, I. (2004). The relationship between anxiety and stuttering: A multidimensional approach. *Journal of Fluency Disorders, 29*, 135–148.

Farroway, J. (2014, September 15). How cognitive behaviour therapy helped me. *The British Stammering Association Newsletter.* Retrieved from https://www.stammering.org/speaking-out/article/how-cognitive-behaviour-therapy-helped-me

Fox, M. D., Snyder, A. Z., Vincent, J. L., Corbetta, M., Van Essen, D. C., & Raichle, M. E. (2005). The human brain is intrinsically organized into dynamic anticorrelated functional networks. *Proceedings of the National Academy of Sciences, 102*, 531–534.

Freeman, A., Pretzer, J., Fleming, B., & Simon, K. M. (1990). *Clinical applications of cognitive therapy.* New York, NY: Plenum Press.

Fry, J. (2013). Therapy within a CBT framework. In C. Cheasman, R. Everard, & S. Simpson (Eds.), *Stammering therapy from the inside: New perspectives on working with young people and adults* (pp. 303–338). Surrey, UK: J & R Press.

Fry, J., Botterill, W., & Pring, T. (2009). The effect of an intensive group therapy programme for young adults who stutter: A single subject study. *International Journal of Speech-Language Pathology, 11*, 11–19.

Helgadóttir, F. D. (2010). *Bridging the gap in internet treatments for mental health: A fully automated online cognitive behaviour therapy for social anxiety for those who stutter* (Doctoral dissertation). Retrieved from https://ses.library.usyd.edu.au/bitstream/2123/7212/1/01fd_helgadottir_2011_thesis.pdf

Hirsch, C. R., & Hayward, P. (1998). The perfect patient: Cognitive-behavioural therapy for perfectionism. *Behavioural and Cognitive Psychotherapy, 26*, 359–364.

Hofmann, S. G., Asnaani, A., Vonk, I. J. J., Sawyer, A. T., & Fang, A. (2012). The efficacy of cognitive behavioral therapy: A review of meta-analyses. *Cognitive Therapy Research, 36*, 427–440.

Ingham, R. (1984). *Stuttering and behavior therapy: Current status and experimental foundations.* San Diego, CA: College Hill Press.

Iverach, L., Heard, R., Menzies, R., Lowe, R., O'Brian, S., Packman, A., & Onslow, M. (2016). A brief version of the Unhelpful Thoughts and Beliefs About Stuttering Scales: the UTBAS-6. *Journal of Speech-Language-Hearing Research, 59*, 964–972.

Iverach, L., Menzies, R. G., O'Brian, S., Packman, A., & Onslow, M. (2011). Anxiety and stuttering: Continuing to explore a complex relationship. *American Journal of Speech-Language Pathology, 20*, 221–232.

Iverach, L., O'Brian, S., Jones, M., Block, S., Lincoln, M., Harrison E., & Onslow, M. (2009). Prevalence of anxiety disorders among adults seeking speech therapy for stuttering. *Journal of Anxiety Disorders, 23*, 928–934.

Joyce-Beulieu, D., & Sulkowski, M. L. (2015). *Cognitive behavioral therapy in K–12 school settings.* New York, NY: Springer.

Karrass, J., Walden, T. A., Conture, E. G., Graham, C. G., Arnold, H. S., Hartfield, K. N., & Schwenk, K. A. (2006). Relation of emotional reactivity and regulation to childhood stuttering. *Journal of Communication Disorders, 39,* 402–423.

Kelman, E., & Wheeler, S. (2015). Cognitive and behaviour therapy with children who stutter. *Procedia—Social and Behavioral Sciences, 193,* 165–174.

Klein, E. R., & Amster, B. J. (2004). The effects of cognitive behavioral therapy with people who stutter. In A. Packmann, A. Meltzer, & H. Peters (Eds.), *Theory, research, and fluency disorders: Proceedings of the Fourth World Congress of Fluency Disorders* (pp. 154–160). Nijmegen, Netherlands: Nijmegen University Press.

Koç, M. (2010). The effect of cognitive-behavioral therapy on stuttering. *Social Behavior and Personality, 38,* 301–310.

Langevin, M., Packman, A., & Onslow, M. (2009). Peer responses to stuttering in the pre-school setting. *American Journal of Speech-Language Pathology, 18,* 264–276.

Manning, W. H. (2001). Locus of Control of Behavior Scale. *Clinical decision making in fluency disorders* (2nd ed.). San Diego, CA: Singular.

Manning, W., & Beck, J. G. (2013). Personality dysfunction in adults who stutter: Another look. *Journal of Fluency Disorders, 38,* 184–192.

Martin, R. (1981). Introduction and perspective: Review of published research. In E. Boberg (Ed.), *Maintenance of fluency.* New York, NY: Elsevier.

McDonald, A. (2012). *Critical review: Is Cognitive Behavioural Therapy (CBT) an effective intervention approach for adults who stutter?* Retrieved from https://www.google.com/search?q=McDonald+2012+Critical+Review%3A+Is+Cognitive+Behavioural+Therapy+%28CBT%29+an+effective+intervention+approach+for+adults+who+stutter%3F&ie=utf-8&oe=utf-8

Menzies, R. G., O'Brian, S., Onslow, M., Packman, A., St. Clare, T., & Block, S. (2008). An experimental clinical trial of cognitive-behavior package for chronic stuttering. *Journal of Speech, Language, and Hearing Research, 51,* 1451–1464.

Menzies, R. G., Onslow, M., & Packman, A. (1999). Anxiety and stuttering: Exploring a complex relationship. *American Journal of Speech-Language Pathology, 8,* 3–10.

Menzies, R. G., Onslow, M., Packman, A., & O'Brian, S. (2009). Cognitive behavior therapy for adults who stutter: A tutorial for speech-language pathologists. *Journal of Fluency Disorders, 34,* 187–200.

Molescki, R., & Tosi, D. J. (1976). Rational-emotive therapy vs. systematic desensitization in the treatment of stuttering. *Journal of Consulting and Clinical Psychology, 44,* 309–311.

Murphy, B. (1999). A preliminary look at shame, guilt, and stuttering. In N. Bernstein Ratner & E. Charles Healy (Eds.), *Stuttering research and practice: Bridging the gap.* Mahwah, NJ: Erlbaum.

Murphy, W. P. (1989). *The school-age child who stutters: Dealing effectively with shame and guilt.* Videotape No. 86. Memphis, TN: Stuttering Foundation of America.

Murphy, W. P., Yaruss, J. S., & Quesal, R. W. (2007) Enhancing treatment for school-age children who stutter. I. Reducing negative reactions through desensitization and cognitive restructuring. *Journal of Fluency Disorders, 32,* 121–138.

Rapee, R. M. (2006). *I think they think . . . Overcoming social phobia.* New York, NY: Guilford Publications with Monkey See Productions.

Reddy, R. P., Sharma, M. P., & Shivashankar, N. (2010) Cognitive behavior study for stuttering: A case series. *Indian Journal of Psychological Medicine, 32,* 49–53.

Riley, G. A. (1994). *Stuttering Severity Instrument for Children and Adults—Third edition* (SSI-3). Austin, TX: Pro-Ed.

Sajatovic, M., & Ramirez, L. F. (2001). The Liebowitz social anxiety scale. In *Rating Scales in Mental Health.* Hudson, OH: Lexi-Comp.

Sheehan, J. (2006). *Effective counseling in stuttering therapy.* Memphis, TN: Stuttering Foundation of America.

Smith, A., & Weber, C. (2016). Childhood stuttering: Where are we and where are we going? *Seminars in Speech and Language. 37,* 291–297.

Smith, A., & Weber, C. (2017). How stuttering develops: The multifactorial dynamic pathways theory. *Journal of Speech, Language, and Hearing Research, 60*, 2483–2505.

St. Clare, T., Menzies, R., Onslow, M., Packman, A., Thompson, R., & Block, S. (2009). Unhelpful thoughts and beliefs linked to social anxiety in stuttering: Development of a measure. *International Journal of Language & Communication Disorders*, 1–14.

Turner, S. M., Beidel, D. C., & Dancu, C. V. (1986). *SPAI: Social Phobia and Anxiety Inventory.* New York, NY: Multi-Health System.

Van Riper, C. (1982). *The nature of stuttering.* Englewood Cliffs, NJ: Prentice-Hall.

Vanryckeghem, M., Brutten, G. J., & Hernandez, L. M. (2005). A comparative investigation of the speech-associated attitude of preschool and kindergarten children who do and do not stutter. *Journal of Fluency Disorders, 30*, 307–318.

Watson, D., & Friend, R. (1969). Measurement of social evaluative anxiety. *Journal of Consulting and Clinical Psychology, 33*, 448–457.

Williams, J. D. (c. 1980). *Stuttering.* Unpublished manuscript, Northern Illinois University, Dekalb, IL. http://www.mnsu.edu/comdis/kuster/jdwilliamslibrary/williamscourse.html

Yaruss, J. S., Coleman, C., & Hammer, D. (2006). Treating preschool children who stutter: Description and preliminary evaluation of a family-focused treatment approach. *Language, Speech, and Hearing Services in the Schools, 37*, 118–136.

Yaruss, J. S., & Quesal, R. W. (2008). *Overall assessment of the speaker's experience of stuttering (OASES).* Minneapolis, MN: Pearson.

APPENDIX 6–A

Automatic Thought Record

Date/ Time	Situation	Automatic Thoughts	Emotions	Cognitive Distortion	Alternative Neutral Response	Outcome

Directions: Use the information and questions below to help complete the automatic thought record. Work across the row for each situation encountered. Use additional paper if necessary.

Date/Time—Provide an approximate date and time when the event or situation took place.

Situation—Describe what happened leading to your upset or emotional state. Who was involved and what did they say or do?

Automatic Thoughts—What thoughts were going through your mind when the situation occurred? How much did you believe that thought to be true at the time from 1 (not much at all) to 10 (absolutely)?

Emotions—How did you feel immediately following the situation? How strong was that feeling from 1 (not much at all) to 10 (absolutely)?

Cognitive Distortion—Which of the following cognitive distortions best fits the situation?

Could you have been engaging in:

All or Nothing Thinking
Not Seeing the Whole Picture
Taking It Personally
Focusing on the Negative
Mindreading
Fortune-Telling
Catastrophizing
Should've, Could've, Would've Thinking

Alternative Neutral Response—Think of a rational and neutral response to your automatic thought. In other words, what's another way to look at the situation? Rate your belief in this alternative response from 1 (not much at all) to 10 (absolutely).

Outcome—How does your alternative explanation make you feel? What is the most realistic outcome? How could changing your thought help you? If another person told you about this same situation happening and had the same thoughts, what would you tell that person?

APPENDIX 6–B

Cognitive Distortions Reviewed in the Educational CBT Model for PWS

All or Nothing Thinking—The person thinks that events, circumstances, attitudes, and the like are divided into two separate categories (excellent or poor) without any shades of gray. PWS may think of themselves as either successes or failures. If their performance is less than perfect, the default is considered a failure. This can apply to any situation and lead to feelings of hopelessness.

Not Seeing the Whole Picture—The person sees a part of a situation negatively while overlooking positive aspects. The PWS who received accolades for a job well done dwells on one negative comment.

Taking It Personally—Individuals assume that others are blaming them for situations for which they were not responsible. They tend to believe that others assume they are responsible for undesirable outcomes or events. A PWS may assume the supervisor's unfriendliness was due to his increased disfluencies during a meeting, whereas that isn't the case at all. In actuality, the supervisor wasn't feeling well that day, which had nothing to do with the PWS.

Focusing on the Negative—The individual focuses on negative aspects of a total situation. For example, the PWS may focus on periods of disfluency during a very successful presentation. When listeners provide positive comments, they are seen as insignificant and/or insincere.

Mindreading—PWS think that others regard them negatively. For PWS it is often related to stuttering. PWS believe they know what others are thinking about them regardless of how the others act.

Fortune-Telling—The person acts as if negative expectations will become reality. The PWS may think he or she won't do well in a situation or won't be given an opportunity because of stuttering.

Catastrophizing—The individual interprets a situation as disastrous and all-encompassing. Instead of putting the encounter in perspective, it is viewed as intolerable and dangerous with serious consequences. The PWS may perceive dire consequences from one less than stellar presentation.

Should've, Could've, Would've—The person believes he/she should have or could have done something differently or better but didn't and regrets it. The range of possibilities is vast, from thoughts of what would have happened if he or she didn't stutter to what could have happened if he or she had acted differently.

CHAPTER 7

Acceptance and Commitment Therapy for Stuttering Disorders

Janet M. Beilby and J. Scott Yaruss

"The real voyage of discovery consists not in seeking new landscapes, but in having new eyes."

—Marcel Proust (1923)

INTRODUCTION

This chapter describes the use of Acceptance and Commitment Therapy (ACT) in the support and management of the psychosocial processes involved in living with stuttering. Stuttering is a multifaceted communication disorder that can have a dramatic effect on an individual's communication abilities. Because communication is central to human social interaction and overall well-being, intervention for stuttering should include multiple components that address the entirety of the speaker's experience (e.g., Yaruss & Quesal, 2004). A recent review of the qualitative experiences of people who stutter concluded that there is "a consensus that emotional factors require attention as well as teaching techniques to improve fluency" (Baxter et al., 2016, p. 15). Smith and Weber (2016) concurred, stating that stuttering involves "heightened emotional reactivity or negative affect [that] would likely benefit from a different treatment strategy" (p. 295) than treatment focused solely on fluency. Smith and Weber further advocated "devising more comprehensive and tailored treatment approaches to effectively address the individual profiles" (p. 296) of clients. This contemporary call for comprehensive intervention that addresses the broad impact of the stuttering disorder sends a strong message to professionals about the future of stuttering therapy. Flexibility will be necessary for challenging and ultimately expanding existing philosophies and treatment practices to include work that directly accommodates individual life experiences.

In treating the entire stuttering disorder, it is important to examine the overt symptoms of the disorder *in addition to* other components. These other components may include the speaker's affective, behavioral, and cognitive reactions; the environmental impact of stuttering, indicated by the difficulty of different speaking situations and the reactions of others; and the overall impact of stuttering on the speaker's quality of life, indicated by limitations in communication activities and restrictions in participation in daily life (Yaruss, 2010). Quality of life, in particular, refers to the well-being of an individual from a multidimensional perspective that includes physical, psychological, social, vocational, and other domains (Frattali, 1998). Many people who stutter have described how stuttering has posed restrictions on their school achievements, career choices, job promotions, participation in social engagements and events, and development of friendships throughout life (Hayhow, Cray, & Enderby, 2002; Hugh-Jones & Smith, 1999; Yaruss et al., 2002). Children and adolescents report negative experiences in the form of bullying and inappropriate teasing (Blood & Blood, 2004; Davis, Howell, & Cook, 2002; Langevin, 1997, 2000; Langevin, Bortnick, Hammer, & Wiebe 1998; Murphy & Quesal, 2002; Murphy, Yaruss, & Quesal, 2007a, 2007b). Such life frustrations may negatively affect a speaker's full participation in vocational and recreational opportunities. Successful treatment must therefore ensure that stuttering does not have such negative effects on a speaker's interaction and engagement.

Many traditional stuttering treatments, particularly fluency modification programs but also some stuttering modification approaches, have attempted to address stuttering by targeting stuttered speech behaviors more or less exclusively (see review in Manning, 2010). It is far from clear that focusing primarily on fluent speech (or even on easier stuttering) leads to the best possible functioning for individuals in their daily living. Other perspectives may also help to reduce overt stuttering symptoms while addressing other aspects of daily life. Indeed, recent research has suggested that a broad-based, functional approach to stuttering that includes a posture of openness and acceptance might lead to less psychological distress as speakers loosen their attachment to the struggle associated with individual stuttered moments (e.g., Beilby, Byrnes, & Yaruss, 2012; Boyle, 2011; Cheasman & Everard, 2013a).

Acceptance and Commitment Therapy is a contemporary and somewhat enigmatic therapy that achieves such engagement. The acronym embraces the main concepts of ACT (Harris, 2009):

A = Accept thoughts and feelings and be present.

C = Choose a valued direction.

T = Take action.

ACT enables people to be in touch with what truly matters in their lives, so that their values can inspire, motivate, and guide their behaviors. The aim of ACT is to help people create a meaningful life while accepting the pain and discomfort that is an inevitable part of living. ACT teaches people necessary skills for handling painful thoughts, feelings, and struggles while clarifying which values are essential and meaningful. From this perspective, people can establish goals that help them to engage in their lives and decrease avoidance in their daily activities and social relationships.

OVERVIEW OF ACCEPTANCE AND COMMITMENT THERAPY

ACT has an empirical base that addresses intimate personal and life values, defusion from problems, and commitment to the experience of compassion while at the same time helping people live in the present moment. Rather than focusing on trying to change or eliminate an individual's negative thoughts and behaviors, as in traditional cognitive-behavioral therapy (CBT), ACT instead tries to reduce frustration through acceptance and mindfulness, and by encouraging individuals to focus on positive experiences in their lives (Beilby et al., 2012). Studies have demonstrated the effectiveness of ACT programs with children, adolescents, and adults in the management of numerous disorders such as chronic pain, depression, and stress (Bohlmeijer, Fledderus, Rokx, & Pieterse, 2011; Wicksell, Kanstrup, Kemani, Holmstrom, & Olsson, 2014). ACT has been described as an "existential humanistic cognitive behavioral therapy" (Harris, 2006) that makes no direct attempt to reduce symptoms. Still it has been shown to achieve just this across a range of debilitating disorders. For instance, a study by Bach and Hayes (2002) demonstrated a 50% improvement in symptoms for schizophrenic patients with just 4 hours of ACT therapy.

The effectiveness of ACT treatment for different disorders has, in recent years, sparked interest in applying ACT as a potential intervention for helping individuals who stutter (e.g., Beilby et al., 2012; Cheasman & Everard, 2013a). One of the main difficulties experienced each day by individuals who stutter is the value placed on their ability to communicate fluently. ACT is an appropriate treatment for this population, as the core processes of the therapy focus on helping individuals identify *other* values that are more attainable and consistent with their true life goals. People can then work toward increasing their participation in daily life through acceptance and mindfulness rather than being preoccupied with trying to be "stutter free" or to hide their stuttering from the world (Beilby et al., 2012).

ACT focuses on increasing psychological flexibility, defined by Hayes, Luoma, Bond, Masuda, and Lillis (2006, p. 7) as "the ability to contact the present moment more fully as a conscious human being, and to change or persist in behavior when doing so serves valued ends." Research studies analyzing ACT treatment with people who stutter have implemented six core processes to increase psychological flexibility. These processes, which will be discussed in detail throughout this chapter, include: self-as-context, defusion, acceptance, mindfulness, values, and committed action. The six core processes should not be viewed as being separate from one another. Indeed, they are often described as six interrelated facets of a "hexaflex," which culminates in psychological flexibility. Following are additional details about each of the components of ACT treatment.

Components of ACT

1. Self-as-Context

Self-as-context focuses on developing the way in which people perceive themselves so that they do not identify who they are purely by an emotion, an idea, or a characteristic. For example, people who stutter may experience a belief that their stuttering defines who they are—that they are, first and foremost, a "stutterer" or "person who stutters." (Note that even the use of person-first language does not diminish the self-identification with the disorder if that identification becomes central or defining.) This is not surprising, given how central communication is to so much of our daily experience as human beings. As people experience ongoing difficulties with communication, they may come to identify themselves with their speaking difficulties rather than recognizing that stuttering is just one facet or aspect of their lives. Stuttering can thereby become an all-consuming, self-defining characteristic, as speakers begin to interpret every experience in the context of how it will affect, or be affected by, their stuttering. Changing this perception can start by helping people recognize the narrow way in which they presently perceive themselves. As they increase their self-awareness, they can evaluate whether there might be other ways to view themselves that do not place stuttering in such a central role.

In this context, self-awareness is promoted through the ongoing process of observing oneself and staying in the present moment during experiences—even unpleasant experiences, such as being in a moment of stuttering, speaking in front of a group, or answering the telephone. The person is taught how the familiar "thinking self," which generates thoughts, beliefs, and judgments, can be viewed as being distinct from the "observing self," which notices how thoughts and feelings can change as we journey through life. By recognizing the difference between the thinking and observing selves, people can better identify when they are viewing themselves through the lens of their emotional biases and when they are viewing themselves as a more objective observer who does not judge or criticize. Observing oneself in a more objective and less judgmental way paves the way for other aspects of the ACT therapy process.

2. Defusion

In a state of fusion, people may perceive that their thoughts must command their utmost attention. They may feel threatened, scared, and anxious. This may cause them to allocate a disproportionate amount of their energy and effort into trying to control their thoughts or to push the thoughts from their mind. For people who stutter, the state of fusion may exist when they experience fears and other negative emotions associated with particular speaking situations or with being identified by others as a person who stutters. It may also be seen in the desire to avoid a moment of stuttering or a speaking situation.

Defusion focuses on helping people identify their thoughts as being no more than thoughts. Speakers can learn that their thoughts are not reality; they are an *interpretation* of reality. Moreover, this interpretation may not actually help them face the true reality. When people are preoccupied with and attached to negative thoughts, those thoughts may become perceived as facts. This makes it more difficult for people to control how they will respond to those thoughts. However, if they are able to recognize that the thoughts are not in fact reality but rather their (potentially skewed) perception of reality, then they have the opportunity to defuse their thoughts or separate their feelings from their thoughts. This helps them choose to respond in a more positive, purposeful way, rather than feeling overwhelmed and reacting with less helpful emotions. For example, people who stutter might learn that their presumption that other people must judge them negatively because of their speaking difficulties is not reality; it is actually just a presumption that can make it harder for them to approach speaking situations. Likewise, they may learn that their belief that they must speak fluently in order to succeed in life is simply a thought; it is not reality but rather their interpretation of reality, and viewing the world in this way actually is making their lives more difficult. Defusion gives speakers the opportunity to recognize that their thoughts may not reflect reality. This opens up opportunities for them to reconsider whether people's reactions to their stuttering are actually as negative as they feared or whether their own reactions to stuttering need to be as negative as they might have become.

3. Acceptance

Acceptance involves recognizing that certain events and experiences in life are not always positive and that coming to terms with those experiences is a normal part of living for all humans. Acceptance allows people to act on their values because they are more open to considering thoughts and feelings that might be painful *without* attempting to deny or negate them. It is understandable for individuals to want to avoid problematic feelings and experiences. However, doing so does not help the negative emotions or events disappear. People who stutter may have difficulty tolerating the fact that they stutter because they feel that they should not do it—or because they feel that they should be able to stop stuttering if they try hard enough or get the right therapy. (Unfortunately, this is a message that has been reinforced by some practitioners in the field over many years.) Research does not support the idea that all people who stutter can stop stuttering, however, so the reality for many people who stutter is that stuttering *is* and *will be* a part of their lives. Self-as-context helps people learn that stuttering does not have to be a central, defining aspect of their lives; defusion helps them learn that stuttering does not have to be viewed as purely negative; acceptance helps people learn that they do not have to completely eliminate stuttering in order to live the life they want to live. Acceptance occurs when individuals embrace the times in their lives that may be challenging so they can come to terms with the emotions, urges, feelings, and sensations that may accompany those many and varied experiences. Letting go of the struggle and the fight to be someone different from who they actually are opens up energy and resources that can be devoted to more meaningful and important choices in life that are more consistent with their values.

4. Mindfulness

Mindfulness encourages individuals to focus on and be aware of the present moment, by paying attention to themselves and to the world around them with openness and curiosity. Mindfulness encourages an awareness of the fullness of each moment. It helps people to acknowledge and accept the present moment rather than being consumed with negative thoughts about the past or worrying about those that might occur in the future. For people who stutter, the value of mindfulness can be seen as they fully experience and live in each situation they face, rather than worrying about prior situations in which they may have stuttered or about future situations in which they may stutter. It can even be reflected in people's experience of each individual moment of stuttering—rather than rushing to get through a stutter so they can move out of an uncomfortable situation, speakers can allow themselves to experience the stutter, thereby learning to recognize their emotional and physical reactions, defuse those negative reactions, and, ultimately, have the opportunity to accept stuttering as a part of their communication—not as something to be feared or avoided but as a part of their daily experience which can be lived and valued.

5. Values

Values reflect people's belief systems, views of themselves and of the world, and priorities for their lives. Clarifying values is essential to exploring life in a more meaningful way. The process of exploring values helps people recognize the areas in their lives that are most significant to them. Examples might include family, recreation, spirituality, or other key aspects of life. The identification of these life priorities helps people establish goals that guide their choices for living, based on achieving and upholding their uniquely personal principles. Clarifying values can be particularly important for people who stutter, as a focus on fluency might cause speakers to become fused to the notion that their speech must be produced in a certain way (fluently). If people recognize that living their values does not actually require the type of "perfect" fluency that they originally thought was necessary, it can be easier for them to realign their behaviors and beliefs about speech to match the life they want to live. Similarly, clarifying values can help people see that avoiding sounds, words, or speaking situations in an attempt to appear fluent actually separates them from being who they want to be; reducing avoidance helps them align themselves with their true values.

6. Committed Action

Committed action encourages individuals to set practical goals to do what it takes in order for them to live according to their values. Any traditional behavioral treatments such as desensitization or skills training can be part of committed action, as speakers pledge to practice and use such techniques (along with other aspects of ACT such as acceptance and mindfulness) to help improve their quality of life. People who have recognized that improving fluency or modifying moments of stuttering is an important part of living their values may take committed action to practice speech management skills. People who have recognized that speaking freely, regardless of fluency, is an important part of living their values may take committed action to focus on strategies for desensitizing to stuttering. Approaching life's changes in this way helps people ensure that the goals they set for themselves, whether in or out of therapy, focus on the types of outcomes they would like to see in their lives. It also helps to ensure that any therapeutic process is consistent with each individual's values and abilities.

COMPARING ACT WITH OTHER TREATMENTS

Comparing CBT and ACT

ACT is based in the behavioral analysis paradigm that also includes traditional CBT. See Chapter 6 in this book for more experiential information on CBT. CBT focuses on teaching individuals to take control of their thoughts, feelings, and behaviors so they can change or eliminate "unhealthy" or "unhelpful" thoughts and behaviors (e.g., Blomgren, 2013; Menzies et al., 2008). CBT has been used for years to target the psychosocial impacts of stuttering, including social anxiety, while decreasing stuttered speech severity. Three domains of CBT have been used when treating social anxiety and stuttering; cognitive restructuring, graded exposure, and behavioral experiments (Menzies et al., 2008). Cognitive restructuring involves individuals identifying and altering any unhealthy or unhelpful thoughts related to their anxiety. Graded exposure relates to desensitization, whereby people are repeatedly exposed to anxiety-provoking situations with the ultimate aim of decreasing their anxiety levels. Behavioral experimentation is implemented in conjunction with graded exposure, as it involves people testing out existing beliefs in comparison with actual results of the situation to which they are exposed.

Early research examined the use of CBT in conjunction with other speech-specific treatments, such as speech modification, speech retraining, and computer-assisted biofeedback programs (Blood, 1995; Craig, Feyer, & Andrews, 1987; Maxwell, 1982). The studies all found reduction in the speech severity of stuttering. The effects on the individual's psychosocial health could not be reliably determined, as these were not empirically assessed or measured. Given that these studies did not evaluate CBT in isolation, it is difficult to determine the benefit that the CBT treatment alone had in relation to the person's stuttering severity (Menzies et al., 2008). As a result, Menzies et al. (2008) conducted a study that evaluated both speech restructuring and CBT separately. The authors found that CBT helped to significantly improve psychological functioning immediately after treatment and that these improvements were maintained at a 12-month follow-up. However, the CBT-only program did not result in any improvements in the participants' fluency overall.

Recent research has looked at implementing internet CBT treatment for targeting fluency and social anxiety related to stuttering. This research has been consistent with previous findings that anxiety levels were reduced; however, there was no concomitant improvement in the clients' stuttered speech severity, which is often a priority for the individual living with the disorder (Helgadóttir, Menzies, Onslow, Packman, & O'Brian, 2014). Other research (reviewed in Chapter 6) has shown that CBT can be useful for helping people who stutter reduce perfectionistic thinking and concerns about stuttering (Amster & Klein, 2008; Klein & Amster, 2004). Thus, CBT can be effective in helping people achieve some of the common goals of therapy for individuals who stutter.

ACT is similar to CBT in some ways, yet different in others. For example, ACT involves a greater focus on awareness, acceptance, and understanding of one's thoughts rather than on direct challenges or changes to those thoughts (Hayes, 2004; Hayes et al., 2006). If one can learn to coexist with and even accept one's thoughts and differences, then it becomes less necessary to try to change those thoughts and differences. The overarching goal of ACT is to promote psychological flexibility by honing the individual's ability to connect with the present moment more fully. The mechanisms underpinning ACT are designed to help people achieve increased consciousness. This in turn helps them change their behavior so it becomes more consistent with their values (Hayes et al., 2006).

Comparing CBT and ACT: The Example of Experiential Avoidance

There has been limited research comparing the treatment intercessors of CBT with those of ACT. Arch et al. (2012) compared treatment outcomes of CBT and ACT therapies for participants with anxiety disorders and specific phobias. Successful outcomes were achieved with both therapies, with experiential avoidance and negative cognitions improving more in the ACT treatment group. This is relevant to the treatment of stuttering, for one of the fundamental aspects of the disorder that is addressed within an ACT framework is experiential avoidance. Experiential avoidance arises from an unwillingness to come into contact with negative private events (e.g., thoughts, feelings, bodily sensations, memories). Experiential avoidance includes attempts to avoid or control the content and frequency of undesirable experiences (Chawla & Ostafin, 2007; Hayes & Gifford, 1997; Hayes, Wilson, Gifford, Follette, & Strosahl, 1996). It restricts psychological flexibility because the desire to avoid discomfort may direct or influence an individual's behavior, sometimes in ways that are not consistent with the person's goals or values. For individuals who stutter, this may mean avoidance of specific words, people, or speaking situations. Such avoidance behaviors may decrease observable stuttering behaviors in the short term. Still, people who avoid speaking situations are eventually compromised in the key activities that are important for their work or social development (Cheasman & Everard, 2013b; Murphy, Quesal, & Gulker, 2007). In addition, they may expend energy through such avoidance, as they seek to change words or to try to find ways around needing to communicate.

Importantly, speakers may also expend energy when employing certain principles of CBT, such as substitution of negative or anxious automatic thoughts with other thoughts, as well as positive self-affirmations. Research has shown that such efforts to eradicate unwanted thoughts may highlight and reinforce them and that this may actually increase stress levels for some individuals (Wegner, 1994; Wenzlaff, Wegner, & Roper, 1988; Wenzlaff & Wegner, 2000). All of this thought, fear, and anxiety may detract from their social engagement with others. This is of concern because these interactions form the core of overall life satisfaction, yet those who stutter report significant stressors in the demands of daily communication. Efforts directed at cognitive avoidance may exacerbate negative thoughts regarding speaking stressors rather than alleviate them.

Similar results have also been observed in relation to another type of experiential avoidance, that of emotion suppression. High emotional suppression has been linked to increased experiences of negative emotions and fewer experiences of positive emotions (Gross & John, 2003). As a result, thought suppression and attempts at emotional self-regulation may increase the amount of control required and exacerbate the inherent struggle a person experiences in daily living. Overt self-control can thereby be seen as a problem that may coexist with negative reactions to stuttering, rather than as a solution to those negative reactions (Hayes et al., 1999). By contrast, ACT proposes a different approach to the management of experiential avoidance and emotional instability. Simply put, the focus is not on attempting to eradicate negative thoughts and feelings; rather, frustration is reduced through acceptance and a focus on valued living.

Mindfulness and ACT

As noted above, mindfulness is a core component of the ACT hexaflex. Recent research has shown that mindfulness can have notable psychological benefits and enhance existing treatment programs (Hayes, 2005). ACT uses mindfulness techniques to help individuals become more aware of their daily situations and of their seemingly automatic reactions to those situations. Both ACT and mindfulness also encourage acceptance of things as they are, even if those experiences are negative. This is supported by seeing thoughts as merely verbal or mental expressions of a belief about an event and not as the actual event itself.

Research has found that adults who stutter may have higher anxiety levels than the general population (Craig, Hancock, Tran, & Craig, 2003). Throughout their lifespans, people who stutter are often subjected to victimization, bullying, and discrimination, and they commonly develop negative attitudes toward certain speech situations (Boyle, 2011). In some circumstances, anxiety disorders can develop, which are characterized by having "significant fear of humiliation, embarrassment, and negative evaluation in social or performance-based situations" (Iverach & Rapee, 2014, p. 69). As a result, approaches such as ACT and mindfulness, which focus on supporting the "whole person" rather than the speech impairment alone, have generated recent interest for clinicians and researchers alike. The concept of mindfulness has been described as "paying attention in a particular way: on purpose, in the present moment, and nonjudgmentally" (Kabat-Zinn, 1994, p. 4). Mindfulness has been shown to improve metacognitive awareness, for it encourages individuals to perceive thoughts as "just thoughts" rather than absolute truths. Benefits of mindfulness can include reduced avoidance of speech situations, improved emotional regulation, acceptance of a disorder, and reductions in anxiety symptoms and depression (Boyle, 2011). De Veer, Brouwers, Evers, and Tomic (2009) conducted a pilot study to investigate the psychological impact of mindfulness-based stress reduction in adults who stutter, using self-reported outcome measures pertaining to stress reactions, anxiety levels, self-efficacy trust, self-efficacy of fluency, locus of control, coping, and attitudes toward speech situations. Both post-treatment and follow-up results showed that participants had a more confident and positive attitude across a range of speaking situations. In particular, there was a notable reduction in anxiety-related outcome measures.

Boyle (2011) noted that the overlap between what is required for effective stuttering management and the benefits of mindfulness are substantial. He therefore recommended that mindfulness practices be actively incorporated into a variety of management programs, including integrated, holistic, ACT-based, and other approaches.

Using ACT with Adults Who Stutter

ACT has generated positive health outcomes across a variety of disciplines, so there is sufficient justification to consider whether this approach might offer relief for people who stutter. Beilby et al. (2012) integrated ACT into speech therapy with 20 adults who stuttered. This research incorporated ACT into 2-hour group and individual therapy sessions for 8 weeks, for a total of 16 hours intervention for each participant. Beilby et al. (2012) incorporated the six core principles of ACT with fluency-enhancing and stuttering modification techniques. As Beilby and colleagues reported, "as the ACT activities for each session were practiced, each participant was encouraged and supported to undertake the discussion and conversation about the activities using individualized speech fluency strategies, negotiated with them based on their pre-treatment assessment" (p. 291). In their position paper regarding the clinical applications of ACT, Palasik and Hannan (2013) wrote that the Beilby et al. results were important because "the results showed that participants experienced significant reductions in the adverse impact of stuttering on their lives . . . an increase in their readiness for change . . . an improvement in their mindfulness skills . . . and a reduction in overall frequency of stuttering" (p. 296). The Beilby et al. (2012) study encouraged the use of a psychotherapy approach to teach clients who stutter how to increase their awareness of thoughts from a neutral and nonjudgmental perspective. That is, clients learned acceptance of their stuttering in conjunction with defusion of negative thoughts about stuttering so they could focus on taking committed action toward living their life values. This differs from classic CBT, which assumes "that clinical improvement depends on changing cognitions" (Springer, 2012, p. 205). ACT does not depend upon cognitive restructuring; rather, it focuses on opening up an individual's awareness of and willingness to engage in contact with the present moment—and by developing less judgmental thoughts through the creation of options-based language.

The Beilby et al. study also highlights a number of measures that clinicians might incorporate into their assessment protocols when using ACT in treatment to ensure that they are documenting their clients' experiences and following the principles of evidence-based practice. Specifically, Beilby et al. collected data using the following tools:

1. The *Overall Assessment of the Speaker's Experience of Stuttering* questionnaire (OASES; Yaruss & Quesal, 2016), which assesses the adverse impact and negative consequences associated with stuttering. These consequences are described in terms of the speaker's general perceptions of the stuttering *impairment,* the speaker's affective, behavioral, and cognitive *reactions* to stuttering, the impact of stuttering on a speaker's *functional* communication in daily situations, and the impact of stuttering on the speaker's overall *quality of life.*
2. The *Modified Stages of Change Questionnaire* (MSOQ), which was developed by

Floyd, Zebrowski, & Flamme (2007) based on work by McConnaughy and colleagues in 1983. The MSOQ measures the four distinct stages of change in therapy for people who stutter: precontemplation, contemplation, action, and maintenance. Floyd et al. (2007) found that confirmatory and exploratory factor analyses of participant responses indicated that the affective, cognitive, and behavioral factors characteristic of stuttering discriminate the stages of change for individuals moving through treatment.

3. The *Mindfulness and Attention Awareness Scale* (MAAS; Brown & Ryan, 2003) is a 15-item scale which assesses the open or receptive awareness of and attention to the present. Using a six-point Likert scale (*almost always* to *almost never*), respondents rate how often they have experiences of being open and receptive to present moment experiences across cognitive, emotional, physical, interpersonal, and general life domains. This scale demonstrates strong psychometric properties and has strong validation.
4. The *Kentucky Inventory of Mindfulness Skills* (KIMS) covers four key areas: observing, describing, acting with awareness, and accepting without judgment in daily living (Baer, Smith, & Allen, 2004). This measure was designed to assess the general tendency to be mindful in daily life, to measure various components of mindfulness and to be understood by general and clinical populations. The KIMS uses a five-point Likert scale, has high internal consistency (range from .76 to .91), and has adequate to good test-retest reliability (Baer et al., 2004).
5. The *Acceptance and Action Questionnaire* (AAQ-II; Bond et al., 2011) assesses psychological flexibility including full awareness of the present moment, including thoughts and feelings, while changing behavior which is consistent with the valued goals. It evaluates the tendency to avoid or control aversive internal stimuli and the inability to take constructive action while experiencing these stimuli. The AAQ-II has been shown to have good internal consistency, a single factor structure, and significant correlations with measures of mental health (Bond et al., 2011).

This integrated ACT intervention for stuttering did not set out to remove or reduce stuttering behaviors, and it did not intervene regarding the validity or helpfulness of the person's beliefs about the causes of stuttering. Instead, the ACT intervention used a variety of activities aimed at altering the client's *relationship* with those symptoms and beliefs. The intended outcome of the integrated ACT intervention was not necessarily that the symptoms (stuttering behaviors) remitted, but that the person was able to act effectively, and with flexibility, even in the presence of symptoms. Improvements in functioning without complete symptom remission provides evidence for the ACT treatment model, as all participants did appear to behave differently in the face of similar symptoms and beliefs about their symptoms. This holistic, integrated treatment led to improvements in quality of life for a range of different people with different outlooks on life.

Fluency and Confidence: ACT and Stuttering Treatment in Practice

As demonstrated above, there are clear benefits to incorporating ACT into the treatment of stuttering, and speech-language pathologists may consider enhancing their current therapy practices with the principles of ACT. Fortunately, there is a considerable amount of helpful resources that clinicians can draw upon as they learn how to apply ACT to their therapy. For example, ACT information and resources are available at http://contextual science.org/ and www.actmindfully.com.au These are excellent and detailed websites for worksheets, handouts, book chapters, videos, and podcasts. The websites also contain information regarding training courses and workshops.

The following stuttering-specific suggestions, derived from content covered in workshops and useful ACT resources referenced (Harris, 2008, 2009, 2012, 2013), can help clinicians implement ACT with clients who stutter. The recommendations are by no means exclusive or exhaustive; they are presented here to demonstrate the integrated nature of ACT and to show how these principles have been used in stuttering management by the first author of this chapter in an approach referred to as "Fluency and Confidence" therapy. This approach, which has been provided at Curtin University in Perth, Western Australia, for many years, is the method that was evaluated by Beilby et al. (2012). Readers will note that this approach includes a particular emphasis on the goal of decreasing experiential avoidance on the part of the person living with stuttering, as ACT provides a novel and useful intervention for managing barriers to engagement and meaningful living (Beilby & Byrnes, 2012).

As with all new therapeutic endeavors, the Welcome and Introduction session is paramount for helping clients and clinicians build a mutual sense of trust and confidence in working with one another for the therapeutic processes that will ensue. We always try to build a sense of excitement and possibility as well, because nearly all people who stutter who participate in therapy have a history of unsuccessful past therapies. Often, the question that is uppermost in their minds during this initial session is, "Why will this be any different?" Clinicians need to explain their professional experience and their philosophy for therapeutic change, as well as practical details regarding timeframes and expected commitment from participants.

Core ACT Processes for People Who Stutter. The six core processes that contribute to psychological flexibility in the ACT model (self-as-context, defusion, acceptance, mindfulness, values, and committed action) are incorporated into Fluency and Confidence therapy in the following manner:

Self-as-context. The self-perception concept for a person who stutters may include perceptions such as "I am a person who stutters," "I am an inefficient communicator," or simply, "I can't talk." If the identity of "I am a person who stutters" has been adopted, the integrated ACT goal would be to assist the client in gaining awareness that "I am a person who stutters" is a thought about the self that triggers certain emotions. Rather than viewing this as a definition of self, this thought can be viewed as simply a description of their speech. (Note that the therapy does not require the speaker to change the definition itself—this is different from cognitive restructuring. Instead, speakers can maintain their belief in that thought; they simply reframe what the thought refers to: not the entire self but only a description of their fluency.)

One way to encourage clients to adopt a more flexible perspective on fluency and their lives as a whole is to conduct an activity in which participants summarize all of the facets of their lives, including family, work, upbringing, belief systems, hobbies, recreational interests, idiosyncrasies, etc. Through such an exercise, speakers can see that stuttering is only one aspect of their lives; they do not need to be defined by their fluency, even if the statement, "I am a person who stutters", is still a statement that they, understandably, believe.

Defusion. The difference between cognitive fusion and defusion can be demonstrated in the difference between saying, "Everyone is noticing my stuttering while I speak" (cognitive fusion) and saying, "I am having a thought that everyone is noticing my stuttering while I speak" (cognitive *de*fusion). Cognitive defusion involves the ability to notice each thought as being just a thought, whereas cognitive fusion requires adhering to thoughts as facts. In therapy, we teach the person that thoughts are not facts; instead, thoughts are just words that express a belief. These words can come and go like the waves of an ocean or leaves flowing down a stream. The activities we use do not require people to push thoughts away or replace them. Rather, we teach our clients to observe their thoughts, acknowledge them, accept them, make room for them, and then move on from them just as they do with other thoughts. One activity that can be used to help clients recognize that thoughts can be held in the mind as just thoughts is to help them recognize the difference between facts and thoughts. When looking out the window, we might notice that it is raining outside. That it is raining can be viewed as a fact. Whether the person likes the rain, on the other hand, can be viewed as a thought. A person may have the thought that he or she likes the rain at some point, and the person may have the thought that he or she does not like the rain at some other point. Thoughts may be consistent, or they may come and go, but they do not reflect reality. Thoughts are different from facts, which are relatively static and do reflect reality. In conducting this exercise, people can see that their thoughts about stuttering are their thoughts only. It is not necessarily a fact that people are noticing their stutter every time they speak, even though they may hold the thought that people are noticing their stutter. Recognizing the difference between thoughts and facts helps speakers defuse their belief systems so they can more flexibly acknowledge or accommodate the existence of other thoughts (e.g., sometimes people are not noticing their stuttering).

Acceptance. Although it is not possible to eradicate the content or occurrence of undesirable experiences, it is possible to reduce their impact through acceptance. Acceptance is particularly indicated when people are avoiding speaking situations that they perceive to be uncomfortable or frightening. Acceptance dilutes the struggle by helping clients recognize that life will necessarily include some uncomfortable situations, and that this is normal. Recognizing the normality of discomfort de-emphasizes the fears associated with stuttering and helps people apply their energies to other aspects of their lives. Discomfort, sadness, unpleasantness, and loss are all just facts of living—for all people. People can learn to accept those aspects of life that are not under their control. They can commit to taking action that improves their lives and their perspectives about stuttering in areas where they can exert some conscious control. When people do this, they recognize that their anxiety does not cease to exist. Instead, they recognize that their anxiety is normal. It is simply the struggle that people engage in as they attempt to not stutter or to not be anxious. This is the crux of the difficulty in communicating. Importantly, anxiety in and of itself is not a problem. The problem arises when speakers try to do something to prevent their stutter from happening, to practice or rehearse scenarios that might increase anxiety, or even to replace negative thoughts with positive ones, for these activities increase the demands on their resources and increase their struggle. In therapy, we talk with clients about the fact that there is no delete button in the brain; people cannot just erase thoughts or eliminate past experiences. Still, they can change their relationship with those thoughts and experiences. Simply put, the focus of acceptance is not on attempting to eradicate negative thoughts and feelings; rather, acceptance means being able to live with those negative thoughts and feelings without struggling with them (e.g., Yaruss, Coleman, & Quesal, 2012). ACT helps people minimize frustration and struggle through acceptance and a focus on valued living.

Mindfulness. As noted above, mindfulness promotes a non-evaluative awareness of, and contact with, the present moment. Mindfulness provides a means of increasing acceptance by helping people coexist with their thoughts and feelings. ACT helps people reorient to the present moment, reminding them that they can have a new or different experience compared with what they have experienced in the past—or compared with what they might expect. The overarching goal of ACT is to promote psychological flexibility by enhancing people's ability to connect with the present moment more fully. Mindfulness encourages increased consciousness, which in turn helps people adjust their persistent negative behaviors to more positive values–based outcomes (Hayes et al., 2006). One simple mindfulness technique for "staying in the moment," which ultimately frees resources for possible fluency strategies, relies on the analogy of "feeling the carpet through your shoes." In other words, individuals are encouraged to experience the moment, allow themselves to fully connect with the sensations and feelings around them, and acknowledge and allow the thoughts that they are experiencing in a given instant. This is quick, simple, and applicable for different ages, as it helps people focus on their experiences in a positive way, rather than worrying about what might be coming, or chastising themselves over what has happened in the past. Mindfulness can thereby help people who stutter manage the negative "mind games" they may have played about themselves and their speech.

Values. Identifying people's values helps them ensure that the steps they take in therapy move them toward being the person they truly want to be. We ask our clients questions about what really matters to them deep in their hearts, what sort of person they want to be, and what personal qualities they want to embody and enjoy. Once values are identified and clarified, goals can be developed that lead to the achievement of these values (Hayes, 2004). In this way, goal-setting helps speakers bring themselves closer to behaving like the person and the communicator they want to become in the future, rather than continuing to act in the way they have been in the past. Personal resources that were previously devoted to the management and avoidance of negative life speaking experiences can then be directed toward living in accordance with and achieving self-defined personal values. These activities help people see that their lives are not restricted because of missed opportunities. And, as they engage in practice, they are experiencing positive social engagement and discourse every week.

Committed action. Ultimately, no change ever occurs in life without action. ACT emphasizes setting practical goals that match each person's current resources, capabilities, and individual life situations. We encourage speakers to choose a practical situation each week in which they can take actions that will reflect their values in their speech, communication, and life as a whole. Such actions may involve facing situations that have previously been avoided, being more open about stuttering, implementing speaking techniques for enhancing fluency, or managing moments of stuttering. *Any* of the strategies that might be used in stuttering therapy can be incorporated into a speaker's action plan, as long as they are consistent with the speaker's values.

In summary, we apply ACT in Fluency and Commitment therapy because it provides a realistic and practical way of viewing and managing the stressors of daily living. Helping clients accomplish this goal also requires that clinicians be willing to take risks in order to embrace new therapies. While this can at times be challenging, it can also be invigorating. As Milton Erikson, the American psychiatrist and psychologist, stated: "Life will bring you pain all by itself. Your responsibility is to create joy."

ACT and the Future of Stuttering Therapy

There has been a long-standing debate regarding different treatments focused on acceptance versus those focused on modification (Nippold, 2011; Yaruss et al., 2012). As many authors have pointed out, however, it is possible to work on both aspects simultaneously (see Yaruss et al., 2012). It is our belief that treatment aimed at acceptance and stuttering modification are complementary, and integrated ACT and stuttering therapy provides one example of how this can be achieved. Speakers can learn to speak more fluently and communicate more effectively *while* living with a greater sense of acceptance and experiencing a reduced burden of stuttering. Integrated ACT therapy can improve psychosocial functioning, as well as speech fluency and overall communication for people who stutter.

The expected outcomes for stuttering symptoms in the ACT also include a reduction in the overall level of stuttering, as acceptance of negative psychological experiences and a focus on valued life domains grow. According to the ACT model, increasing acceptance should precede lessening of symptoms, because speakers will be less likely to struggle in their efforts to avoid words, speaking situations, moments of stuttering, or life circumstances. Successful treatment is associated with a more positive overall engagement in life and expansion of resources available for using management strategies (if the person chooses to implement them).

Case Study: ACT in Action

Of course, every person who stutters experiences stuttering differently, just as every person in therapy experiences therapy differently. Individual flexibility is one of the key components of ACT therapy. The implementation of the six core principles of ACT ensures that each client considers his or her own values, thoughts, feelings, experiences, and actions. Still, several themes can be identified in the following case study that reflect some of the common aspects of the stuttering disorder for many speakers. These are offered here to show readers how people who stutter might think about their experiences and how ACT can help individuals achieve desired changes in their overall quality of life through therapy.

I'm not sure how to characterize my stutter. On the one hand it is not bad because many people I know are unaware of it. I often manage to hide it with circumlocutions and a few helpful techniques from speech pathologists. On the other hand, when I do stutter I tend to block rather than have a lot of repetitions. I seem to remember the speech pathologists saying that blocking was the most severe kind.

I have observed that when I get tired or stressed, my stuttering gets worse. I suppose this makes sense because controlling my stutter is an effort. Sometimes I feel like I can't be bothered and I want to stutter with impunity. Fortunately my wife loves me anyway!

Outside of stuttering, I am a software engineer with nearly 10 years' experience. I currently lead a team of about 15 engineers. I try to balance my work with my home life and coach my son's soccer team. As you can see, my stutter hasn't really stopped my doing anything. It probably just makes me a little more quiet and reserved.

I was recently invited by a corporate software development company to fly to Sydney for an interview with them for a role in the U.S. These large tech companies pride themselves on a grueling interview process. An interview is akin to a series of computer science exams in which you also have to be polite and cheerful. I was told to be prepared for a four-hour grilling. Eat first, they told me.

One of the things that bothers me most about stuttering is that people will think I'm a poor communicator or, worse, just plain stupid. In fact I think I'm a good communicator and I'm pretty sure I'm not stupid.

The interview was bothering me for a few reasons. Firstly, good communication skills are required and clearly appearing stupid is not an option. Secondly, there are particular terms that are correct to use in a technical conversation and this often rules out circumlocutions. Let's say I block when I try to describe the technologies I use on my current project. It probably looks like I don't even know what technologies I use!

And so it was that I ended up in a hotel in the red-light district of Sydney reading a textbook, feeling nervous, and wondering if I could explain Djikstra's algorithm without stuttering. Fortunately I also had J. B., my speech pathologist, on the other end of the phone line.

I had asked for her help because, although I know some strategies, I'd been struggling to apply them. I wanted someone to talk me through it. J. B. helped me practice some techniques. For example, being nervous I was talking at a million miles an hour, so it was good to practice slowing down.

Important though the techniques are, J. B. also took the focus away from my stutter. I think this was of even greater help. She reminded me why I had been invited to interview in the first place: because of my skills and experience. A stutter was simply a speech characteristic. "Fluency is not the goal," she told me. This was a bit of a revelation to me. To that point my aim had been to complete the interview stutter free, an unlikely aim given that I was almost guaranteed to be tired after 4 hours. Now I could focus on me and not my stutter.

The interviews were organized into four consecutive one-hour interviews. I decided to use "voluntary disclosure" at the start of the first interview, one of J. B.'s ideas. I explained that I sometimes stutter and made the interviewer aware that that was what was happening if I seemed to pause inexplicably.

The first interview went well, from both a candidature and a stuttering perspective. At the start of the second interview I felt relaxed enough that I didn't need to do another voluntary disclosure. I even started to enjoy the interviews because we were talking about topics that interested me. I left the interview feeling positive about how it went. I felt like the stuttering was a non-issue. Sure, I stuttered a little but everyone has occasional speech errors. More importantly I was reasonably happy with how I handled the questions and engaged with the interviewer.

I slept soundly and contentedly that night, despite the noise of the red-light district outside the hotel window. In many ways the interview was the easy part. I am now considering the finer points of a move to Seattle. (F.B., 2016)

SUMMARY

In summary, Acceptance and Commitment Therapy (ACT), and the psychological flexibility it promotes, can help people who stutter develop the ability to resolve challenging thoughts, accept personal experiences for what they are, stay in touch with the present moment, make valued life outcomes, and build patterns of committed action in pursuit of these positive results (Hayes, Strosahl, Bunting, Twohig, & Wilson, 2004). The principles of ACT can be meaningfully integrated into other aspects of a comprehensive approach to stuttering therapy, and existing data, though preliminary, reveal that ACT can enhance treatment outcomes across a range of relevant domains for individuals who stutter.

REFERENCES

Amster, B. J., & Klein, E. R. (2008). Perfectionism in people who stutter: Preliminary findings using a modified cognitive-behavioral treatment approach. *Behavioral and Cognitive Psychotherapy, 36*, 35–40.

Arch, J. J., Eifert, G. H., Davies, C., Vilardaga, J. C. P., Rose, R. D., & Craske, M. G. (2012). Randomized clinical trial of cognitive behavioral therapy (CBT) versus acceptance and commitment therapy (ACT) for mixed anxiety disorders. *Journal of Consulting and Clinical Psychology, 80*(5), 750–765.

Bach, P., & Hayes, S. (2002). The use of Acceptance and Commitment Therapy to prevent the rehospitalization of psychotic patients: A randomized controlled trial. *Journal of Consulting and Clinical Psychology, 70*, 1129–1139.

Baer, R. A., Smith, G. T., & Allen, K. B. (2004). Assessment of mindfulness by self-report: The Kentucky Inventory of Mindfulness Skills. *Assessment, 11*, 191–206.

Baxter, S., Johnson, M., Blank, L., Cantrell, A., Brumfitt, S., Enderby, P., & Goyder, E. (2016). The state of the art in non-pharmacological interventions for developmental stuttering. Part 1: A systematic review of effectiveness. *International Journal of Language & Communication Disorders, 51*(1), 3–17.

Beilby, J. M., & Byrnes, M. L. (2012). Acceptance and commitment therapy for people who stutter. *Perspectives on Fluency and Fluency Disorders, 22*, 34–46.

Beilby, J. M., Byrnes, M. L., & Yaruss, J. S. (2012). Acceptance and Commitment Therapy for adults who stutter: Psychosocial adjustment and speech fluency. *Journal of Fluency Disorders, 37*(4), 289–299.

Blomgren, M. (2013). Behavioral treatments for children and adults who stutter: A review. *Psychology Research and Behavior Management, 6*, 9–19.

Blood, G. W. (1995). A behavioral-cognitive therapy program for adults who stutter: Computers and counseling. *Journal of Communication Disorders, 28*, 165–180.

Blood, G. W., & Blood, I. M. (2004). Bullying in adolescents who stutter: Communicative competence and self-esteem. *Contemporary Issues in Communication Science and Disorders, 31*, 69–79.

Bohlmeijer, E. T., Fledderus, M., Rokx, T. A. J. J., & Pieterse, M. E. (2011). Efficacy of an early intervention based on acceptance and commitment therapy for adults with depressive symptomatology: Evaluation in a randomized controlled trial. *Behavior Research and Therapy, 49*, 62–67.

Bond, F. W., Hayes, S. C., Baer, R. A., Carpenter, K. M., Orcutt, H. K., Waltz, T., & Zettle, R. D. (2011). Preliminary psychometric properties of the Acceptance and Action Questionnaire–II: A revised measure of psychological inflexibility and experiential avoidance. *Behavior Therapy, 42*, 676–688.

Boyle, M. P. (2011). Mindfulness training in stuttering therapy: A tutorial for speech-language pathologists. *Journal of Fluency Disorders, 36*, 122–129.

Brown, K. W., & Ryan, R. M. (2003). The benefits of being present: Mindfulness and its role in psychological well-being. *Journal of Personality and Social Psychology, 84*, 822–848.

Chawla, N., & Ostafin, B. (2007). Experiential avoidance as a functional dimensional approach to psychopathology: An empirical review. *Journal of Clinical Psychology, 63*, 871–890.

Cheasman, C., & Everard, R. (2013a). Embrace your demons and follow your heart: An Acceptance and Commitment Therapy approach to work with people who stammer. In C. Cheasman, R. Everard, & S. Simpson (Eds.), *Stammering therapy from the inside: New perspectives on working with young people and adults* (pp. 267–302). Guildford, UK: J & R Press.

Cheasman, C., & Everard, R. (2013b). Interiorized (covert) stammering—The therapy journey. In C. Cheasman, R. Everard, & S. Simpson

(Eds.), *Stammering therapy from the inside: New perspectives on working with young people and adults* (pp. 125–160). Guildford, UK: J & R Press, Inc.

Craig, A., Feyer, A. M., & Andrews, G. (1987). An overview of behavioral treatment for stuttering. *Australian Psychologist, 22*, 53–62.

Craig, A., Hancock, K., Tran, Y., & Craig, M. (2003). Anxiety levels in people who stutter: A randomized population study. *Journal of Speech, Language, and Hearing Research, 46*(5), 1197–1206.

Davis, S., Howell, P., & Cook, F. (2002). Sociodynamic relationships between children who stutter and their non-stuttering classmates. *Journal of Child Psychology and Psychiatry and Allied Disciplines, 69*, 141–158.

De Veer, S., Brouwers, A., Evers, W., & Tomic, W. (2009). A pilot study of the psychological impact of the mindfulness-based stress reduction program on people who stutter. *European Psychotherapy, 9*(1), 39–56.

Floyd, J., Zebrowski, P. M., & Flamme, G. A. (2007). Stages of change and stuttering: A preliminary view. *Journal of Fluency Disorders, 32*, 95–120.

Frattali, C. (1998). Measuring modality-specific behaviors, functional abilities, and quality of life. In C. Frattali (Ed.), *Outcome measurement in speech-language pathology* (pp. 55–88). New York, NY: Thieme Medical.

Gross, J., & John, O. (2003). Individual differences in two emotion regulation processes: Implications for affect, relationships, and well-being. *Journal of Personality and Social Psychology, 85*, 348–362.

Harris, R. (2006). Embracing your demons: An overview of Acceptance and Commitment Therapy. *Psychotherapy in Australia. 12*, 2–8.

Harris, R. (2008). *The Happiness Trap: How to stop struggling and start living.* Boston, MA: Trumpeter.

Harris, R. (2009). *ACT made simple.* Oakland, CA: New Harbinger.

Harris, R. (2012). *The reality slap: Finding peace and fulfillment when life hurts.* Oakland, CA: New Harbinger.

Harris, R. (2013). *Getting unstuck in ACT: A clinician's guide to overcoming obstacles in Acceptance and commitment therapy.* Oakland, CA: New Harbinger.

Hayes, S. C. (2004). Acceptance and commitment therapy, relational frame theory, and the third wave of behavioral and cognitive therapies. *Behavior Therapy, 35*, 639–665.

Hayes, S. C. (2005). *Get out of your mind & into your life.* Oakland, CA: New Harbinger.

Hayes, S. C., & Gifford, E. (1997). The trouble with language: Experiential avoidance, rules, and the nature of verbal events. *Psychological Science, 8*, 170–173.

Hayes, S., Luoma, J., Bond, F., Masuda, A., & Lillis, J. (2006). Acceptance and commitment therapy: Model, processes and outcomes. *Behavior Research and Therapy, 44*(1), 1–25.

Hayes, S. C., Strosahl, K. D., Bunting, K., Twohig, M., & Wilson, K. G. (2004). What is Acceptance and Commitment Therapy? In S. C. Hayes & K. D. Strosahl (Eds.), *A practical guide to Acceptance and Commitment Therapy* (pp. 3–29). New York, NY: Springer-Verlag.

Hayes, S. C., Strosahl, K. D., & Wilson, K. G. (1999). *Acceptance and commitment therapy: An experiential approach to behavior change.* New York, NY: Guilford Press.

Hayes, S. C., Wilson, K. G., Gifford, E., Follette, V., & Strosahl, K. (1996). Experiential avoidance and behavioral disorders: A functional dimensional approach to diagnosis and treatment. *Journal of Consulting and Clinical Psychology, 64*, 1152–1168

Hayhow, R., Cray, A. M., & Enderby, P. (2002). Stammering and therapy views of people who stammer. *Journal of Fluency Disorders, 27*, 1–17.

Helgadóttir, F. D., Menzies, R. G., Onslow, M., Packman, A., & O'Brian, S. (2014). A standalone internet cognitive behavior therapy treatment for social anxiety in adults who stutter: CBTPsych. *Journal of Fluency Disorders, 41*, 47–54.

Hugh-Jones, S., & Smith, P. K. (1999). Self-reports of short- and long-term effects of bullying on children who stammer. *British Journal of Educational Psychology, 69*, 141–158.

Iverach, L., & Rapee, R. M. (2014). Social anxiety disorder and stuttering: Current status and future directions. *Journal of Fluency Disorders, 40*, 69–82.

Kabat-Zinn, J. (1994). *Wherever you go, there you are: Mindfulness meditation in everyday life*. New York, NY: Hyperion.

Klein, E. R., & Amster, B. J. (2004). The effects of cognitive behavioral therapy with people who stutter. In A. Packmann, A. Meltzer, & H. Peters (Eds.), *Theory, research, and fluency disorders: Proceedings of the Fourth World Congress of Fluency Disorders* (pp. 154–160). Nijmegen, Netherlands: Nijmegen University Press.

Langevin, M. (1997). Peer teasing project. In E. Healey & H. F. M. Peters (Eds.), *Second World Congress on Fluency Disorders: Proceedings* (pp. 169–171). Nijmegen, Netherlands: Nijmegen University Press.

Langevin, M. (2000). *Teasing and bullying: Unacceptable behavior. The TAB Program*. Edmonton, Alberta, Canada: Institute for Stuttering Treatment and Research.

Langevin, M., Bortnick, K., Hammer, T., & Wiebe, E. (1998). Teasing/bullying experienced by children who stutter: Toward development of a questionnaire. *Contemporary Issues in Communication Science and Disorders, 25*, 12–24.

Manning, W. (2010). *Clinical decision making in fluency disorders* (3rd ed.). New York, NY: Delmar Cengage Learning.

Maxwell, D. (1982). Cognitive and behavioral self-control strategies: Applications for the clinical management of adult stutterers. *Journal of Fluency Disorders, 7*, 403–432.

Menzies, R. G., O'Brian, S., Onslow, M., Packman, A., St. Clare, T., & Block, S. (2008). An experimental clinical trial of a cognitive-behavior therapy package for chronic stuttering. *Journal of Speech, Language, and Hearing Research, 51*, 1451–1464.

Murphy, B., Quesal, R. W., & Gulker, H. (2007). Covert stuttering. *Perspectives in Fluency and Fluency Disorders, 17*, 4–9.

Murphy, W. P., Yaruss, J. S., & Quesal, R. W. (2007a). Enhancing treatment for school-age children who stutter. I: Reducing negative reactions through desensitization and cognitive restructuring. *Journal of Fluency Disorders, 32*, 121–138.

Murphy, W. P., Yaruss, J. S., & Quesal, R. W. (2007b). Enhancing treatment for school-age children who stutter. II: Reducing bullying through role-playing and self-disclosure. *Journal of Fluency Disorders, 32*, 139–162.

Nippold, M. (2011). Stuttering in school-age children: A call for treatment research. *Language, Speech, and Hearing Services in Schools, 42*, 99–101.

Palasik, S., & Hannan, J. (2013). The clinical applications of Acceptance and Commitment Therapy with clients who stutter. *SIG 4 Perspectives on Fluency and Fluency Disorders, 23*, 54–69.

Smith, A., & Weber, C. (2016) Childhood stuttering: Where are we and where are we going? *Seminars in Speech and Language, 37*, 291–297.

Wegner, D. M. (1994). Ironic processes of mental control. *Psychological Review, 101*, 34–52.

Wenzlaff, R. M., & Wegner, D. M., (2000). Thought suppression. *Annual Review of Psychology, 51*, 59–91.

Wenzlaff, R. M., Wegner, D. M., & Roper, D. (1988). Depression and mental control: The resurgence of unwanted negative thoughts. *Journal of Personality and Social Psychology, 55*, 882–892.

Wicksell, R. K., Kanstrup, M., Kemani, M. K., Holmstrom, L., & Olsson, G. L. (2014). Acceptance and Commitment Therapy for children and adolescents with physical health concerns. *Current Opinion in Psychology, 2*, 1–5.

Yaruss, J. S. (2010). Assessing quality of life in stuttering treatment outcomes research. *Journal of Fluency Disorders, 35*(3), 190–202.

Yaruss, J. S. (2012). What does it mean to say that a person "accepts" stuttering? In P. Reitzes & D. Reitzes (Eds.), *Stuttering: Inspiring stories and professional wisdom* (pp. 97–101). Chapel Hill, NC: StutterTalk Publications.

Yaruss, J. S., Coleman, C. E., & Quesal, R. W. (2012). Stuttering in school-age children: A comprehensive approach to treatment. Letter to the editor submitted to *Language, Speech, and Hearing Services in Schools, 43*, 536–548.

Yaruss, J. S., & Quesal, R. W. (2004). Stuttering and the International Classification of Functioning, Disability, and Health (ICF): An update. *Journal of Communication Disorders, 37*, 35–52.

Yaruss, J. S., & Quesal, R. W. (2006). Overall Assessment of the Speaker's Experience of

Stuttering (OASES): Documenting multiple outcomes in stuttering treatment. *Journal of Fluency Disorders*, *31*, 90–115.

Yaruss, J. S., & Quesal, R. W. (2016). *OASES: Overall Assessment of the Speaker's Experience of Stuttering.* McKinney, TX: Stuttering Therapy Resources.

Yaruss, J. S., Quesal, R. W., Reeves, L., Molt, L., Kluetz, B., Caruso, A. J., . . . McClure, J. A. (2002). Speech treatment and support group experiences of people who participate in the National Stuttering Association. *Journal of Fluency Disorders*, *27*, 115–135.

CHAPTER 8

Experiential Therapy for Adults Who Stutter

Principles and Methods

C. Woodruff Starkweather and Janet Givens

INTRODUCTION

Experiential therapy is an amalgam of methods derived from the authors' experiences. Woody Starkweather is a speech-language pathologist (SLP) who worked therapeutically with people who stutter (PWS) for 40 years. Most of what he knows about stuttering he learned from his clients. One thing he learned is that during a moment of stuttering, PWS do not usually feel that it is something they are doing; it feels like something that is happening to them. This experience follows from the highly automatic nature of speech production, which has evolved so that speakers can attend to the thoughts they are communicating. Observers see the stuttering behavior; PWS feel it as an experience but are only partially aware of their behavior. And the experience usually includes emotional reactions ranging from frustration or fear to embarrassment or shame. Their attempts to minimize the experience through avoidance and denial, although understandable, complicate the process of recovery.

Janet Givens is a PWS whose path to recovery began in a yoga class with the discovery that one does not always have to make discomfort go away; one can actually play around with it. Years later, while doing work on self-awareness, she discovered that when she was open about her stuttering, when she "played around with it," she spoke more easily. She began welcoming the stuttering events as opportunities for her to get to know her stuttering better. Unexpectedly, over time, her stuttering gradually diminished until it was no longer significant to her.

Both authors were trained in Gestalt psychotherapy and have found its methods and principles useful in providing group therapy sessions for people who stutter and the therapists who treat them. Janet studied with Maria Fenton Gladys and her colleagues at the Pennsylvania Gestalt Center in Malvern, PA; Woody was trained by the faculty of the Gestalt Therapy Institute of Philadelphia. Although there were differences in the two 3-year training programs, both emphasized the importance of accepting the reality of whatever was happening. From their work, they developed the Awareness, Acceptance, Change model, which is the foundation for their approach to Experiential Therapy for Stuttering (Starkweather & Givens-Ackerman, 1997).

PRINCIPLES

Those of us who do not stutter see the disorder from the outside, and it is tempting to believe that stuttering is what you can see and hear. But it's not that simple. Stuttering is more than what is on the surface. Indeed, the surface behavior is less important than what's going on inside.

Repetitions, blocks, and prolongations are bad enough, but the dread of anticipated difficulty, the shame of exposing a "defect," the fear of seeing a listener's eyes widen in disbelief and shock, the anger and frustration at not being able to say what you want to when you want to, are worse, leading to the belief that almost anything, even silence, would be better.

These reactions begin at onset, usually in children of preschool age. At this age, children react in typical ways. First they are frustrated, and in a typical frustration pattern (Amsel & Roussel, 1952) try to push and force the word out or speed up the tempo of repeated elements, truncating syllables to do so (Bloodstein, 1960).

The family reacts too, and then the child reacts to the family. Developmental stuttering is a dynamically shifting set of problems that become more and more complicated as layers of emotions and behaviors are added to earlier layers until the earlier layers are buried and forgotten, and only the current symptoms present themselves.

We define fluency as the relative effortlessness of speech (Starkweather, 1987). Normal speech requires only a little muscular and cognitive effort. Fluency is thus a variable of human speech; it is not the absence of stuttering. Normal speech can be more or less fluent, and so can stuttering.

The goal of experiential therapy is less effortful speech, a reduction of the behaviors, thoughts, and feelings that PWS have and want to remove. So the first step in experiential therapy is listening and observing.

Listening Well Is Key

Listening seems easy, and speech therapists[1] trained in the medical model (and that is most of them) feel that they are not earning their pay when they are "just" listening. They feel that they should be *doing* something—showing the person how to talk, fixing. But PWS already know how to talk. They know how to pronounce words and form sentences. The problem is how they hear themselves and how they listen to themselves. Their experience of the act of talking is different than that of non-PWS. It takes more effort and is often overlaid with multiple emotions and a false belief that they lack skill in a basic human function: communication. The experiential therapist helps them learn how to hear themselves more constructively.

Therapists who listen with curiosity and compassion but without judgment model attitudes that help PWS hear their own speech. PWS have seen listeners turn away, blink, stare incredulously, offer "helpful" suggestions, fill in words, and try to show them how to talk. And those are the ones trying to be helpful; others can be downright rude. So, on first meeting an SLP, they often expect the worst.

It is exhilarating to meet an SLP who listens well, respects their opinion, follows the thread of their ideas, and attends patiently, during long and difficult blocks. But the real value of listening lies in the effect it has on the PWS's sense of worth. By listening this way, therapists show PWS that they too can listen to themselves with curiosity and compassion —a springboard to more fluent speech.

[1] We use the term "therapist" because we think it is more accurately descriptive of what we do in therapy.

The Cause Is Irrelevant

From the moment stuttering begins, it starts to change. And the way it changes determines the form it takes later on. By the time the PWS is an adult, the disorder's original form has faded into obscurity. The present constellation of behaviors, emotions, perceptions, and beliefs that constitute the disorder is the product of its development over the years since childhood. In experiential therapy, the therapist's and the PWS's attention is focused on the present.

The Therapist's Reactions Are Also Important

SLPs are typically trained to set aside their feelings and reactions and focus objectively on the client. But, therapists may feel angry, bored, amused, frustrated, confused—or any one of many other reactions—by something a client has said or done. Their hearts might race, their palms sweat, or their attention wander. Therapists may articulate these feelings or not, but they need to be aware of them and accept them without judgment. The therapist's reactions can provide useful material in the conversation that therapy becomes.

Control Is Not the Goal

Many PWS see their disorder as a problem of control. In the midst of stuttering they feel that they have lost control of their speech mechanism. To regain control they may talk with stiffened lips and jaws or monotone voices. Or they just stop talking. Effort expended in trying to control the uncontrollable is exhausting. Similarly, ignoring something that can be changed is a wasted opportunity. The trick is to discover what can be changed and work on that.

Respect Resistance

PWS often resist treatment. It seems odd to the neophyte that people who have come for treatment voluntarily will nonetheless resist the treatment the therapist offers. But it is common. It is hard to admit that stuttering is a problem one cannot solve on one's own. Some PWS resist the very idea that they need help.

PWS also resist because what therapists ask them to do is difficult. To recover, PWS must look their stuttering squarely in the eye, see it for what it is, handle it, taste and feel it, embrace it, and come to grips with it, even though they may have a history of avoidance and denial.

How the therapist handles resistance when it first occurs is crucial to the therapeutic relationship and the future of their therapy together. A careful examination of the resistance, made jointly by the PWS and the therapist, and without judgment, will set the right tone.

Most adult PWS have developed many defense mechanisms that have helped them cope with the disorder over the years. Working through them as they arise by respecting their power and appreciating their connection to the PWS's identity will enable the PWS to re-examine attitudes and beliefs about stuttering that hinder recovery. Here again, curiosity and compassion are key.

METHODS FOR INCREASING AWARENESS/ COUNTERING DENIAL

In the following sections we have supplemented some of the descriptions with verbatim examples of actual therapy. They are taken from sessions with a number of different PWS over the years and are reconstructed from notes and modified for simplicity and coherence.

Denial takes many forms. Some PWS just try hard not to think about it. Or they tell themselves, "Someday I'll outgrow it" or "It really isn't that bad." Others literally blank out, in what Charles Van Riper called "la petite mort" (the little death) during moments of stuttering (Heite, 2001). Momentarily absent from the scene, they are protected from the shame and humiliation.

Denial, though, is like a blanket that protects us from cold. The therapist has to "warm" things up so the PWS will feel able to remove the protection. By showing understanding and compassion, the therapist creates an atmosphere of safety so PWS can look at aspects of the disorder that they may have tuned out.

The Awareness Interview

The awareness interview is simply a conversation with the PWS about stuttering as it happens. Often, talking about stuttering is a new experience, and a conversation about it can relieve the shame produced by the "conspiracy of silence." But, the conversation begins gradually.

In an awareness interview, therapists rely on their own feelings of curiosity in the PWS's thoughts, feelings, and behaviors. Curiosity leads to questions that take the interview forward.

As the PWS and therapist talk, the therapist comments on some aspect of the PWS's behavior and asks what it feels like, if there is a specific reason for doing it, or an emotion or thought accompanying it. The therapist may also comment on empathetic reactions he or she might feel in response to the muscular tension, struggle, or attempts to hide or avoid. These straightforward, but gentle, comments make the conversation honest, straightforward, and accepting.

Experiential Therapy Verbatim—The Awareness Interview

Therapist: *Did you have trouble getting here this morning, what with the snow and all?*

PWS: *Nnnnno, nnnnnot really. I-, I-, I- just t,t,t,t, took mmmmmy time.*

Therapist: *You seem to be stuttering a little more than usual today.*

PWS: *Yyyyyes. I- I- I-, think it's gggggoing to, uh, to, uh, to, uh bbbe a bbbbbbbad day.*

Therapist: *Do you think the idea that it is going to be a bad day came first, or did some unusually bad stuttering come first, so you thought you were going to have a bad day?*

PWS: [shrugs] *I don't know.*

Therapist: *I noticed, when you were stuttering back there on the word "yes" that you pursed your lips together like this* [demonstrates], *and I have seen you do that often when you are stuttering, at least on certain sounds.*

PWS: *Yes, I know. I-, I-, I-, do that.*

Therapist: *What does it feel like?*

PWS: *I can feel some tension in my lips. I am pushing a little.*

Therapist: *How are you pushing?*

PWS: *I dddddon't know.*

Therapist: *Do you feel some tension anywhere else?*

PWS: *Yyyyyyes, I think so. There, yyyyyyes, I did it again when I said yyyyes. I am pushing the word out. I can feel it in my stomach.*

Therapist: *I see. And when you are pushing the word out, you purse your lips. Does that make it easier?*

PWS: *I am trying to make a channel for the words to come out.*

Therapist: *A channel? By pursing your lips?*

PWS: *Yyyyyyes. I started dddddoing that a llllllong time ago. I-, I-, I-, think it wwwwwwas in gggggrammar school.*

Therapist: *And how did you decide that pursing your lips like that would make a channel for the words to come out?*

PWS: *I-, I-, I-, I-, I don't know. It just seems that, wwwwwwhen I make my llllllips rrrr-round like that, the wwwwwwords will be a-, a-, uh, wwwwwwill come out mmmm-mmmore easily.*

Therapist: *That's very interesting. From my point of view, pursing your lips like that might make it harder for the words to come out.*

This conversation goes on and leads to an "experiment" in which the client inhibits the lip pursing behavior during stuttering. "*What will it feel like to stutter without that particular behavior? How strong is the pull to use that behavior as a way to help get the words out?*" are other possible questions. The compulsion to perform an avoidance behavior can be quite powerful and hard to resist, but most PWS learn, with awareness and practice, that these behaviors can be abandoned, and that it is easier to talk without them.

The word "experiment" is used here in an unusual sense. Its goal is to create an experience that makes a behavior, thought, or feeling vivid for PWS, increasing their awareness of a pattern. Not all experiments "work." That is why they are called experiments. Nevertheless, they help to develop a flavor of "let's try this and see what happens" that assists the course of therapy.

The One Finger Exercise

This exercise reveals when, and if, PWS become aware that they are stuttering or are about to. Therapists ask clients to raise a finger as soon as they realize they are stuttering or are about to. Using a signal helps the flow of speech, although some interruption may be necessary at first. This exercise is more than a diagnostic tool; it is a first step for PWS look objectively at the disorder.

Experiential Therapy Verbatim—The One Finger Exercise

Therapist: *While we are talking this afternoon, I want to ask you to signal to me whenever you realize that you are about to stutter, or when you realize that you actually are stuttering, whichever comes first. So, the moment you know you are going to stutter or are actually stuttering, raise your finger like this* [demonstrates], *so I will know what is going on.*

PWS: *OK.*

Therapist: *What have you been working on in school lately?*

PWS: *Oh, we, uh* [signals], *we are read-* [signals] *ing a bbb* [signals] *book called Ssssss*[signals]*Silas M, uh* [signals], *Marner. Like that?*

Therapist: *Yes, that's fine. You are signaling very clearly to me as soon as you know you have stuttered. It looks to me as though you don't usually know before you stutter that you are going to.*

PWS: *Sometimes I do.*

Therapist: *OK. Let's keep going. Maybe I will see that. What is the book about?*

PWS: *Um* [signals], *I-,* [signals] *it is, is,* [signals] *is a-, about...*

Therapist: *OK, that time it seemed to me that you were signaling while you were repeating "is" but you were thinking that you were going to stutter on the word "about." Is that right?*

PWS: *Yeah.*

Therapist: *Good, I really learned something about your stuttering from that.*

PWS: *What?*

Therapist: *That when you repeat whole words, it is sometimes because you are thinking you are going to stutter on another word later on. That is just the kind of detail we want to get to.*

PWS: *OK. Bbbbbut, I-, I dddddon't think that repeating the word like that, when I am waiting, putting off, waiting for time to pass, before I say thththththth wwwwword thththth-that I am going to sssssstutter on that that is, is, is, uh, sssssstuttering.*

Therapist: *Oh I see. To you, repeating the word like that, in anticipation of a hard word, that isn't stuttering. What is it, do you think?*

PWS: *Well, that's just trying to say the word.*

Therapist: *The later word, the hard one.*

PWS: *Yes.*

Therapist: *OK. So for you, saying the word over and over is something you do to prevent stuttering.*

PWS: *Yes.*

Therapist: *I can see why you wouldn't think of it as stuttering. But it is a part of the whole pattern, isn't it?*

PWS: *Yes.*

Therapist: *I would like to put it down as something you do, but make a distinction between things you do to cope with the stuttering and the other behaviors that are more the stuttering itself. In a sense they are both part of the stuttering pattern, but they are also different.*

PWS: *OK.*

The Two-Finger Exercise

This exercise helps PWS gain a clearer sense of the timing of their behavior. People tend to be polite and try to ignore stuttering when they see it, lulling some PWS into a kind of fantasy that "no one has noticed." Also, listeners may become so used to the presence of stuttering that in fact they do not notice it. Many PWS do not know what their listeners see and hear. Some think that people do not hear it, even though it may be obvious, while others believe that stuttering is all their listeners see, even though it may be mild and unobtrusive.

In this exercise, the PWS signals the occurrence or expectation of stuttering (finger #1), and the therapist signals to the PWS when the therapist first sees it (finger #2), making clear just when listeners can see or hear their stuttering. As a result, PWS gain a more realistic perspective on what listeners actually see and hear.

The one- and two-finger exercises do something else, too. Most PWS try to hide the disorder. For some, severity is so great that hiding is not an option, but for most, some hiding is possible, and it can develop into a well-established habit. In the one-finger exercise, PWS are not trying to minimize the disorder; they are signaling "Here it is" repeatedly. When, in addition, the therapist signals back during the two-finger exercise, they receive a confirmation, "Yes, I saw it." There is then a complete, two-way openness about the occurrence of stuttering behaviors, something quite new for most PWS.

Examining Patterns

Examining patterns is another way to begin gradually. It is a joint exploration of the "places"—situations, words, sounds—where stuttering occurs. Most PWS do not find this difficult; many already know these places. The exploration process not only teaches the therapist; it tells the PWS that he or she has important knowledge. It is often done in traditional therapy to assess severity, but in experiential therapy it begins a conversation about the PWS's experience. The therapist doesn't just note that words beginning with /p/ are hard, but might ask what impact the pattern has. "Well, it means that I can never order pizza," or "I can't introduce my girlfriend because her name is Patricia." In experiential therapy, the influence of these patterns on the person's experience is made known.

Experiential Therapy Verbatim—Examining Patterns

Therapist: *Can I ask you a little about the times when you stutter? I mean by that the places or situations where you stutter or the sentences, words, or sounds that you stutter on?*

PWS: *OK.*

Therapist: *Are there any particular places or situations where stuttering is a particular problem for you?*

PWS: *Um, y-, yes. I-, I stutter real bad when I-, talk to, to, to, uh, to ssssssomeo-, one, someone I don't know.*

Therapist: *So, talking to strangers is a situation where you are more likely to stutter?*

PWS: *Yes.*

Therapist: *OK. That's one. What's that like for you?*

PWS: *It's like being shy, but I'm not shy!*

Therapist: *What do you mean, 'It's like' being shy?*

PWS: *People think I'm shy. I seem shy, but I'm not.*

Therapist: *That sounds hard to me. Sad.*

PWS: *I look like someone else. I hate that.*

Therapist: *Oh, wow. Where else are you more likely to stutter?*

PWS: *Um. I-, I ha-, ha-, have a ha-, hard time wwwwwwhen I-, I call mmmmmmy, uh, girlfriend.*

Therapist: *Is it the phone, or . . .*

PWS: *Yeah, sure. The, uh, the, the, uh, the phphphphphone ha-, has always been ha-, hard for me, but..*

Therapist: *So, we can add talking on the phone to the list of situations in which you are more likely to stutter?*

PWS: *Yeah, yeah, but, um, but it's also, um, it's, I-, I also sssssssstutter on, on her name.*

Therapist: *What's her name?*

PWS: *Um, um, um, uh, a P-, uh, P-, uh, PPPPPPatricia.*

Therapist: *OK. I'm remembering what it was like to be a teenager calling a girlfriend. It was very hard for me and I didn't stutter. When you stutter on her name, would you be talking to her parents?*

PWS: *Yeah.*

Therapist: *And what's that like?*

PWS: *I don't know what they think. Maybe that I'm not good enough for her. Or something worse; I dunno.*

Therapist: *It must be very difficult. I think we want to see what we can do to make it easier for you to say her name.*

PWS: *Oh, yeah, I'd like that.*

After this conversation, the experience of stuttering has been changed. The disorder is less amorphous, less mysterious and unpredictable. And less painful. Now, it can be dealt with.

Listing False Beliefs

This is another way to begin work. PWS often have false beliefs about themselves and about their stuttering, beliefs that do not serve them well. A short list of typical false beliefs is given below. (We return to this list later when we discuss positive affirmations.)

There is something wrong with me.

I am responsible for others' feelings.

I can control what others think or feel about me and how they treat me.

I can't handle pain.

If I am vulnerable, I will be hurt.

I must not get angry.

I cannot make a mistake.

Fluency is the most important thing.

People don't want to listen to me.

Most PWS will not find it difficult to create a list of their own. These beliefs are "false" not just because they are untrue. They are also false because they lead the PWS into behaviors and feelings that make the problem worse rather than better. They get in the way, interfere with life, motivate avoidance and struggle, and lead to social withdrawal.

Listing Values

Our values direct our choices, our behavior. They are the force that runs the show. When "not stuttering" is the PWS's main value, or the most important thing in his life, recovery is harmed. Chasing the fluency god, as it has been called, just decreases effective communication.

A high value on the opinion of others will intensify feelings of embarrassment and motivate avoidance, while other values, such as perseverance and courage, can be helpful.

METHODS FOR INCREASING ACCEPTANCE/ COUNTERING AVOIDANCE

Two kinds of acceptance can be identified: acceptance of self and acceptance of stuttering.

The Acceptance of Self

Some people feel accepted by others but still do not feel accepting of themselves. Some PWS say, "If they really knew me, they wouldn't like me so much" because of a deeply internalized sense of shame. They do not feel worthy, lovable, complete, whole, etc. Such a sense of inadequacy is probably related to childhood experiences, which have been traumatic for many PWS. Nevertheless, they may still influence current behavior.

Healing the Wounded Inner Child

The "inner child" is a metaphor for psychological injuries done in the past that still hurt. Reactions that seem "out of proportion" to the reality of the moment often indicate that these old experiences are still impacting our present life. As Bradshaw (1990) describes it, "We first see the world through the eyes of a little child, and that inner child remains with us throughout our lives, no matter how 'grown-up' and adult we become." If childhood experiences of stuttering were humiliating or shaming and there was no opportunity back then to express those feelings and move on, this "unfinished business" may still be present and affecting present life. Healing the inner child means recalling these events and finishing the unfinished business.

Certainly, psychotherapy can be useful for this type of healing, but sometimes a simple exercise, such as the one described below, can provide an opportunity to heal. At least it may help the PWS realize that it is time to pursue this healing with a more psychologically trained professional, or obtain the training for themselves.

There are many exercises available for healing the wounded inner child. Left hand/right hand journaling is one and can easily be undertaken on one's own. In this exercise, the person conducts a dialogue with his or her inner child by using first the dominant hand as the adult, then answering with the non-dominant hand as the child. The feeling of writing with the uncoordinated non-dominant hand helps to "tap into the more creative, less logical side of the brain and makes it easier to get in touch with the feelings of your inner child" (Bradshaw, 1990).

The PWS can try this for twenty minutes each day for a month before deciding if it is useful, or needs to be modified. Some people prefer drawing to writing, alternating between the dominant and non-dominant hand. For more information on the inner child concept, see Whitfield (1987) and Bradshaw (1990).

Positive Affirmations

An affirmation is a positive statement, stated as if it were a fact, in the present tense, and focused on countering some aspect of self that has been identified as a negative belief. For example, a PWS who wants to stop changing words might affirm, "I can say what I want to." Making an affirmation is also a change technique, but PWS who want to stop feeling ashamed and be more accepting of themselves can affirm "I am enough" or "I am complete and whole."

Previously, we suggested listing false beliefs. A positive affirmation can be constructed for each item on the list. For example, rather than the original, "There is something wrong with me," the new positive affirmation might be a simple "I am enough." Here are eight more examples:

> "I am responsible for others' feelings" becomes "I am responsible for my own feelings."
>
> "I can control what others think of me or feel about me and how they treat me" turns into "I can only control my own reactions and thoughts."
>
> "I can't handle pain" becomes "Pain is a part of life; I can handle it."
>
> "If I am vulnerable, I will be hurt" turns into "Feeling vulnerable reminds me I'm human."
>
> "I must not get angry" becomes "I have a right to all my feelings, even my anger."
>
> "I cannot make a mistake" turns into "Mistakes are the price we pay to learn new things."
>
> "Not stuttering is the most important thing" becomes "The most important thing is being true to myself."
>
> "People don't want to listen to me" turns into "People want to hear what I have to say."

Once a positive affirmation is identified, PWS need to say it to themselves often, reminding themselves of its veracity. "Trying on" new behaviors, attitudes, and beliefs is an opportunity to explore again any remaining resistance the PWS has to the old belief. A discussion around what it was like to "try it on" can be helpful.

Guided Imagery

A guided imagery, or visualization, is a prepared text with suggested images that lead the individual to imagine. The therapist presents the elements, but the PWS does the imagining.

No two listeners imagine the same thing, so the method can be used in a group. Most guided imageries are healing, if not soothing, but some can be challenging and emotionally powerful.

"Morphing"[2] is a guided imagery that was originally written to have additional and personal affirmations written into the script as it is being read. It creates a setting in which the affirmations can be taken very seriously.

The Acceptance of Stuttering

When the acceptance of stuttering leads to less stuttering, it may seem almost miraculous, but it is really very simple. Most of the behaviors that PWS perform are things they are doing to get through, hide, minimize, stifle, or divert attention from their stuttering. As acceptance grows, there is less need for these avoidance behaviors, and they slowly fall away.

Avoidance behaviors make up far more of stuttering than most people recognize. Some are obvious, as when a PWS crosses the street to avoid talking to someone, or changes words, alters sounds, orders unwanted food, or, on a larger scale, seeks a career that involves little talking. These are recognizable avoidance behaviors. But so too is backing up, changing vocal pitch, or saying a word slowly and carefully to get through it without getting stuck.

This type of avoidance is embedded inside the repetitions and prolongations that traditional SLPs label as "core behaviors" (Van Riper, 1982). Few PWS would repeat a sound, e.g., the /t/ in the word "time," slowly and easily, "tuh, tuh, tuh, time." That is not the way most PWS talk. Instead, they may (1) speed up the /t/ to get past it as quickly as possible, (2) try to push the sound out with air pressure, (3) truncate the syllable to t-,t-,t- (a different way to speed up), (4) tense oral muscles to stiffen movement and inhibit extraneous repetition, or (5) say the word quietly so listeners will not hear it. Experiential therapy holds that even in these "core" behaviors, most of the effort is in the hiding, the struggle, or the forcing—behaviors that, with increased acceptance of the person's stuttering, fade away.

Reducing avoidance behaviors has an immediate payoff in better communication, but it can't be done without addressing the original fear that motivates it. A host of studies make it clear that to reduce fear, one must experience the feared entity in the absence of negative consequences. This doesn't work very well for stuttering. In phobias, the feared entity—spiders, heights, or germs, for example—is only remotely dangerous and it is relatively easy to have the patient imagine being near a spider or high on a ladder or covered in dirt without experiencing negative consequences. But for PWS, the fear is not irrational. In their experience, stuttering has resulted in unpleasant reactions both in themselves and in their listeners (Siegel, 1970).

Voluntary Stuttering

One of the oldest and best-known methods for avoiding avoidance is voluntary stuttering. The method has several different forms and a number of different uses. One use is to increase acceptance of stuttering as it occurs. Since the fear that motivates most avoidance behaviors is the fear of stuttering itself, it follows that stuttering on purpose can reduce fear. But most PWS resist the idea at first, so therapists start it in a safe environment, after a sense of trust has been established. Therapists begin slowly, asking for just one brief sample of voluntary stuttering, and then talk about it to see if the experience was vivid. Soon, the PWS will be able to do more and will begin to feel the power of performing a behavior

[2]A copy of "Morphing" can be obtained by sending an email to woody.starkweather@gmail.com.

that was once frightening. And then, gradually the PWS can be helped to perform voluntary stuttering outside in the real world, first with relatively safe people, "Designated Listeners" (DLs), then with more and more difficult listeners. Once PWS see the value of voluntary stuttering, they are usually excited and eager to use it. The PWS can begin to practice "avoiding avoidance."

Even if fear has been reduced, a tendency to perform avoidance behaviors remains. The reason is that avoidance behaviors suppress the fear that motivates them. For example, you are approaching a busy intersection and see cars whizzing by. The light is red, so you apply the brakes. This is an avoidance behavior. But well-practiced drivers do not feel any fear because they are confident that the brakes will stop the car. So too with PWS. They know that if they do not say the feared word but instead use some other word, they will probably not stutter.

PWS need to understand that they aren't going to immediately get completely rid of the fear. They won't be able to wait for the fear to go away before they try something new. They need to "do it anyway." The PWS needs to actively inhibit the tendency to perform the avoidance behavior, and as long as the fear has been reduced or is absent, this inhibition is possible. The therapist helps by identifying avoidance behaviors and witnessing and celebrating triumphs.

Advertising

Advertising is being as open as possible about one's stuttering. PWS advertise by mentioning the fact that they stutter, talking about stuttering whenever they can, and stuttering openly and obviously. Classic, traditional voluntary stuttering is a form of advertising. A good place and time to advertise is answering the telephone. On answering the phone, it is expected in the United States that one says "Hello." This expectation of a specific word makes answering the phone difficult for many PWS. A PWS who has laryngeal blocks has a particular problem, because no sound at all comes out, and the caller has no idea what is happening.

For the PWS, the caller's confusion only makes matters worse. Voluntary stuttering in saying "hello" solves the problem. The caller knows a PWS has answered the phone, and will then likely wait until the PWS gets the word out.

Self-Imitation

In self-imitation, the PWS learns to hear and feel the difference between real and voluntary stuttering. Often, this experience makes it clear just what the real stuttering consists of, such as an area of tension in the tongue, lips, jaw, or vocal mechanism. Being aware of this focus can be helpful later in therapy when working on changing from stuttering to normal disfluency.

Easy stuttering is a step between real stuttering and normal speech. It shows the PWS that there is more than one way to stutter, which introduces the possibility of change, and that some ways are better than others, with less muscular tension, less struggle, less avoidance. Easy stuttering is simply the stuttering pattern that the individual presents but with as little struggle as possible. Behaviorally, easy stuttering is real stuttering from which the struggle has been removed.

Talking about stuttering ensures that stuttering is not a forbidden topic. Most PWS find that when they talk about their stuttering, they stutter less.

Experiential Therapy Verbatim—Self-Imitation

Therapist: *Hi. I wanted to show you something a little different today. We have worked on different forms of voluntary stuttering—*

bouncing and gliding—and you seem to find those useful.

PWS: *Yes.*

Therapist: *Now, I want to show you a form of voluntary stuttering that is called self-imitation. Simply put, you just stutter voluntarily in the same way that you do when you are stuttering involuntarily.*

PWS: *I see.*

Therapist: *Would you like to try it out and see what happens?*

PWS: *I am not sure that I can do that.*

Therapist: *Would you like to try? Tell me about that book that you brought with you.*

PWS: *OK. Ththth- uh, th- I don't know. I can't seem to do it.*

Therapist: *I see. Can you say more?*

PWS: *No, it just seems too hard.*

Therapist: *All right. My sense is that I am asking you to do something that seems really wrong for you, at least now. Maybe we could take a look at that. It will help me understand.*

PWS: *OK.*

Therapist: *When you started to imitate yourself—I think it was on a word beginning with th* (/ð/)*—what can you tell me about that moment?*

PWS: *I had a strong reaction.*

Therapist: *Can you tell me something about that reaction?*

PWS: *What do you want to know?*

Therapist: *Well, where did you feel something? Where in your body?*

PWS: *In my ch,ch,ch,ch,chest, it was, yes. It was in my chest.*

Therapist: *And what was the feeling in your chest?*

PWS: *I dunno. A kind of tightness I th,th, th,th,think.*

Therapist: *Is that a feeling you have had before?*

PWS: *Yes, when I am afraid.*

Therapist: *OK. So, would it be fair to say that when I asked you to imitate yourself, you felt afraid?*

PWS: *Yes.*

Therapist: *Well that in itself is helpful. Let's try something similar, and see if we can get a little closer to that feeling.*

PWS: *OK.*

Therapist: *Try to say a sentence about the book you brought and stutter on the first sound in the sentence in the way that you would typically stutter.*

PWS: *I, I, I, am reading a book on gardening. But that wasn't a sound I would usually stutter on.*

Therapist: *Well, try to think of a sentence that begins with a sound you would usually stutter on.*

PWS: *OK. Th, th, th, th — uh, OK. Th, th, that's very real. It's not voluntary stuttering. It's real stuttering.*

Therapist: *OK. So, when I ask you to imitate yourself, you start to do it on purpose, and it turns into a real stutter.*

PWS: *Yes, and I don't like it. It f,f,f,f,feels like, like I am about to step into a hole.*

Therapist: *Oh, I see. So impending disaster. That kind of feeling.*

PWS: *Yes.*

Therapist: *OK. Well that's very helpful. Let's go on to something else. But I would like you to pay attention to that feeling in your chest during this coming week, before our next ses-*

sion. If you feel that feeling again, make a note, a mental note or in your diary, about what it was like, where you were, what was going on. We need to get a little deeper into that feeling. It is an important feeling for you.

PWS: *OK.*

The Empty Chair

This method provides the opportunity to move from *talking about* to *talking to*.

Stuttering can create much misery, and most PWS understandably hate the disorder. But hatred is alienating, and the PWS who hates the disorder may find it difficult to even think about it. Stuttering is the enemy. This attitude, understandable as it is, is unhelpful. A dialogue with one's stuttering brings it closer and may achieve a kind of rapprochement that makes it easier to deal with.

Experiential Therapy Verbatim—The Empty Chair: Dialogue with Stuttering

PWS: *It-, It-, It's aaaaaawful cccccccold out there tttttttoday.*

Therapist: *It sure is. It's been a bad winter, hasn't it?*

PWS: *Yyyyyyyeah.*

Therapist: *I notice that when you stutter like that, there seems to be a lot of muscular tension. I can see some tremoring and a lot of tightness.*

PWS: *Yes.*

Therapist: *What does that feel like?*

PWS: *It ffffffeels very ssssssssstiff, like a bbbbbboard al-, al-, almost.*

Therapist: *If you were to picture your stuttering, what would you see?*

PWS: *I'm, I'm, nnnnnnnot sure whwhwhwhwhat yyyyyyou mean.*

Therapist: *Well, you said before that your mouth felt stiff like a board. Close your eyes and imagine looking at that, what do you see?*

PWS: *I sssssssee a mmmmmmouth made out, out, out of wwwwwwood.*

Therapist: *OK.* [waiting] *Do you see anything else?*

PWS: *There is a nose above the mouth and eyes.*

Therapist: *Are they all made out of wood?*

PWS: *Yes.*

Therapist: *OK. Now, just imagine, in a general way, that there is a body below the head, so that you can see your stuttering as if it were an entire person. Can you see that?*

PWS: *Yes.*

Therapist: *Let's imagine that that person, your stuttering, is sitting right there in that chair.*

PWS: *OK.*

Therapist: [waiting] *What else can you tell me about what you see?*

PWS: *Well, thththththere are lllllllines rrrrrrrunning up and ddddddown in the face, lllllllike grooves.*

Therapist: *Like the grain in the wood?*

PWS: *Yes.*

Therapist: *What color is it?*

PWS: *Bbbbbbbrown. The nnnnnnose is broken.*

Therapist: *OK. Good. That's a nice piece of detail.* [waiting] *Can you say anything more about that?*

PWS: *Yes, whwhwhwhwhen I wwwwwwwas a bbbbbbboy, I broke my nose.*

Therapist: *OK. Does that help us know that this is YOUR stuttering, not someone else's?*

PWS: *Yyyyyyes.* [Sits quietly]

Therapist: *Would you like to say something to your stuttering, while it is sitting right there in the chair? Is there anything you would like to say?*

PWS: *Um, um, um, I-, I-, I-, I ddddddon't know.*

Therapist: *What comes to your mind?*

PWS: *I hate it.*

Therapist: *Talk to your stuttering, right TO it. "I hate you."*

PWS: *I hate you.* [Said flatly, without much emotion]

Therapist: *Say it again. More like you mean it.*

PWS: [louder] *I hate you.*

Therapist: *Once more. Say it the way you feel it.*

PWS: [yelling a bit] *I hate you!*

Therapist: *I HATE YOU!* [Modeling what a loud angry voice sounds like]

PWS: *Yes. I hate you. I HATE YOU. YOU HAVE RUINED MY LIFE!*

Therapist: *There you go. How did you feel doing that?*

PWS: *Whew! I-, I-, dddddidn't expect to yyyyyell that lllloud.*

Therapist: *What did it feel like to do that?*

PWS: *I, I, IIt, It, ffffelt good actually. Maybe powerful, strong. I don't know*

Therapist: [smiles in agreement] *Now I want you to go sit in the empty chair yourself.*

PWS: *OK.* [Moves to the other chair]

Therapist: *When you were sitting over here, you shouted "I hate you." What does your stuttering say back to you?*

PWS: *I-, I-, knknknknow.* [catching on quickly now] *It's bbbbbbecause I hurt yyyyyou.*

Therapist: *Now, back to this chair. What do you say to that?*

PWS: *Whwhwhwhwhy do you want to hurt mmmmmme so mmmmmmuch?*

Therapist: *Good; now back over there.*

PWS: *Bbbbbbecause thththththat's who I am.*

Therapist: *OK. Now come sit back here where you started.* [Sits quietly for a moment while PWS gets settled] *What was that exercise like for you?*

PWS: *A little weird but OK. I am surprised. I never knew I could yell like that.*

Therapist: *This is just a beginning. We will do this again and often and see what more we can learn.*

PWS: *OK.*

After several sessions using this technique, the PWS may begin to see things from the stuttering's point of view. This change from complete hostility toward a more accommodating relationship between the PWS and the stuttering reduces anger, fear, or sadness that the stuttering has created and helps the person find an easier way to talk. But in the first few dialogues, the gain will be increased awareness, as in the example above when the client became more aware of how angry he was.

Moving Forward—One Transition at a Time

This technique is a way for PWS to talk with little or no stuttering behavior, after emotional work is under way. But it is also a way to increase acceptance. Each time PWS move forward through syllables without struggling, even with the fear that they might stutter, they are learning to accept. Hence, it is in this section.

To use this technique, PWS have to be aware of their behaviors and feelings. The avoidance behaviors—speeding up, rhythmic movements, ballistic movements, etc.—should have already been removed from the stuttering pattern. Increased acceptance will allow the person to stutter more easily. From the one- and two-finger exercises, the PWS will know when stuttering is about to occur. The therapist then encourages moving forward to the next sound, whether or not stuttering will occur. Often, because of increased acceptance, there will be no stuttering. There will be the expectation, but no stuttering. Eventually the expectations will diminish. Furthermore, by "not pushing" as a comfortable way to deal with stuttering that does occur, the emotional consequence of that eventuality is also lessened. Moving forward leads to a discussion about transitions.

Experiential Therapy Verbatim—Moving Forward/Transitions

Therapist: *Hi. How has it been going?*

PWS: *Good. I feel that I have been able to drop almost all of the whole word repetitions. Sometimes I forget, but mostly I remember not to do it.*

Therapist: *OK. Now I want to take this one step further. When you feel that you are about to stutter on the word, I want you to go ahead and stutter on it. Don't pause. Just go right into the stuttering. We have done enough stuttering on purpose so that you ought to be able to do this.*

PWS: *OK. I cccccan dddddo that, even if I have to ffffffake it.*

Therapist: *Well, it might be good to fake it for a while, just to get used to the new rhythm, but then I want you to let yourself have real stuttering that is not preceded by a stall for time.*

PWS: *OK. Let's practice it.*

Therapist: *Great. I really like that kind of attitude.*

PWS: *Well, the* [brief pause] *ppoint is to ggget better.*

MORE PRACTICE

Therapist: *How did those feel?*

PWS: *I think I stutter less when I dddon't pause, than when I dddo.*

Therapist: *I think so too. That pausing by holding back the air with your vocal folds was creating a lot of tension throughout your vocal tract.*

PWS: *Yes! I can feel that there is less tension in the stuttering when I don't pause.*

Therapist: *And what is also important, because you are neither pausing nor repeating words, AND your actual stuttering repetitions are shorter because they are less tense, you have gained a whole lot of speech time. Your new way of stuttering takes up much less time than the old way. You are moving forward instead of waiting.*

After more practice, inside and outside the therapist's office, the PWS was ready for the next step.

PWS: *This ppast week has bbbeen ggreat. I am stuttering about as often as I used to, bbbut I can feel myself moving forward much more rapidly. I feel almost as if I am not stuttering anymore.*

Therapist: *And how is that for you?*

PWS: *Great!*

Therapist: *What does it feel like?*

PWS: *Like I am suddenly part of the human race.*

Therapist: *And before you were just . . . what?*

PWS: *Just stuttering me. Yes. I think that I miss that old me a little too.*

Therapist: *That is to be expected, and later, when your speech is even more normal, you may find that it is even more difficult. We are all more comfortable with the familiar.*

PWS: *Oh.*

Therapist: *I want to try taking the moving forward strategy just a little bit farther today.*

PWS: *OK.*

Therapist: *Have you ever noticed that when you stutter on a word, that you aren't actually stuttering on the first sound? For example, when you say the word "dog" and stutter on it by repeating the /d/, you really aren't having any difficulty saying the /d/ sound. You say it just fine; in fact, you say it several times, and each time you are pronouncing it exactly as it is supposed to be pronounced.*

PWS: *But too many times.*

Therapist: *Right. The problem is not in saying the /d/, it is in moving from the /d/ to the vowel that follows it. The problem is not in the first sound, but in the transition from the first to the second. In your case, moving from a consonant to a vowel is your stuttering.*

PWS: *That is interesting, and very helpful. I can see more clearly where the problem is. Why didn't I ever notice that before?*

Therapist: *Speech is so fast. It is hard even to think about such brief events. Now what I want you to do is concentrate on moving from the first sound to the second. So, you are going to feel as though you will stutter, you are going to let yourself stutter, as we have been doing, but you are not going to repeat the sound. Instead you are going to move smoothly from the first to the second sound. It might help if you make this transitional movement more slowly at first.*

PWS: *OK. I am going* [prolonging the transition from the /g/ to the /o/] *to keep moving forward* [prolonging again] *instead of repeating.*

Therapist: *Good. Let's keep talking so you can practice some more.*

PWS: *Alright. This* [again] *feels quite different* [again] *from the way I am used to talking* [again].

Therapist: *I am not surprised. What does it feel like?*

PWS: *It feels* [again] *a lot like that sliding* [again] *technique you showed me a while back* [again].

Therapist: *I think it is the same in terms of what you are doing, but it is a little different in the way we approach it. Also, as soon as you feel used to talking in this way, I want you to try to shorten the transition. Right now you are slowing down while you make the transition so that you can feel it happening. But you will not need that little crutch in a while and you will just be able to move forward in real speech time. I need to warn you about something as you practice this way of talking. It is going to feel as if you are not stuttering at all, and in one sense you are not. You will really not sound as though you are stuttering, but in fact you are still stuttering, just in a very easy, comfortable, and unobtrusive way. People are going to tell you that you have been cured. You have not been cured; it just sounds that way. You can tell people anything you want to, but I think it is helpful to remember that you are still stuttering.*

METHODS FOR CHANGE

Changing Attitudes and Feelings

We are all a little rigid and need to be seized by the shirtfront and shaken from time to time.

Change can be frightening, and fear is at the heart of many forms of rigidity. But, as awareness increases and acceptance grows, small changes occur. We begin to see that change is not only possible, it is liberating. We become open to change.

Cultivating an attitude of gratitude helps make change possible. Gratitude for the good things in life is easy. How about gratitude for our mistakes? Our struggles? Our challenges? Nobody wants to make mistakes, but mistakes are often how we learn. Be grateful for them. When PWS apply this idea to their stuttering, they begin to see each stuttering event as an opportunity to learn, to try something new.

Many PWS are emotionally exhausted by the disorder, particularly if there has been a long series of unsuccessful therapies. The idea of trying something new can be intimidating. Just going to a therapist can feel like an admission of failure. Even PWS who are already seeing therapists have to make this same leap just to come to their scheduled appointment. But speech therapy is like dentistry; it helps with the problem, but it is not fun.

Letting Go

PWS may be trying to control the uncontrollable. Not just speech movements, but trying to hide the stuttering by using very short sentences, or by not talking, only create new problems. The antidote to these counterproductive attempts to control the uncontrollable is rightly called "letting go." It is an important part of experiential therapy for stuttering.

Experiential Therapy Verbatim— Letting Go of Struggle

Therapist: *We've been working for several months now, and I have been very pleased to see you willing to try new things. You have even learned how to feel comfortable thinking about your stuttering in a very different way from what you are used to.*

PWS: *Ththththanks. I lllllike the way thththththis feels. I ffffeel, uh, uh, ffffffreeer than I used to.*

Therapist: *Let's do a little more work today directly on your stuttering behaviors. You know, I really appreciate how patient you have been about this. When you come in, of course, you want to be able to talk more fluently, but there are a lot of things to do before we even approach that possibility.*

PWS: *OK. What do we do?*

Therapist: *I know we have done this before, but I want you to talk to me about what it feels like when you stutter.*

PWS: *OK. Today, I came fffffffrom wwwwwork, uh . . . I felt some tension that time in my lips.*

Therapist: *OK. Anything else?*

PWS: *I was holding back ffffffrom pushing the wwwwwword out. I wwwwanted to pppppush on it to get it over wwwwith.*

Therapist: *Good. You have really learned how to pay attention when you are stuttering.*

PWS: *I ththththink also I wwwwwas fffffeeling a little, um, affffraid.*

Therapist: *Can you tell what you were feeling afraid of?*

PWS: *No. It's lllllike an old tape, something that isn't even there anymore.*

Therapist: *I would like to try an experiment. Are you up for it?*

PWS: *Sure.*

Therapist: *I want you to try to let go of your stuttering. Don't try not to push. Don't bother with pushing, either. Just let the stuttering happen however it is going to happen. You may feel fear; I think you will. But try to remember that you are safe.*

PWS: *OK. Let's see, I need to talk about something. I had a little run-in wwwwww, wi, wi, wi, ooh, that just sort of ran away with itself.*

Therapist: *OK.*

PWS: *Anyway, I had a confrontation www-wwith my boss. I ththththink I told you that he doesn't lllllike the wwwway I do things.*

Therapist: *Are you trying to let go of the control?*

PWS: *Yes. And it is ffffeeling easier. That ffffffirst repetition wwwent off, but now it fffeels kind of nice.*

Therapist: *OK. Keep going. Try to get a good sense of what it feels like not to fight with it.*

PWS: *OK. Well my bbbbbboss— I really let that one go; I wwwanted to push it out— my bbbboss wwwas very critical of mmmmy wwwork, and I had to deffffend myself a little. It wwwas hard bbbut I did it, and I fffelt good about it afterwards. I lllike the wway this feels. It takes mmmmuch less effort to talk this way. I think I could talk more—I mmean fffor a longer time—if I talked mmmore like this. I wwouldn't get so tired.*

Therapist: *I am sure that's true.*

PWS: *Can we keep doing this fffor a wwhile?*

Therapist: *Sure. Tell me more about that boss of yours.*

Letting Go of Attempts to Hide Stuttering

Some PWS try to hide their stuttering by closing the vocal folds. The hope is that the "moment" will pass and the stuttering will remain hidden from the listener. But vocal fold closure stops speech completely, creating a moment of silence that radiates tension. It is no less deviant than the stuttering it is designed to hide. It is simply another form of stuttering.

Another way to hide stuttering is simply not talking at all, inhibiting the natural urge to communicate but sacrificing contact with others. Many PWS carry this strategy so far that they would be considered covert PWS. They may be keeping their stuttering a secret, but a deep sense of shame often develops from keeping such a big secret, from presenting themselves as other than they are.

Experiential Therapy Verbatim—Letting Go of Fear

Therapist: *I would like to work today on something you told me about with great feeling the last time we met. You told me how you learned as a child not to talk when you thought you would probably stutter and that you still hold back from talking when you think you are going to stutter. What is it like for you not to talk when you really have something to say?*

PWS: *Well, it's, it's very hard. I, I, I, have a lot to, to, say. I, I know I am smart. And, and, and when I do that, just keep quiet, I always feel angry afterwards.*

Therapist: *Who do you feel angry with?*

PWS: *Just myself. I, I, I, feel very mad at myself. But I still don't dare let people see me stutter.* [Tears well up]

Therapist: *This is a tough place for you to be in, isn't it?*

PWS: *Yes, I feel kind of trapped. There is no way out of it. Either I expose my worst characteristic, or I don't get to, to, to be who I really am. I, I lose, lose, either way.*

Therapist: *I have noticed that you aren't afraid to talk in here.*

PWS: *I don't think I will stutter in here. And even if I do, you are the only one who will hear it.*

Therapist: *That's interesting. What is it about me that makes it OK to stutter in front of me?*

PWS: *Well, you, you see a lot of people who stutter. It's no big deal to you.*

Therapist: *That's certainly true. I wonder how big a deal it is to other people. Who can you talk freely to?*

PWS: *Really only my sister. And I am not completely free with her either.*

Therapist: *Maybe we can expand that. Could you have a conversation with her this week about your stuttering?*

PWS: *Oh, I don't know. I feel comfortable with her. She certainly knows I stutter. We have even mentioned it a few times. But a conversation about my stuttering sounds difficult.*

Therapist: *Well, you can tell her that I asked you to do it. Sometimes that helps with the little awkwardness when you haven't had that kind of a conversation before.*

PWS: *I think I can do that.*

Therapist: *Good. You will still feel fear, but I would like it if you go ahead with the conversation anyway. Could you do that?*

PWS: *I'll try.*

Therapist: *Good. Then we can talk about it the next time.*

Changing False Beliefs About Stuttering

Many PWS see their stuttering as a barrier to talking. They believe that stuttering makes it hard to talk. Their resulting struggle confirms the belief. Or they may believe stuttering is awful, perhaps worse than not talking at all. This too is circular, causing the PWS to dread any talking. The mental and muscular tension this belief creates colors the speech act with an acidic wash of fear, making it an awful experience.

To counter these vicious cycles, the PWS needs to examine and question the origins of the belief, and then re-experience speaking with a different belief, creating a contrasting memory to help weaken the earlier false one.

Experiential Therapy Verbatim—Negative Self-Talk

Therapist: *We have been working together for quite awhile now, and you have made a lot of progress in how you stutter. The struggle behaviors that you used to use routinely as you spoke are now pretty much a thing of the past. May I ask you how these changes in your behavior have changed the way you feel about your stuttering?*

PWS: *I really like the way I sound, and I am very relieved to find that I can talk so much more easily. I used to get very sharp pppains in my jaw if I had to talk for any length of time. Now, I don't stutter anywhere near as often, and when I do, it is easier to do, so I don't get these pains anymore.*

Therapist: *That's wonderful. So, how do you actually feel when you are in a situation where you think you might stutter?*

PWS: *It's funny. Even though I know that I don't have to struggle and fight with it so much, I still feel apprehensive when I get into a situation that has always been hard for me.*

Therapist: *You say "apprehensive." Can you say a little more?*

PWS: *I still feel the way I used to. Maybe not so much. Not so intense, but I still feel afraid that I am going to stutter, and I have to work hard to keep that fear from getting a grip on me.*

Therapist: *And what might happen if you stutter?*

PWS: *I, I, I am not really concerned anymore about being embarrassed. I gave that up a while ago. But talking has just always been very difficult for me. It has been frustrating and at times physically painful. So, when I am about to do a lot of talking, I have a kind of "Oh shit, here we go" kind of feeling.*

Therapist: *It sounds to me as though you are bracing yourself.*

PWS: *Exactly. I can almost hear myself saying, "Here it comes. Get ready."*

Therapist: *So you have the expectation that it is going to be difficult, even though your recent experience with stuttering is that it is not so difficult.*

PWS: *Sure. I guess I know that it doesn't have to be difficult, but I still feel that it is, or that it could be.*

Therapist: *OK. I think it may be helpful if we try to replace your self-talk—when you say "Here it comes. Get ready" with something else, something more like the current reality. Then, we'll see how that feels to you.*

PWS: *OK.*

Therapist: *One of the situations you have found difficult in the past is a business meeting. Do you have this "brace yourself" feeling just before these?*

PWS: *Yes, that is probably the hardest situation for me, and I still feel anxious just before one. I still get that sinking feeling.*

Therapist: *Instead of saying, "Oh shit. Here it comes. Get ready," what could you say that would more accurately reflect the fact that you don't stutter with much struggle anymore?*

PWS: *Something like, "I'm going to stutter. I don't have to struggle. It will be OK."*

Therapist: *And "I will be OK."* [client nods in agreement]. *How about, "I can deal with this," to put it in a positive way.*

PWS: *I don't like that. I would rather say, "I can stutter easily."*

Therapist: *Yes, I like that much better, too. It was great that you rejected my phrase. Yours is much better for you.*

PWS: *OK. I'll try it.*

Changing Behaviors

Stuttering Differently

The end goal of all therapy for stuttering is to help the person speak more easily, that is, more fluently. But since most stuttering behaviors are performed in order to minimize, hide, or avoid stuttering, it would make very little sense to simply try to speak without stuttering; it would only produce more of the same behaviors that are already present. To get around this problem, the technique of learning to stutter in a different way was developed many years ago (Van Riper, 1973).

From our point of view, this technique is a way for PWS to alter the experience of stuttering. Most PWS feel "out of control" when stuttering because they have always tried not to stutter. Stuttering differently produces a new experience. The PWS suddenly has some control—he or she can stutter in a different way without trying not to stutter. Stuttering differently breaks the logjam.

At first, the PWS may simply stutter in any different way—faster, slower, blocking instead of repeating, or repeating instead of blocking, voluntarily instead of involuntarily, with longer or shorter stuttering duration—it doesn't really matter much. The goal is simply to experience what it feels like to do something different with the stuttering. It might be overwhelming at first, but breaking it down into a series of smaller tasks helps. The therapist can identify different components and suggest one to work on. One change, even a small one, can open a door to another change, and so on until the pattern is substantially altered.

One way to begin is for PWS to have a dialogue with some part of their speech mechanism. Most PWS have developed a hostile relationship with their speech mechanism. It has become their nemesis, as if it were not a part of them, or a part that has become uncooperative. A recurring dialogue with the mouth, tongue, or throat, weird as it may sound, can get them back on the same team. Many PWS are focused on one part: their tongue, or jaw, or voice, or lips. The dialogue can be with that part. The goal is reintegration.

Experiential Therapy Verbatim—Dialogue with Your Jaw

Therapist: *I want to try something now that is a little different. It may feel very odd to you, but bear with me. I think you will find that it has beneficial results.*

PWS: *OK.*

Therapist: *You have told me before how you feel a lot of tension in your jaw when you stutter, particularly when the block is a severe one that you can't seem to get out of.*

PWS: *Yes.*

Therapist: *Can you picture your jaw, as large as you need it to be, in that chair over there? Can you visualize such a thing?*

PWS: *Yes.*

Therapist: *Now, I want you to think of something that you would like to say to your jaw. Pretend that it is listening to you.*

PWS: [laughing] *OK.*

Therapist: *Go ahead. What would you like to say to it?*

PWS: *Why do you tense up so much when I am trying to get a word out?*

Therapist: *Try not to ask, "Why." It doesn't usually help much.*

PWS: *OK. What should I ask?*

Therapist: *You don't need to ask anything, just say what is on your mind.*

PWS: *OK. I don't like it when you tense up.*

Therapist: *Good. What else?*

PWS: *I think you are trying to keep me from saying what I want to.*

Therapist: *OK. What else?*

PWS: *You have it in for me. You are trying to hurt me.*

Therapist: *Good. How do you feel about that?*

PWS: *It makes me angry.*

Therapist: *Tell him.*

PWS: *It makes me angry when you do that.*

Therapist: *Say "I am mad at you."*

PWS: *I am mad at you.*

Therapist: *Louder.*

PWS: [shouting] *I am mad at you!*

Therapist: *Good. What did that feel like?*

PWS: *Good.*

Therapist: *OK. Now why don't you sit over there in the chair and be your own jaw for a while. It is, after all, a part of you.*

PWS: *OK.* [moving over to the other chair and adopting a devilish smirk] *I am going to get you.*

Therapist: *What do you mean?*

PWS: *I am going to trip you up. When you least expect it, I will stiffen up and stop you from going forward.*

Therapist: *Say more about that.*

PWS: *I want to hold you back. You are too big for your own britches. I am going to show you that you are not in charge.*

Therapist: *Very good. Anything else?*

PWS: *No.*

Therapist: *OK. Come back over here now. How was that?*

Not Fighting with Yourself

Some stuttering behaviors can be considered forms of fighting with oneself—speeding up to get past the "stuttering moment," forcing the mouth to move in the "right way," or speaking with as little movement as possible. Probably the most common struggle behavior is trying to push the word out.

Experiential Therapy Verbatim—Giving Up Struggles

Therapist: *I want to try an experiment. We have talked before about how you try to push your words out when you stutter, and you have become very good at feeling the air pressure build up in your chest when you do that. I want you now to talk and when you stutter, just let the stuttering go on. Don't try to push the word out. Let the stuttering happen. Be a passive observer. Can you do that?*

PWS: *I'll try.*

Therapist: *Tell me what happened at work last week. You were going to have an important meeting the last time we met.*

PWS: *Yes. We had it, and for a change I did speak up. I thought I had a good idea for this new account we are working on, so I wwwwwwwas motivated. Whew! I thought that /w/ would never stop.*

Therapist: *But you didn't push.*

PWS: *No. It seemed to go on forever.*

Therapist: *In the end it did stop, didn't it?*

PWS: *Yes, but I don't like it when the stuttering lllllllasts—that too, but it was a little better.*

Therapist: *Keep trying to let the stuttering come out when it is ready. Don't force it.*

PWS: *OK. Well, anyway, I said what I meant to say, and I did stutter, but it was OK.*

Therapist: *Did they like your idea?*

PWS: *Yes. They are going to use it in the next campaign.*

Therapist: *That must feel good.*

PWS: *It does. I nnnnnnnnneed to—whew! There is another long one. I nnneed to remember ththat—those were much shorter—that I have ssomething to sssay.*

Therapist: *I think if you keep trying not to push you will find that over time, the stuttering diminishes. It should happen less often and it should not last so long, although in the beginning it may last longer. Just keep trying not to push.*

PWS: *OK. It also feels easier to talk. You know I get really tired when I ssstutter a lot. This way, I don't think I will get so tired.*

Therapist: *I have heard other PWS say the same thing. Let's practice doing this some more.*

Changing Feelings

Like behaviors and thoughts, feelings change through a progression of awareness and acceptance. Change is the natural consequence of accepting a long-denied reality.

When feelings are too painful, we may numb ourselves to them, making it hard to identify them. A place to start is to consider the "big five"—anger, sadness, joy, fear, and shame. Most feelings fall into one of these categories. Of course, there are hundreds of different emotions, and we generally don't have just one at a time. But for therapy, it is simpler to identify one at a time, name it, own that it is indeed theirs, and then decide how best to "honor" it so that it supports their needs.

Identifying the emotion, naming it—particularly feelings that have been long denied—takes practice. Bodily sensations help. *Is your chest tight, your palms sweaty, your heart beating fast?* Emotion always shows up in the body and locating it helps.

Once identified and named, the feeling needs to be "owned." When we feel nervous talking in front of a group, it is our nervousness; the group did not "give it to us." If you feel angry, statements like "She makes me so angry" don't help.

Finally, it is vital that whatever the emotion, it is seen to the end. It is acted upon. Grief needs to be fully felt (and usually many times); tears are vital. Anger needs to be channeled; joy expressed; fear acknowledged; shame examined and returned to its source. These are crucial steps and are not to be undertaken lightly or superficially.

Experiential Therapy Verbatim—Dealing with Grief

Therapist: *How are you today?*

PWS: *Fine, thththththththanks. Its, Its, Its, IIIIIIIIts a bbbbbbbeautiful ddd, ddd, ddday, isn't it?*

Therapist: Yes. Later I am going to get out, I think.

PWS: *MMMMMMy pppppplan is, is, is, tttt, tttt, ttt, tttttttto work in the gg, gggg, gg, ggggggarden.*

Therapist: *Has your stuttering always been as severe as it is now?*

PWS: [tears welling up in his eyes] *YYYYYYes, ever ssss, sssssssince I can re, re, re, remmmmmember.*

Therapist: *What was it like for you as a child with stuttering that was so severe?*

PWS: *IIIIIt wwww, wwww, wwwwwww-was awful, hhhhhorrible.*

Therapist: *Tell me more about that.*

PWS: *WWWWWell, I, I, I, I, rrrrrrre-member once wwwwwhen I wwww, wwwas about ttt, tttt, tttttten I think. I, I, I, had wr, wr, wr, written an eeeeessay, and it, it, it, it wwwwwon a kkkkkind of ccccontest that the ssssssssssschool had. The, the, the, thththththing was that, that, that, the ww, wwww, wwww-wwwinner wwww, wwwwwwas sss, sss, ssup-pose to rr, uh, rrrrread the ww, wwwinning es, es, uh, essay outllllloud to the whwhwhwhole ssschool, bbbbbut whwhwhwhen it www, wwww, uh, wwwwwwwas ttt, tttttime for me to rrr, rrread my essssay, they had thththe bbb, bbb, un, bbbboy [tears running down his cheeks] who had cccc, ccccccccome in sss, sssssssecond read his in, in, instead.*

Therapist: *You mean they changed the rules because of your stuttering, and they didn't let you read your essay, even though you had gotten the first prize?*

PWS: [a little angry now] *Yes!*

Therapist: *Can you tell me a little about what that felt like?*

PWS: *Well, I, I, I, I have to sss, sssssay that I, I, I, I, wwww, wwwwas kind of rrrr, rrrrrrre-lieved that, that, that, I ddd, uh, ddddddidn't have to rrrrr, rrrrread it, bbbut, bbbut, it was, was, wasn't fff, ffffair either. I, I, I, I, I shsh-shshshould have been al, al, al, alllowed to rrrrread mine.*

Therapist: *Of course. It makes me feel sad just to hear that story.*

PWS: [obviously sad] *I, I, I, I, I'll nn, nnnnn, uh, nnnnnnever forget that, that, that mmm, mmmm, uh, mmmmoment.*

Therapist: *Just stay with that feeling of sadness. Feel how unfair and awful that was.*

PWS: [putting his head down and sobbing hard]

Therapist: *Good. It was a terrible loss to you. You were entitled to feel good, even triumphant, because you had written such a good essay, but instead you had to listen to the runner-up reading his essay.*

PWS: [nodding, still crying]

Therapist: *Say "It wasn't fair."*

PWS: [through tears, voice choking] *It wasn't fair!*

Therapist: *Say it again.*

PWS: [clearer, stronger] *It wasn't fair!*

Therapist: *One more time.*

PWS: [very loud] *It wasn't fair!*

Therapist: *Good. Thank you for sharing that with me.*

PWS: [calmer] *OK.*

FINAL THOUGHTS

Coping with Fluency

Many PWS find it disconcerting to talk without noticeable stuttering. They may feel that something huge is missing. Stuttering was an old enemy, but it was familiar, part of who they were, usually the most important thing about them. It can be hard to lose it.

Most PWS are surprised by this feeling of loss. They expected to feel wonderful, but instead they feel as if they have lost a limb. This is a normal reaction, and therapists can help by giving them permission to mourn the loss and helping them focus on other aspects of themselves. Stuttering may have defined them in the past, but it was not the entire definition, only a big part of it. Now, they can realize that their intelligence, humor, seriousness, diligence, free-spiritedness, playfulness, carelessness, forgetfulness, all their strengths and weaknesses, are still present even though the stuttering is gone. Listing all their characteristics, both "good" and "bad" can help. With continued work, a better perspective on the loss of stuttering can be gained. But, perspective or not, the loss needs to be acknowledged, fully felt, and accepted.

Change always produces repercussions. Life is a web of connections, not a set of separate compartments. When one aspect changes, it affects other aspects connected to it. Changes usually produce stress, even when the overall change is for the better. Sometimes a change for the better produces a loss in another area. Anyone with a disability may learn to use it to further his/her own interests, and its usefulness is lost with recovery. There are many "secondary gains" from stuttering: getting attention from the opposite sex, excusing failures, being excused from certain activities, such as unpleasant social obligations, etc. Occasionally, the loss of these secondary gains during therapy creates resistance. A close examination of the resistance and the feelings accompanying it will uncover the loss, or the fear of loss, of a secondary gain. Once this dynamic is understood, the PWS can choose between recovery from stuttering or the continued use of the secondary gain. It is important for therapists to remember that the choice is, in the end, always the PWS's to make.

We change most easily and completely when change brings us closer to our real selves, not some constructed other. The paradoxical theory of change (Beisser, 1970) suggests that forcing a desired change is not really possible. The problem is that the adult PWS has been trying not to stutter for years. "Trying not to" is, in fact, an important part of the disorder. So, a good way to begin is for PWS to become more aware of how hard they are trying not to stutter, to feel the frustration of pushing words out, the guilty feeling of hiding the stuttering from others. These aspects of stuttering need to be fully felt and experienced vividly. Change is most likely to come, passively or not, once this awareness and the acceptance of its reality are fully taken in.

We all have our own tempo and pace. When PWS first decide to take steps to recover from stuttering, their first thought is naturally about speaking without stuttering. And, if they come to a professional therapist, they often believe that the therapist is going to do something to them that is going to help them not stutter. Recovery from stuttering is not like that, and it takes some time for the person to realize that recovery is different from what they thought it would be. It is probably best to let this realization occur at a comfortable pace. Some PWS "get it" very quickly; others not. It is, in our opinion, the PWS, not the therapist, who determines how quickly recovery will occur.

REFERENCES

Amsel, A., & Roussel, J. (1952). Motivational properties of frustration: I. Effect on a running response of the addition of frustration to the motivational complex. *Journal of Experimental Psychology, 43*, 363–368.

Beisser, A. R. (1970). The paradoxical theory of change. In J. Fagan & I. Shepherd (Eds.), *Gestalt therapy now* (pp. 77–80). Palo Alto, CA: Science and Behavior Books.

Bloodstein, O. (1960). The development of stuttering: I. Changes in nine basic features. *Journal of Speech and Hearing Disorders, 25*, 219–237.

Bradshaw, J. (1990). *Homecoming: Reclaiming and championing your inner child.* New York, NY: Bantam Books.

Heite, L. (2001). *La Petit Mort* (Unpublished master's thesis). Temple University, Philadelphia, PA.

Siegel, G. M. (1970). Punishment, stuttering, and disfluency. *Journal of Speech and Hearing Research, 13*, 677–714.

Starkweather, C. W. (1987). *Fluency and stuttering.* Englewood Cliffs, NJ: Prentice-Hall.

Starkweather, C., & Givens-Ackerman, J. (1997). *Stuttering.* Austin, TX: Pro-Ed.

Van Riper, C. (1973). *The treatment of stuttering.* Englewood Cliffs, NJ: Prentice-Hall.

Van Riper, C. (1982). *The nature of stuttering* (2nd ed.). Englewood Cliffs, NJ: Prentice-Hall.

Whitfield, C. (1987). *Healing the child within.* Deerfield Beach, FL: Health Communications.

CHAPTER 9

Avoidance Reduction Therapy for Stuttering (ARTS®)

Vivian Sisskin

INTRODUCTION

"Your fluency won't help you and your stuttering won't hurt you."

—Joseph Sheehan

Good Day, Bad Day

I am the parent of an adult child with autism. Years of daily notes in communication books from teachers and caregivers have taught me that we tend to judge success and failure based on single, key behaviors, those identified as the problem behaviors. The presence of these behaviors (bad day) and the absence of them (good day) are the basis for a binary judgment of the entire day. The truth is, these behaviors occur every day, but our binary judgment system keeps us from noting important changes, insight, or growth because we struggle to get past the observation that these behaviors are present. Sometimes I wonder if anyone notices that my son demonstrates newfound resilience or acts in a way to promote problem solving and self-efficacy. He might even do this on a bad day, but I would never know.

Some people who stutter also make binary judgments about each and every speaking situation—good interaction, bad interaction. I might ask my school-age client how the oral report went: "Good! I didn't stutter." Even for some clients who have evolved beyond the notion that fluency is good and stuttering is bad, the dichotomy is still there, but with more "therapy-correct" semantics: "Not good. I struggled more than I wanted to." I have learned to ask questions that help my clients evaluate the quality of their experiences by identifying something they value or how their listeners made them feel: "I gave my opinion, and that felt good" or "I think the interviewer liked my sense of humor." I find that I continually discover new outcomes of treatment, such as letting go of binary judgments of success and failure related to communicative interaction. However, there was a specific instance when my group therapy clients taught me the most important outcome and the true value of the therapy. I was preparing a workshop that I was to present with a dozen of my clients at a stuttering conference. I decided to group the presentations for a semblance of structure, and I asked each client to select a topic he or she wanted to talk about. The choices included Avoidance Reduction Therapy for Stuttering (ARTS) concepts, such as reducing struggle, confronting fear, and dealing with shame. One of the topics

I suggested was "joy of communication." It was just one on the list. When the votes were tallied, it was unanimous; everyone wanted to talk about the *joy of communication.* Though my clients achieved greater fluency through therapy, what mattered most in the end was their ability to express themselves spontaneously and joyfully—to live free of judging success based on the presence or absence of stuttering.

This chapter serves as an overview of Avoidance Reduction Therapy for Stuttering (ARTS), including the historical and inspirational roots of the treatment approach created by Joseph Sheehan. Quotes from Sheehan himself are sprinkled throughout—some found in his writings, and some recalled from memorable moments during my work with him. His analogies resonate with people who stutter, young and old, and provide a window into his wit, charm, and sense of humor. Basic principles of treatment are presented, followed by a selection of treatment goals, their rationales within the framework of ARTS, and sample treatment activities to help translate principles to practice.

WHAT IS AVOIDANCE REDUCTION THERAPY FOR STUTTERING (ARTS)?

"Grant me the serenity to accept the things
I cannot change, courage to change the things
I can, and the wisdom to know the difference."

—Adapted from the Serenity Prayer
by Reinhold Niebuhr

No Tools Required!

Common stuttering treatments are often divided into two groups: those that aim to increase fluency by changing the way one speaks, fluency enhancement, and those that aim to change the way that one stutters, stuttering modification (Guitar, 2006). In this dichotomy, ARTS would be considered a stuttering modification approach, with outcomes that include both spontaneous fluency and comfortable stuttering. The focus of many treatment targets is the moment of stuttering, modifying it to be less struggled, resulting in less reactivity on the part of the person who stutters. This is not a new idea. Most stuttering modification approaches would aim for similar outcomes (e.g., Breitenfeldt & Lorenz, 1989; Van Riper, 1973). Many treatment approaches, both those that aim for increased fluency and those that aim for comfortable stuttering, include *techniques* that the client employs to achieve desired outcomes. Clinicians often refer to these as *tools*, used to *manage* stuttering. On the other hand, we might consider that the person who stutters is not broken and does not need to be fixed. Instead of managing stuttering with techniques, ARTS eliminates efforts, past and present, used to manage and control stuttering.

Disfluency in stuttering may not be fully explained but is currently understood in the framework of a multidimensional model combining motor, linguistic, and psychosocial factors (e.g., Conture, 1990; Smith, 1999; Smith & Cooper, 1990; Starkweather, Gottwald, & Halfond, 1990). As the child grows and copes with stuttering moments, the *problem* of stuttering becomes one of struggle—reactivity to the moment of disfluency, including physical tension, feelings of loss of control and embarrassment, and thoughts of negative listener reaction. Rather than changing speech to achieve fluency, or doing something "to" the moment of stuttering, clients who practice ARTS aim to do *less*—eliminate learned escape behaviors, emotional reactions, and unhelpful thoughts that lead to struggle. Disfluency itself need not be changed, as it ceases to be problematic for effective communication once struggle is eliminated. Clinicians who understand the parameters of normal speech fluency (Logan, 2015; Starkweather, 1987), and the multidimensional problem of stuttering, are fully equipped to treat stuttering using principles of ARTS. No additional tools are required.

The Roots of Avoidance Reduction Therapy

The roots of ARTS are found in the pioneering work of Joseph Sheehan, a professor of psychology at the University of California, Los Angeles, who was my mentor from 1974 until his death in 1983. During that time and beyond, I worked closely with his wife, Vivian Sheehan, a speech-language pathologist in Southern California. The Sheehans applied concepts from Conflict Theory (Miller, 1944) and Role Theory (Sarbin, 1943) to formulate an explanation for the behaviors and paradoxes observed among those who stutter (Sheehan, 1953, 1970, 1975; Sheehan & Sheehan, 1984).

Conflict Theory

As described by Sheehan (1970, 1975), the experience of stuttering can be compared to an "approach-avoidance conflict," whereby desires toward competing goals—to both speak and hold back from speaking—result in oscillation, the moment of blocking. The very act of stuttering releases the fear that elicited it, and the speaker cannot finish the word. Sheehan referred to the approach-avoidance conflict in describing why some people who stutter can be fluent when angry (strong approach drive, weak avoidance drive) or silent in a group discussion (strong avoidance drive, weak approach drive). Negative thoughts about potential listener reactions combine with fear of speaking and/or stuttering and lead to avoidance at many levels: word/sound avoidance, situational avoidance, and avoidance impacting relationships and life choices. Avoidance reduction (approaching feared situations), on the other hand, resolves the conflict.

Role Theory

People who stutter experience periods of fluency: "Sometimes I stutter, and sometimes I don't." The experience of fluency leads to hope for sustained fluency. "Playing the role" of someone who is fluent requires false role behaviors (Sheehan, 1975), such as pretending to think, speaking in odd ways, or taking on an air of false confidence. When stuttering is inevitably revealed, one is thrust into the role of a person who stutters. Role conflict ensues, resulting in shame, that is, negative feelings about "self." Conversely, enacting the role of a person who stutters (planning to stutter) may reduce the anticipatory anxiety that triggers stuttering. This kind of role congruency aids in self-acceptance as a person who stutters.

Exposing the Iceberg

Stuttering has been compared to an iceberg (Figure 9–1), as much of the problem is below the surface and invisible from view (Sheehan, 1970).

Surface features of stuttering, including repetitions, prolongations, and silent blocks, are apparent for some people who stutter. For others, the surface features include physical concomitant behaviors (loss of eye contact, facial grimaces, hand movements) or linguistic escape behaviors (filler words, pauses, phrase repetitions, unintended words) learned as efforts to hide stuttering-like disfluencies. For many older children and adults, the larger part of the problem is below the water level. These covert features of stuttering include feelings related to showing stuttering (fear, shame, embarrassment), avoidance, and false role behaviors. According to Sheehan (1975,

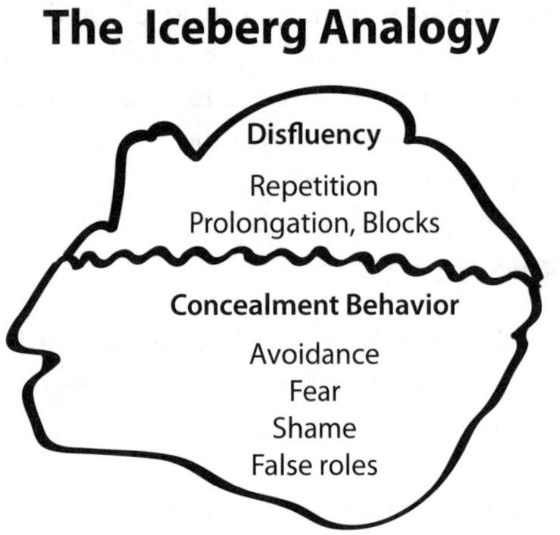
The Iceberg Analogy
Disfluency
Repetition
Prolongation, Blocks
Concealment Behavior
Avoidance
Fear
Shame
False roles

Figure 9–1. The iceberg analogy demonstrates covert and overt features of the stuttering profile. Concealment behaviors are below the surface. Exposing stuttering transforms guilt into shame, which can be reconditioned. *Source:* Adapted from Sheehan, J. G. (1970, p. 15). *Stuttering: Research and treatment.* New York: Harper and Row.

p. 15), when covert shame is converted into overt guilt it can be reconditioned. In keeping with the analogy, when shame below the surface is exposed, it is reduced as if it were melted by the sun.

The Central Theme of Suppression

"The successful suppression of stuttering is what maintains and perpetuates it."

—Joseph Sheehan

The Habituation of Secondary Escape Behaviors

"The stutterer becomes a walking museum or a talking museum of all of the things he has tried to avoid stuttering."

—Joseph Sheehan

The control and suppression of stuttering may appear to be desirable outcomes for stuttering treatment, but they are alien to ARTS (Sheehan, 1970, 1975, 1984). Control and suppression evoke visions of struggle: force, antagonism, tension, and efforts to hold back. Suppression begins during the earliest stages of avoidance, when children find that unintended distractions, such as looking away or a slight jerk of the jaw, result in the release of the momentary disfluency.

Mowrer (1947) used a psychological learning theory model to describe the development of emotional and behavioral factors in anxiety. His Two-Factor Theory demonstrated how classically conditioned negative emotion may become the stimulus for instrumentally conditioned problem-solving responses, or coping mechanisms. Two-Factor Theory has been applied to psychological disorders such as phobias, to explain the role of operant conditioning in the development of avoidance and escape from fear (Buck, 2010). Brutten and Shoemaker (1967) used Two-Factor Theory to explain the development and maintenance of stuttering within a learning theory paradigm, inviting some controversy over the role of punishment in the development of stuttering (Hegde, 1995). Current neurophysiological research no longer supports a learning theory model for the cause of stuttering. However, in a retrospective of Brutten's contributions to current understanding of stuttering, Hegde points out that environmental input can disrupt a neuromotor system and concludes that the role of emotional conditioning in stuttering cannot be discounted (Hegde, 1995, p. 223).

I draw upon the work of the early learning theorists to help explain how secondary behaviors in stuttering may be developed and habituated through an operant model. Figure 9–2 provides a graphic to demonstrate how anticipated negative emotion or production of uncomfortable disfluency (stimulus) may accidentally or intentionally evoke a behavior (response) distracting enough to trigger *escape* from negative emotion or shameful

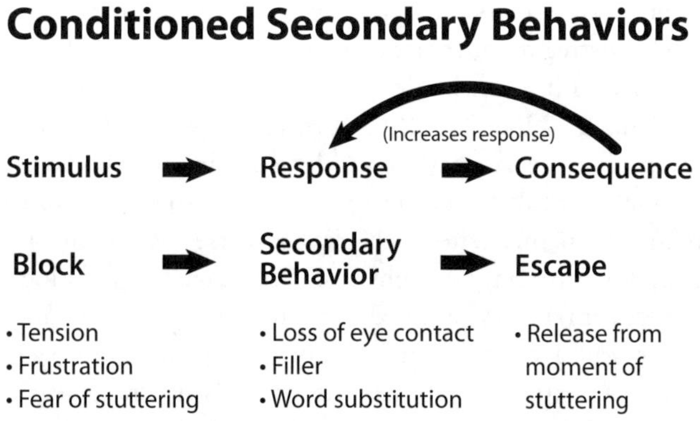

Figure 9–2. The operant conditioning paradigm demonstrates a learning theory explanation for the development of secondary struggle behaviors, conditioned through negative reinforcement. *Source:* Adapted from Brutten, G. J., & Shoemaker, D. J. (1967). *The modification of stuttering.* Englewood Cliffs, NJ: Prentice Hall.

disfluency (consequence). For the person who stutters, there is probably nothing more desirable than escape/concealment, and as a result, the response increases through the process of negative reinforcement.

Escape behaviors are most powerful when they are new and novel. As adaptation takes hold, the person who stutters must employ new behaviors, perhaps the insertion of an interjection "um" or a quick inhalation. As novelty wears off, escape behaviors become less effective. The person who stutters must come up with new ones. Furthermore, because sometimes they "work" and sometimes they don't, they function on an intermittent reinforcement schedule, which naturally makes any behavior stronger. Escape behaviors become habituated, even when they no longer serve their original function, to escape from unpleasant stimuli.

The Disruption of Parameters of Normal Talking

"The goal, then, is not to reduce or to stop something called 'stuttering.' It is to change the way the speaker talks, so that he does more and more things that most people do when they talk."

—Dean Williams

Dean Williams (1957, 1979), out of the Iowa school of thought, helped clients see that they were doing things to interfere with normal talking. The "doing" was the important concept. Struggle was not happening "to" the speaker; rather, the speaker was doing something that made up the struggle (Quesal & Yaruss, 2000). It follows, if the speaker is doing something, he or she can do something else.

Even without having acquired a host of escape behaviors (secondary behaviors), stuttered speech is often struggled. In this case, the inefficiency comes from habituated reactivity, or learned efforts to move through disfluencies as quickly as possible. The irony is that efforts to hide what some might consider a potential "ugly stutter" are the very behaviors that make the disfluency struggled. Williams describes this reactivity as being motivated by fear: fear of stigma, communicative failure, and feeling out of control (Williams, 1979). Through both anticipatory reactions and efforts to escape, the person who stutters alters the normal processes of speech: airstream, movement, placement of articulators, timing, tension levels, and voicing (Williams, 1979, p. 253).

Close observation of stuttering patterns reveals the various ways that speakers interfere with the above parameters in their efforts to avoid, control, or suppress stuttering. A slight inhalation (adjust in airstream) prior to a feared word can distract from and avert the anticipated block. However, as explained above, behaviors learned through negative reinforcement cease to "work," become habituated, and develop as a feature of one's stuttering pattern. Efforts to push through a disfluency are accompanied by tension during release. Again, in an operant learning model, tension present at release of the disfluency will habituate, as it is paired with escape from the disfluency. The approach-avoidance conflict can illustrate interference with the normal talking process. The desire to "hold back" from speaking, coupled with the desire to speak, may manifest as a silent block, whereby the person who stutters alters normal parameters of voicing, tension, airstream, and movement.

When Stuttering Goes Underground

"Stuttering is a role-specific self-presentation disorder."

—Joseph Sheehan (1970, p. 11)

During one of my group therapy sessions, group members were engaged in a spirited discussion of who suffered more emotionally, someone with an overt profile of stuttering or someone with a covert profile of stuttering. The arguments on both sides were compelling. Those who stutter overtly spoke about the intense shame and embarrassment they felt during the moment of communicative failure. The awkwardness, frustration, and interruption in communicative connection added to ongoing feelings of failure and incompetence. Those with a covert profile, who could "pass" as fluent in the outside world, spoke of constant worry and dread, every moment of every day worrying that their ability to hide stuttering would fall apart. They described the emotional exhaustion and vigilance of pretending to be someone they were not, and even worse, being told by friends and even speech-language pathologists that they didn't stutter. One group member settled the discussion: "Let's face it, for everyone who stutters, it all boils down to fear and shame." Well-meaning family members, friends, and clinicians may encourage someone who stutters to go ahead and talk, to participate. They may even have a story of someone they know who overcame the problem of stuttering by just talking. They might give advice or a speech assignment to "go ahead and stutter. You'll see, maybe you won't feel awkward or different." It can be difficult for those who do not stutter to understand the power of fear and shame and the lengths that people who stutter will go to in order to avoid these feelings. Silence is the most effective; if you don't talk, you don't stutter. Suppression of stuttering permits suppression of feelings, as well as the thoughts that evoke the feelings, "He won't want to date me" or "She'll think I am stupid."

For many, the fear of presenting oneself as someone who stutters exceeds the fear of the actual stuttered moment. Hiding one's identity as a person who stutters can take its toll. Many people who are successful at hiding their stuttering for years may eventually seek out treatment, as false role behavior leads to guilt, poor self-esteem, and significant life impact.

PREPARING THE CLIENT AND FAMILY FOR ARTS

The Problem of Stuttering

Stuttering looks quite different in young children near onset than it does in older children and adults. Using the iceberg analogy, early stuttering may reveal very little below the surface. However, with increasing awareness, efforts to escape or push through disfluency, and fear of negative listener reaction, stuttering develops into a multidimensional problem impacting not only speech efficiency but social and psychological well-being with significant life impact (Healey, Trautman, & Susca, 2004; Yaruss, 2007). Researchers and clinicians commonly use the ABCs of stuttering (Cooper & Cooper, 1985), based on concepts from Cognitive Behavioral Therapy (Beck, 1997), as a counseling tool to aid in understanding the complexity of the stuttering problem. *Affective* (feelings), *Behavioral* (actions), and *Cognitive* (thoughts and beliefs) components of stuttering do more than describe the problem; this framework sheds light on the interaction among these components. Thoughts about what others may think trigger negative feelings about oneself and influence behavior: "If I stutter, he will judge me as incompetent (thought). I will be humiliated (feeling). I will ask my co-worker to present my work (behavior)."

The Problem of Stuttering Chart, Figure 9–3, can be an effective counseling tool to help both clients and parents understand how the ABCs of stuttering interact, leading to avoidance and poor self-esteem. The first column lists *affective* components of the stuttering problem and provides a sample of negative feelings associated with the experience of stuttering. *Behaviors* in the middle column provide examples of actions, including physical and linguistic escape, choices to hold back from speaking, and false role behavior. The third column lists *cognitive* components, thoughts or beliefs about what others might be thinking and what that would mean for one's own self-image. Imagine a school-age child who is motivated to respond to a teacher's question in class. Just prior to raising his hand, a brief thought that his peers would think he is "stupid," and perhaps even glance at his friends

The Problem of Stuttering

What PWS Feel

- Fear
- Shame
- Guilt
- Embarrassment
- Anger
- Frustration
- Anxiety
- Dread / Apprehension
- Out of control / Panic

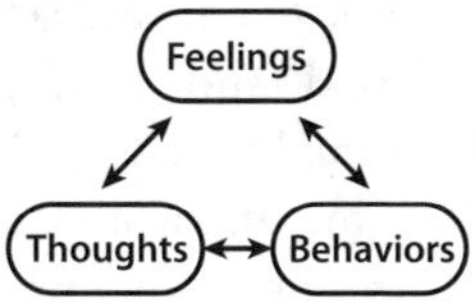

What PWS Do

- Loss of eye contact
- Eye closure, blinking
- Jaw / head jerks
- Hand / foot movements
- Facial grimaces
- Inhalation during speech production
- Retrying words
- Repeating phrases
- Using fillers ("uh", "um")
- Word substitution
- Circumlocution (talking around a word)
- Stopping / giving up
- Pretending to think
- Cutting conversation short

What PWS Think

People will think I'm ...

- Stupid
- Nervous
- Shy
- Not confident

He/she wouldn't want to ...

- Be my friend
- Talk to me
- Be associated with me

I couldn't ...

- Ask him/her
- Volunteer for that
- Say that
- Go there
- Participate in that

Figure 9–3. The Problem of Stuttering Chart can be a helpful counseling tool to demonstrate the multidimensional aspects of the stuttering experience. Columns represent the ABCs of stuttering, what the person who stutters (PWS) feels (affective), does (behavioral), and thinks (cognitive).

and smirk, leads to feelings of embarrassment and rejection. The child decides not to raise his hand, which in turn, leads to feelings of frustration or guilt.

This visual can help clients and families understand that the problem of stuttering is not limited to disfluent speech but includes those things that develop in response to it. The relationship among the ABCs can also illustrate positive scenarios during the treatment process, when we begin to observe cognitive shifts that lead to changes in both feelings and behavior. Given the same desire to respond to the teacher's question, imagine this time that the school-age child cues himself with a cognitive message: "I am going to answer the question and will likely stutter. My classmates already know I stutter, and it's OK if they hear me stutter, that's just what I do." This leads to participation and feelings of pride that come from self-advocacy. His classmates see he knows the answer—"I can be smart and stutter."

Disfluency Versus Struggle

Clients and families might ask what techniques or strategies are learned in ARTS to achieve efficient, comfortable, and joyful communication. Unfortunately, sometimes doing *more* will not improve communication; it will only lead to more struggle. The process of therapy is concerned with doing *less.* With a growing understanding that stuttering is genetic and neurological, we may not be able to eliminate stuttering. It is essential for clients and families to understand that just because someone may stutter does not mean that he or she will *struggle*. It can be helpful to conceptualize stuttering as the name of a communication disorder, an umbrella term for both disfluency and struggle. It's the struggle, however, that is the problem of stuttering.

If we can distinguish between disfluency (spontaneous breaks in continuity, including repetitions and prolongations) and struggle (everything else), then clients and families can more easily distinguish among behaviors targeted for reduction and the behaviors that are to be left alone. Figure 9–4 depicts this "sorting" of symptoms associated with stuttering. The goal of ARTS is to reduce all the characteristics noted under "struggle." Disfluencies themselves are not a target of therapy, as they shrink in both frequency and intensity as a by-product of reducing struggle. As mentioned above, clients will need to do less—less to both suppress and control their disfluency.

The Culture of ARTS

When someone transitions to a new culture, there is often a period of culture shock consisting of distinct stages leading to acceptance (Oberg, 1960). Initially there is a "honeymoon" period, characterized by fascination and excitement. Soon a stage of "crisis" sets in, during which the differences between the old and new culture create anxiety, frustration, and anger. Eventually, there is a period of "adjustment" when the individual becomes more comfortable and establishes a positive perspective. The new culture makes sense as he develops problem-solving skills to deal with new situations and frustrations. Finally, he enters the stage of "adaptation," where he can view both cultures more objectively and consider the advantages and disadvantages of each (Oberg, 1960; Winkelman, 1994).

It appears that an individual progressing through ARTS passes through similar stages. Initially, it requires one to rethink basic beliefs, reassign labels of "good" and "bad," and redefine success and failure. In therapy, the person who stutters will be moving from a culture of suppression of stuttering to one of openness and acceptance. There is the initial excitement when one can visualize being free of the burden to conceal stuttering and anticipate easy,

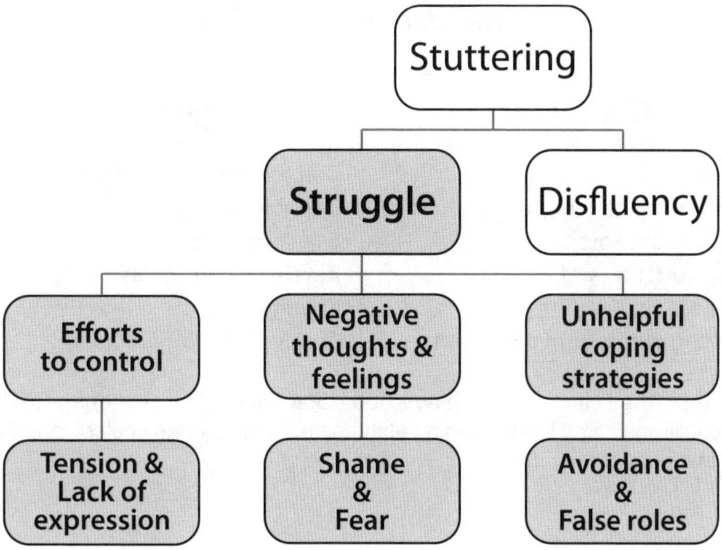

Figure 9–4. The goals of Avoidance Reduction Therapy for Stuttering (ARTS) are designed to decrease struggle and its consequences. Comfortable disfluency will remain.

comfortable stuttering. Soon internal conflicts arise when faced with the reality that changing old habits and attitudes may result in feeling shame, facing listener reactions, and examining one's deepest fears: "This is harder than I thought." The new behaviors are not hard to achieve, but the ensuing culture clash takes time to work out. Change becomes easier as one adapts to the culture and makes choices based on this new biculturalism. This is often easier in the context of group therapy, where the individual can observe others who have made this transition successfully.

While Sheehan did not talk about culture shock as a problem of adjusting to new values in ARTS, he did mention an analogy of swimming across a lake. The shoreline where one initially is standing represents the culture of suppression, while the culture of openness is across the lake. The person who stutters begins swimming enthusiastically, reaches a point in the middle, and becomes conflicted. There is a choice to make: reverse direction and swim back to suppression, or keep swimming (as hard as it might seem) to the other side. This period of conflict, when the individual is splashing around in circles, feeling like he is drowning, seems to be the stage of crisis in the context of culture shock. I have found very few clients who choose to go back to the shore of suppression.

The process of ARTS involves both attitudinal and behavior change reflecting new cultural values. These values, listed in Figure 9–5, may be counterintuitive not only to the person who stutters, but to his family, support system, and the community at large.

Fluency

"Fluency is a fair-weather friend that deserts the stutterer when he needs it most."

—Joseph Sheehan

It is commonly understood among those who stutter that the harder one tries to be fluent, the more one stutters. The quest for fluency seems to be culturally "hard-wired." One client

The Culture of ARTS

Not Valued	Highly Valued
• Fluency	• Comfortable, forward moving speech
• Reduction in frequency of disfluencies	• Struggle-free speech
• Control (of any sort)	• Exercising choice
• Hiding stuttering well	• Revealing yourself as a PWS
• "Practice"	• Change
• Protecting others from discomort	• Connecting with others

Figure 9–5. The culture of Avoidance Reduction Therapy for Stuttering (ARTS) may initially challenge some long-standing attitudes about stuttering, including the value of fluency and control of stuttering.

told me that he was on board with *whatever* it would take to achieve comfortable disfluency and self-acceptance as a person who stutters: "I am willing to feel shame, show struggle, and allow others to think what they will, if that is what it takes to be fluent." He eventually learned that when he truly gave up the quest for illusive fluency, fluency fell into his lap. The irony is that when a person who stutters values alternatives to fluency, including comfortable disfluency and stuttering well, fluency is inevitable.

Frequency of Disfluency

"You have a choice as to 'how' you stutter. You do not have a choice as to 'whether' you stutter."
—Joseph Sheehan

A common measure of stuttering severity is frequency of words (or syllables) stuttered. This is calculated by computing the percentage of disfluent words out of total intended words in a sample of spontaneous speech. Typical speakers generally have some disfluency in their speech; therefore, mild stuttering might be designated at 3% words stuttered, for example. Stuttering treatments often regard the reduction of percentage of words stuttered as a measure of progress in therapy, and furthermore, treatments with good evidence behind them can demonstrate an arbitrary low percentage of words stuttered—for example, no more than 5%. The problem with valuing low frequency of stuttering is that it does not necessarily correlate with the problem of stuttering or life impact from stuttering. When I present workshops on ARTS, I like to demonstrate this rather dramatically. I produce speech with nearly 50% words stuttered; however, moments of disfluency are free of reactivity (including tension). I am speaking spontaneously without signs of control, and I am clearly confident and joyful in the delivery of my message. I then contrast this to a sample of fluent speech, marked by just one disfluent word. This one word is full of tension, struggle, attempts to escape, and body language riddled with shame and panic. This moment is painful for the audience, but I explain that someone who speaks this way would not be identified as a person who stutters through assessment measures that use frequency of stuttering as their defining criteria. Counting disfluencies is useless for measuring progress in ARTS. Qualitative measures that assess efficiency and comfort in communication are more applicable. The shift to valuing these outcomes, rather than outcomes related to frequency, is an important cultural component.

Control

"Without the effort to control his speech, the stutterer would be able to speak quite naturally and normally."

—Joseph Sheehan

We refer to a couple of "seven-letter dirty words" during our group therapy sessions. The first is *fluency* and the second is *control*. They are not forbidden in the culture of ARTS; they are just not valued. A common treatment outcome for many stuttering therapies is for the client to learn to control or manage stuttering. A quick glance at "control" in a thesaurus will bring up the terms *dominance*, *restraint*, *overpower*, and other language that conveys the message that stuttering is something to be battled and defeated, or at least tamed. The change in values from controlling stuttering to exercising choice about *how* one stutters is an important cultural shift for success in therapy. Only by letting go of control speech can speech be free of effort, which is essential for comfortable communication.

Concealment

"Misrepresentation of self to others is always representative of guilt."

—Joseph Sheehan

A new group therapy member with an overt stuttering pattern was intrigued by the report of a home assignment from someone with a covert pattern of stuttering. The report included multiple successes related to talking about stuttering to others and showing disfluency to a new friend in a social situation. The new member commented, "Wow, if I had the choice to hide my stuttering, I probably wouldn't be here." The client with the covert pattern explained that she used to feel just that way, but when she could no longer hide, she hit "rock bottom." "I still occasionally experience an intense desire to hide my stuttering, but now I feel guilt and disappointment when I do. Hiding is no longer of much value to me," she said. Willingness to show stuttering is a gradual process that parallels self-acceptance. As noted with the iceberg analogy, reduction of concealment behavior leads to reduction of negative feelings and attitudes and an increase in "open stuttering." Those who have made progress in this cultural shift value open stuttering over false fluency.

Change

"You are changed by what you do, not what you think about, read about, talk about, write about, intellectualize about, or emote about."

—Joseph Sheehan

Practice is an essential ingredient in treatment approaches that employ techniques to control stuttering. Practice does have its place in habit reduction, but not as an essential value in ARTS. I might even add practice to the list of things that don't lead to change in the Sheehan quote above. The kind of change that is needed for success in ARTS requires the person who stutters to risk feeling that dreaded feeling or face that ever-present fear of showing stuttering. The group cheers with excitement for someone who has stepped out of his comfort zone to do something different. That could be anything from "showing up" someplace previously avoided, saying more than required in an interaction, or taking the initiative to engage in small talk. None of these successes requires practice.

Connection

"The single biggest problem in communication is the illusion that it has taken place."
—George Bernard Shaw

Joyful communication involves speaker and listener connection. The give and take in this kind of interaction can be compared to a satisfying handshake or a perfect waltz. Each person "gives weight" so that movement is balanced, based on the nonverbal communication from subtle physical cues. When the connection is broken, the flow of communication is interrupted, and that conversation, handshake, or dance becomes less satisfying. When success in stuttering therapy is based on protecting the listener from awkwardness related to one's stuttering, the connection is broken because the person who stutters is thinking about the potential thoughts of his communicative partner rather than the content of his message. The speaker is no longer in the moment, but in his own head. The cultural shift from valuing connection above the judgment of others is a significant change that leads to spontaneity in communication, one of the most important outcomes of ARTS.

The Lifestyle of ARTS

Once engaged within the culture of ARTS, clients who make rapid and consistent progress follow certain principles that are part of the fabric of group or individual therapy. These principles—Action, Support, Semantics, Problem Solving, and Assignments—together appear to be the engine of change.

Action

Therapy is action oriented. The content of a therapy session might include expressing feelings related to the experience of stuttering or sharing with other group members the lengths to which one has gone to hide stuttering, including changing one's name during an introduction or ordering the item on the menu that one can say rather than what one wants. These activities are valuable in the therapy process and may contribute considerably to motivation for change or movement from a stage of change characterized by considering or "contemplating" change to a stage of change in which one is actively involved in change (Prochaska, DiClemente, & Norcross, 1992). However, the "doing" is the success in ARTS. The clinician and client work together to find something that the client is excited to do. This might be telling a close friend or family member about the decision to enter treatment or going to a place where one fears speaking, even if speaking is not part of the plan. Just "showing up" is a success, as it is something that one *does*. It represents action.

Support

Action-oriented therapy involves facing fears and stepping out of one's comfort zone. It requires risk taking. The clinician and client work together to find a risk located somewhere low on the client's "fear hierarchy." This is where desensitization takes place (Wolpe, 1958). If the client aims too high, the fear can be increased; if too low, progress can be stalled. Support is essential for risk taking. Group therapy is an effective avenue of support. A suggestion from a clinician can result in change, but it can't compete with the experience of observing a veteran group member formulate a challenging assignment and return the following week to report on his success, glowing with the confidence he has gained. Role models develop naturally within the group. The acts of giving and gaining support are equally valuable for promoting change. One client admitted, "If I give you advice, then I better do it myself. I don't want to be a hypocrite!"

Healthy competition also takes place within the group setting: "Let's see if we can both do at least one 'shame-busting' assignment each day this week, and check in during the week." Without the benefit of a built-in support system that the group provides, those participating in individual therapy are encouraged to identify a support person with whom they can check in. Online communities where members can interact with others who have either gone through ARTS or are in the process can broaden the circle of support to include people of all ages around the world who share the culture of ARTS.

Semantics

Wendell Johnson's ideas about stuttering evolved from Semantic Theory, the notion that the words we use influence our interpretation of events and behavior (Johnson, 1946). This includes the labels we attach to things and ideas. If we label "fluent" speech as a success, then disfluent speech (stuttering) is a failure. As mentioned earlier, attributing failure to something we can't change is not usually helpful. However, if we label "comfortable" speech as a success, then perhaps struggled speech would be the logical failure. Struggle can be changed, reduced, and even eliminated.

Semantic Theory can also account for our interpretation of situations and conditions based on our choice of actor and agent in our descriptions. Sheehan encouraged people who stutter to use the "language of responsibility" (Sheehan, 1970, 1975) as a prerequisite for change. As he would say, if we are doing something, then we can change what we are doing. He enjoyed catching instances of "non-responsibility" in the group therapy setting to point out these semantic subtleties. When a client reported that filler words were "creeping back into my stuttering pattern," Sheehan stopped the group so that members could visualize the personification of "uh" slowing creeping along and jumping into the client's sentence. The inevitable rewording of the sentence followed, shifting responsibility for the behavior back to the client: "I am using those annoying filler words again." The idea is that internal and external loci of control, the extent to which we have control over the events that happen in our lives (Rotter, 1966), may shift toward the internal end of the continuum with use of language of responsibility. This may have implications for maintenance of change from therapy, as a shift toward internal locus of control has been associated with less relapse after therapy (Craig, Franklin, & Andrews, 1984).

Problem Solving

Independent problem solving on the part of the client, regardless of age, is an important principle of ARTS. The theme of "becoming your own clinician" is reflected in treatment goals, therapeutic activities, and teaching strategies employed by the clinician. This is vital, as generalization occurs not in the therapy room, but in the outside world. We encourage clients to identify escape behaviors on their own, allowing them several weeks to identify something that perhaps the clinician observed during the initial meeting. I encourage young school-age children to explore, identify, and "own" their behavior through self-observation: "There is something that you are doing with your tongue when you stutter; I can't really figure it out, but maybe you can." That same child also will be encouraged to verbalize, in his own words, the rationale for maintaining eye contact during a disfluency. Each treatment target (some discussed in subsequent sections) has a very specific rationale within the framework of ARTS. When children or adults can verbalize the rationale, their language will influence their interpretation of the situation or condition. They are better able to act in ways that promote attaining treatment goals, educating the people in their support system, and progressing to their desired outcomes.

Assignments

Planned assignments are the mechanism for change in ARTS. Assignments are developed and evaluated by the client, initially with clinician guidance. A plateau in progress, a slump in motivation, or frustration with one's own work habits are most often traced back to problems with assignment formulation, execution, and evaluation. First, clients should not work on speech targets all day long. Instead, three to five specific assignments are advised. In this case, more is not better. While impromptu assignments are sometimes successful, more often they result in failure. This is because the person who stutters may be enacting the assignment to avoid struggle or embarrassment in the moment. The thought is, "Let me try to 'open stutter' or 'voluntary stutter' here so that I don't block; I hate blocking!" In this case, the fear is high and the selected target is likely off the mark. Second, a vague assignment to "work on my speech" lacks a specific target, and therefore, there is no plan of action. In this case, the client will evaluate the success of the assignment on an outcome such as fluency or comfortable stuttering, neither of which has a clear target, something to *do*. Finally, the evaluation of success must not drift from the target. This is easier said than done. It appears to be human nature to discount what went well and instead focus on the features of the experience that did not go well. The classic example is the client who plans a specific assignment to do two times at the table during an upcoming dinner party. Despite being clear on the target (to say something), he reports on the disappointment and shame he experienced because his speech was struggled when he spoke. This tendency to "bait and switch" prevents the client from gathering successes that provide momentum to move through the therapy efficiently. The mnemonic device in Figure 9–6 is helpful for encouraging healthy work habits among clients. If they can remember "TOAST," they can remember the steps to effective assignments. First, select a specific *t*arget; second, identify *o*pportunities for carrying out the assignment; next, *a*ct by carrying out the assignment; then, count the *s*uccess; and finally, evaluate the assignment according to the *t*arget expectations, not other features of the stuttering pattern or resulting listener reactions.

TREATMENT OUTCOMES, GOALS, AND ACTIVITIES

Outcomes of ARTS include efficiency, comfort, spontaneity, and joy in communication. They are subjective concepts, not easily measured by counting or evaluating speech disfluency. While these qualities of communication are taken for granted by most people who do not stutter, people who do stutter long to experience these things. Similarly, we who do not stutter may decide that we long to experience happiness, love, or inner peace, which are also not easily measured. However, if we chase these things, we never seem to catch them. Sometimes when we cease to value these things for their own sake, they end up in our laps. It may be the case that "fluency," whatever it means to those who believe they don't have it, will be right in front of them when they stop chasing it.

The outcomes of ARTS are by-products of the treatment. They are indirect consequences of the changes made through treatment. For my clients, change is not always apparent as they are making it. It is mostly visible on reflection, when looking back through the rearview mirror. I observe change in my clients through their narratives. The semantics of their stories shift from binary themes of

1. Select your **TARGET**	**Be specific...** • Say one extra thing • Self-disclose
2. Identify an **OPPORTUNITY**	**Consider home, schools, friends, work...** • Ordering food • Conference call
3. Carry out your **ACTION**	**Think...** • You are changed by what you *do* • Seize the opportunity!
4. Count your **SUCCESSES**	**Focus on...** • The target • Staying in the moment
5. Accept **THOUGHTS**	**Accept non-target observations...** • But I struggled • I got a "pity" look

Figure 9–6. The mnemonic device "TOAST" can be a useful strategy for successful assignment development and completion.

fluency and stuttering (good-day, bad-day) to themes of confidence in communication and self-acceptance as a person who stutters.

An attempt to operationalize the process of ARTS has led me to concrete goals that highlight benchmarks for behavioral changes and attitudinal shifts. Some examples of *long-term goals* are featured in boxes throughout this section, along with their rationales within the framework of ARTS. Examples of treatment activities to meet specific *behavioral objectives* in each goal area are also included in the boxes. The *targets*, or actions, identified in behavioral objectives are used to formulate *assignments* and activities. The following example will help clinicians conceptualize the flow from goals and objectives that tend to be formulated by the clinician to assignments and activities that tend to be formulated by the client.

- Outcome/By-product: Spontaneity in communication
- Long-Term Goal: To say all that I want to say when out with my friends
- Behavioral Objective: Will initiate communication in three social situations per week, in two out of three weeks
- Activity/Assignment: Will make a comment (or introduce myself) to one new person who comes to the bike club meeting this week

Treatment to Improve Efficiency and Comfort in Communication

Goals and activities in this section are aimed at reducing physical struggle, including motor and linguistic escape behaviors, and developing a comfortable, forward-moving speech pattern, which usually includes disfluency. Efficient speech is straightforward and includes the entire intended message. It is devoid of word substitutions and additions, revisions, phrase repetitions and filler words that are used to avoid disfluency. It is also devoid of timing devices, attitudinal "tricks," and false roles that suppress stuttering. Speech rate (number of intended words spoken per minute) will generally increase with improved efficiency. While many people who stutter, as well as their listeners, perceive speech rate of stuttered speech to be too fast, it is often slower than average. Speech rate most often increases once inefficiencies are eliminated.

Becoming an Expert (Figure 9–7)

The first step in therapy is to demystify stuttering. Early in therapy, clients view the problem of stuttering as a gestalt concept, a single unit without component parts or variables. They have not considered changing it in ways that are less struggled. They have only considered eliminating, managing, or fixing it. During this time, clients become experts on their own stuttering pattern, understand how they learned and habituated struggle behaviors, and begin to see that disfluency itself is not the enemy. They pay attention to their own speech, in spontaneous conversation and monologue, to identify specific behaviors they use to hide or escape from stuttering (Van Riper, 1973). These are known as "tricks," or false role behaviors (Sheehan, 1970, 1975). They are intended to fool the listener into believing that the speaker is not a person who stutters. It is sometimes difficult to admit to tricks, because it will mean eventually giving them up. Bargaining is not uncommon in the group setting: "I don't think that my lack of small talk is a trick; I have always been a shy person. It's just who I am." Clients will begin to evaluate their behaviors honestly when the clear definition of a trick is provided: *A trick is something you do to hide or conceal your stuttering or your identity as a person who stutters. The only way to know if it is a trick is to consider your intent. If your intent is to hide, it is likely a trick.* Clients are always the best judges of their own intentions.

Activities that generate lists of behaviors that can be sorted into categories of "helpful" or "harmful" for comfortable speech can be used with clients of all age levels. Young children can draw pictures of the things they do to "help" when they get "bumpy" or "stuck," which later become their collection of tricks. Once eliminated from their speech pattern, they can perform a ceremony of "tricks to the trash" and throw away the picture or symbol of the escape behavior that used to make talking hard. Creative symbols have included cars looping on a track to symbolize phrase repetitions or a glitter-lined eyeball to symbolize loss of eye contact during disfluency. Older children talk about their stuttering fingerprint. Everyone's fingerprint is different and

GOAL:
Becoming an expert on your stuttering pattern

Concept or Rationale	The problem is not *if* you stutter, it's *how* you stutter.
Treatment Activities	• Stuttering fingerprint • Helpful vs. unhelpful behaviors

Figure 9–7. Sample treatment goal: Becoming the expert.

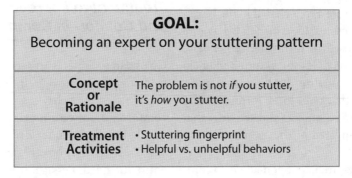

it follows that people stutter differently. These children learn that their stuttering pattern is mostly made up of the things they learned to do to stop stuttering, but now they make talking worse. Adults resonate with a delightful Sheehan metaphor paraphrased here: "The stutterer becomes a walking museum, or talking museum, of all of the things he has learned to avoid stuttering." An inventory of the museum's holdings can be an effective analogy (Sheehan & Sisskin, 2001).

Verbalizing Rationales (Figure 9–8)

Most clinicians would agree that it is important for clients to understand the reasons behind treatment goals and activities. If treatment is meaningful, it will increase the likelihood of engagement. However, ARTS goes a step farther than understanding the rationales of therapy concepts and strategies by requiring the client to verbalize those rationales. This skill will develop independent problem solving, improve generalization, and strengthen support systems important for lasting change.

Struggle increases with fear of stuttering, self-imposed time pressure, high cognitive or emotional load, and a host of other variables. Clients will need to adjust targets for assignments in the moment to work toward gathering successes. One client explains: "I gave myself the assignment to allow myself to show stuttering and not to use my 'uh' when I ordered my burrito. But as soon as the server asked me what I wanted, I knew I wasn't going to get anything out, and I threw in the towel. I used a ton of 'uh's' just to say 'burrito.' Instead of walking away a failure, I decided that this situation was way too feared for my original assignment. I changed my assignment to just saying all the ingredients I want on the burrito (with my tricks). I guess my success was that I was eating exactly what I wanted!" The successful problem solving demonstrated by this young teen could only occur if he was clear on the rationale for his target, that changing words increases the fear of saying those words, as well as the priorities for his own speech work. Successful generalization of speech targets also requires generalization of attitudinal targets. This teen generalized a concept discussed in group therapy: Saying feared words will eventually reduce the fear of saying them. Having said that aloud within the group therapy context at some point in time increased his chances of making a "healthy choice" in the moment of fear. Older children and teens are most often not accompanied by a parent in the therapy room where they learn about the rules that govern their stuttering behavior and new options they might select when faced with fear. They are reinforced for the choices

GOAL: Verbalizing the rationales for treatment concepts and strategies	
Concept or Rationale	If you understand *why* and *how*, you can adjust assignments, teach others, and make choices that lead to success.
Treatment Activities	• Identifying circle of support • Mentoring others

Figure 9–8. Sample treatment goal: Verbalizing treatment rationales.

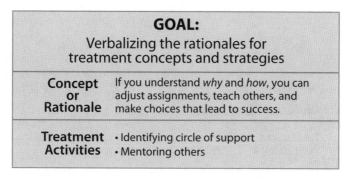

that lead to comfortable speech by the clinician as well as by their peers in group therapy. Unfortunately, parents can fall behind in this learning process. They have not had the opportunity to desensitize to their own shame as their children have. Without adequate counseling and opportunities to understand the rationales behind ARTS, their praise may be aligned with previous values. They may be unable to see that positive change is not equivalent to fewer moments of stuttering. "It drives me crazy when my dad tells me my speech is great when I am using all my covert strategies. He thinks I am getting worse when I show my stuttering." Effective activities and assignments in this goal area include "teaching parents how and why." An appropriate home assignment for a young child on the first day of therapy might be to teach his mom something that he learned about his talking that day in therapy. He might be able to explain to his mom, "Some of the things I do when I get stuck are helping me and some are not," a success within this goal area.

Reducing Escape and Avoidance (Figure 9–9)

At this point, most clients are eager to get rid of escape and avoidance behaviors that have become the face of their stuttering patterns. They feel as though they are chained to unwanted, habituated physical and linguistic behaviors that no longer can be counted on to hide stuttering. But how? Identification activities have long been a staple of stuttering modification approaches based on the work of Van Riper (1973). With active monitoring through planned assignments, secondary escape behaviors are reduced on their own (Sheehan, 1970). Monitoring is the act of "catching" oneself in the process of using a target behavior and noting it, bringing it to consciousness. Adults are successful with a simple raise of a finger when they observe a selected trick; children tend to do better by dropping a chip in a cup or similar voluntary action. In many cases, children may need to learn the skill of monitoring prior to monitoring an escape behavior. This can be accomplished using a non-speech behavior—for example, catching the clinician's intentional cough as an initial step, gradually moving to words by catching the clinician's use of "um," and then together as a team, catching the child's use of "um."

While monitoring is effective in reducing an escape behavior, there are consequences. Escape behaviors are initially used to hide stuttering, and eventually become habits. By removing them, real disfluency on the feared or intended word/sound will often result as

GOAL: Reducing escape and avoidance behaviors	
Concept or Rationale	They were initially learned to escape (help), but have become habituated, and are now a source of struggle.
Treatment Activities	• Monitoring • Reinforcement of incompatible behavior

Figure 9–9. Sample treatment goal: Reducing physical and linguistic escape/avoidance behaviors.

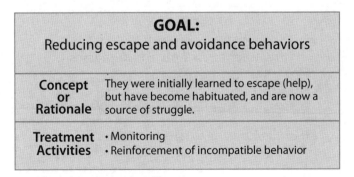

a replacement behavior. We call this "open stuttering," a great success and an important milestone in the process of ARTS.

Desensitizing to "Open Stuttering" (Figure 9–10)

"Open stuttering," simply stated, is stuttering directly on the intended sound or word. I advise my clients to put the disfluency where it belongs—on the feared word. Concealing this very behavior has been the motivation for all learned escape behaviors up to this point. The benefits of "open stuttering" are explained by behavioral therapy, specifically Systematic Desensitization, or Exposure Therapy. John B. Watson, known as the father of behaviorism, was responsible for the famous "Little Albert Experiment," whereby a child was classically conditioned to fear a white rat contingent upon pairing it with a loud noise (Watson & Rayner, 1920). However, it is Mary Cover Jones who was credited with the first experiment in desensitization with her "Little Peter Experiment." She reduced fear of white rabbits in a 3-year-old boy by gradually introducing the boy to the rabbit and pairing the presentation with candy (Jones, 1924). Systematic Desensitization, or Graduated Exposure Therapy, is credited to Joseph Wolpe, who treated phobias and anxiety disorders by working gradually through a hierarchy (Wolpe, 1958). The use of fear hierarchies for desensitization has become a staple of stuttering treatments over the past 50 years to reduce fear of speaking and/or stuttering.

In this stage of ARTS, the client gradually desensitizes to "open stuttering" by pairing this behavior with a cognitive message—for example, to *plan* to feel shame or *plan* to feel awkward, depending on the feeling that the client would prefer to suppress. Shame is experienced quite differently if one plans to feel it, rather than hoping not to. Certainly, exposure on its own would lead to desensitization; however, clients are more likely to independently carry out assignments to "open stutter" if they utilize a strategy that changes their perception of that experience. ARTS utilizes a variety of strategies from mindfulness therapies to support clients in developing assignments that aid in desensitization to "open stuttering" (Bailey, Ciarrochi, & Hayes, 2012; Fodor & Hooker, 2008; Hayes, 2005; Semple, 2011). Dialectical Behavioral Therapy, for example, offers strategies to increase the ability to identify triggers that lead to reactivity and develop coping skills to aid in cognitive and emotional regulation (Linehan Institute, 2012). Riddoch and Eggers Huber Christensen (2009) offer examples of child-friendly assignments to help develop a "wise

GOAL: Desensitizing (tolerating) "open stuttering"	
Concept or Rationale	A block may represent "holding back" from open stuttering. Showing and tolerating it will reduce reactivity and struggle.
Treatment Activities	• Stuttering directly on the feared sound/word • Planning to feel shame per the fear hierarchy

Figure 9–10. Sample treatment goal: Producing and desensitizing to "open stuttering."

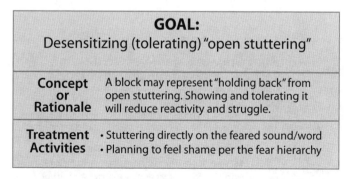

mind"—for example, employing the concept of "opposite action." If the child is feeling sad, the urge is to be alone; the opposite action is to be around others. An adaptation of this exercise for a child who stutters encourages the child to identify the *emotion*—embarrassment from struggling in front of others; next, identify the *urge*—escape by using a "trick"; finally, identify the opposite action—"open stutter"—and count it as a success. Chapters 6 and 7 in this book offer specifics relating to Cognitive Behavioral Therapy and Acceptance and Commitment Therapy that can be helpful for pairing cognitive/emotional strategies with speech assignments for positive outcomes.

Open stuttering is a milestone for clients in the process of ARTS, though initially not welcomed. It exposes the very behavior they have learned to hide: "My name is, um, um, my, uh name is Vivian." The escape behavior, interjections, and phrase repetition allowed me to say my name without disfluency on my name, a success prior to therapy. Now the success looks very different: "My name is Vi-vi-vi-vivian." The clinician must be sensitive to the client's reactivity to "open stuttering." Even without anticipation of negative listener reaction (in the group setting, for example), it is natural to retreat from this kind of "raw" disfluency, as it is sometimes struggled while the client navigates through his or her approach-avoidance conflict—wanting to be open, but at the same time, wishing that "open stuttering" had evolved to the point where it was comfortable and forward-moving. The reality is that initially "open stuttering" can be more struggled than the former collection of escape behaviors. Helping the client to understand that repeated exposure to "open stuttering," by carrying out assignments that move slowly through a fear hierarchy, will reduce reactivity and related struggle. I often advise clients not to "be a hero" in speaking situations when the shame and negative thoughts that result from "open stuttering" are too bombarding to receive the benefit of desensitization.

Adjusting Parameters of Normal Fluency (Figure 9–11)

Once disfluency is "clean," free of linguistic and physical escape and avoidance behaviors in at least some speaking contexts, modification strategies can be successful. I explain to clients that "open stuttering" offers something to change, something to mold into comfortable disfluency. At this point, clients begin to identify the features of "open stuttering" and the corresponding parameters of "normal talking" (Williams, 1957) that are interfering with comfortable disfluency. Clinicians and clients together develop teaching strategies to help the client adjust an identified parameter. This becomes a speech target for modification of

GOAL: Adjusting speech parameters to develop comfortable, forward-moving disfluency	
Concept or Rationale	Open stuttering may contain irregularities in voicing, tension, airflow, movement or timing. Adjustments improve efficiency and comfort.
Treatment Activities	• Identify multiple adjustment strategies • Practice according to linguistic complexity, cognitive load, and emotionality of content

Figure 9–11. Sample treatment goal: Making choices to adjust parameters of "open stuttering."

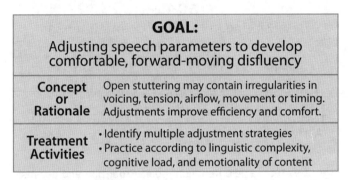

"open stuttering." Figure 9–12 provides examples of teaching strategies that I have used with school-age clients to help make modification targets more concrete.

In a scenario in which the "open stuttering" pattern consists of tight prolongations on initial consonants, "Vvvvvvivian," the parameters identified could be *tension* and *movement.* The client is not moving to the intended vowel. It is likely that the prolongation is serving the function of a "filibuster." That is, the client is holding the sound until he or she feels it is safe to move to the vowel without sounding "out of control" or as some of my clients might joke, like "a bleating sheep." The desire to simultaneously move ahead and hold back leads to tension. The target to "resist self-imposed time pressure" will be helpful in reducing tension in this case, reducing the approach-avoidance conflict that elicits it. I might say, "Take the time to stutter well." Another target might be "vowel busting," a fun label for stuttering on the feared sound, the vowel in this case. I might encourage this by saying, "Get to the vowel and put the disfluency where it belongs."

Treatment to Develop Confidence and Joy in Communication

Goals in the sections to follow are essential for supporting change in speech. In fact, goals that focus on attitudes, thoughts, and emotions are paired with goals for speech efficiency in the process of assignment development. An assignment to say the intended word (and not substitute) while placing a food order could lead to overt disfluency, as an unintended and unwanted consequence. However, the addition of a cognitive assignment, "plan to let the waiter think I am 'weird,' " increases the likelihood of success. In this case, feeling shame or embarrassment due to the potential thoughts of others is now a success, rather than a failure. Feeling feelings, rather than suppressing them, is part of the culture of ARTS.

Approaching/Entering Feared Speaking Situations (Figure 9–13)

Aforementioned goals addressed escape and avoidance in the stuttering pattern. Here, we address situational avoidance. In accordance with a client-developed fear hierarchy, assignments are developed first to enter low-feared situations. The first step here is "showing up." Attending a networking event, accepting an invitation to a party, and walking into a store are examples of risks, even without any expectation of speaking to someone. We might later pair this situation with the target of "saying something to one person." Assignments are designed to be functional and meaningful, and involve some risk.

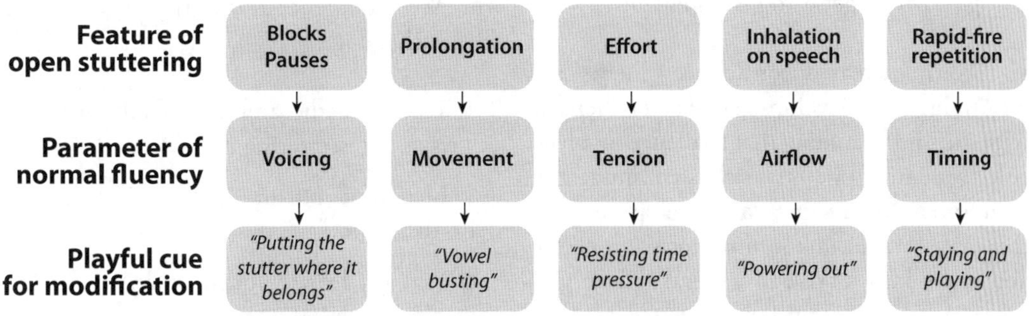

Figure 9–12. Examples of playful treatment targets to help make modification strategies concrete.

GOAL: Approaching feared speaking situations	
Concept or Rationale	If stuttering is a conflict between going ahead and holding back, then increasing the approach drive will resolve the conflict.
Treatment Activities	• Entering feared situations • Risk-taking; "Running stop signs"

Figure 9–13. Sample treatment goal: Increasing "approach" and reducing "avoidance" in daily activities and life choices.

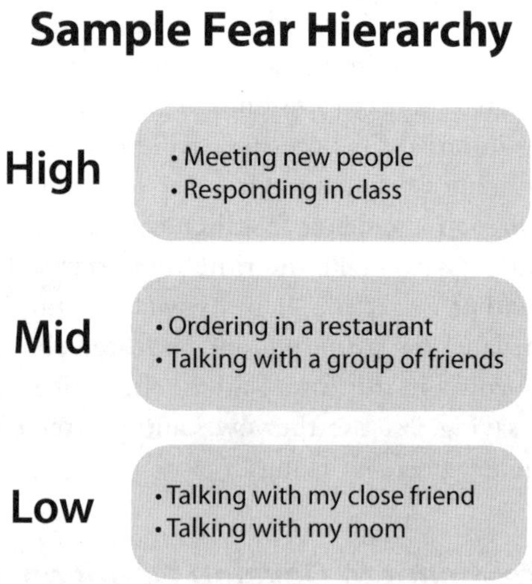

Figure 9–14. This chart is a product of a counseling activity to create a personalized fear hierarchy later used for individualized assignment development.

Figure 9–14 provides an example of a client-designed fear hierarchy. It is a general rule that clients leave the therapy session with a clear idea of their specific assignments in low-, mid-, and high-feared situations. Specific assignments for a school-age child might include the following:

Low-Feared Situation

- Open stutter (without a trick) with Mom in the car after school. Plan for her to think you are stressed out.

Mid-Feared Situation

- Monitor my "backups" (phrase repetitions) for the first two minutes during lunch with my friend Joe. Plan to talk about something that I don't need to think too much about.

High-Feared Situation

- Go to the movies with my friends on Friday night. My target is to just "show up."

With increased confidence, clients are encouraged to develop personal challenges with the understanding that challenge involves risk. Evaluating potential risk is an important component of assignment development in this case. I might talk to my adolescent client about the idea of risk in general. He might take a risk to ask a girl for a date, to drive his car to school, to enter a contest he might not win. We then generate the risks involved in speech challenges:

> If I increase the amount of talking I do, I risk . . . ("stuttering more")
>
> If I let go of control, I risk . . . ("struggling on disfluency")
>
> If I say my feared words, I risk . . . ("being stuck, forever!")

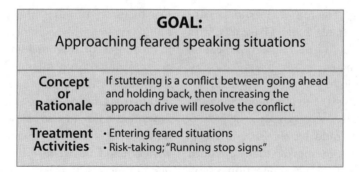

I might ask this teen if he is willing to take any of these risks. If the answer is "no," then we need to select something less risky. If the answer is "yes," then we proceed to develop the details of the assignment.

Letting Go of Efforts to Control (Figure 9–15)

The culture of ARTS encourages letting go of both avoidance and control. We have seen how efforts to hide stuttering lead to struggle through the conditioning of secondary behaviors, and efforts to control the expression of "open stuttering" lead to tension from "holding back" (Van Riper, 1937; Williams, 1957). This goal area addresses efforts to control what others think, the motivation behind most maladaptive reactive behavior. Though futile, it is human nature to attempt to control the thinking of others. White lies are typically told to avoid hurting someone's feelings. We may say we are late due to traffic, in the hope that a friend will think that we did not intend to make him wait. Despite our efforts, we can never control the thoughts of others, and we never really know what others are thinking. While those who stutter are well aware of this reality, they persist in reinforcing maladaptive struggle behaviors in their attempts to influence the thinking of their listeners: "If I show stuttering, he will think I am nervous and incompetent"; "I would rather the teacher think that I don't know the answer than think that I stutter." Aaron Beck, the father of Cognitive Behavioral Therapy (CBT), explains that whether the disorder is psychological or behavioral, when patients get better, there is improvement in their attitudes and in the way they think (Beck, 1997). Exercises and behavioral experiments from Cognitive Behavioral Therapy are effective in helping clients identify dysfunctional thinking and challenge maladaptive beliefs (Menzies, Onslow, Packman, & O'Brian, 2009). Judith Beck (2011) provides detailed exercises to guide clients through the process of cognitive restructuring, including identifying and evaluating automatic thoughts, developing coping statements, and modifying beliefs.

Cognitive restructuring is essential for lasting behavior change through ARTS. Paradoxical assignments are developed by the client that are both fun and challenging. Begin with open-ended sentences that lead clients to share their desire to control the thoughts of others. Work up to challenging assignments by first exploring and evaluating automatic thoughts through CBT exercises especially for children (Stallard, 2003). It is often helpful to explore potential assignments, even if the client is not ready to carry them out. Client responses are conveyed in parentheses below:

GOAL: Letting go of efforts to control what others think	
Concept or Rationale	Fear of negative listener thoughts and reactions leads to use of false fluency and exhausting mental gymnastics.
Treatment Activities	• Predicting best and worst outcomes (CBT) • Paradoxical challenges, e.g., getting someone to grimace or hang up on you

Figure 9–15. Sample treatment goal: Letting go of control.

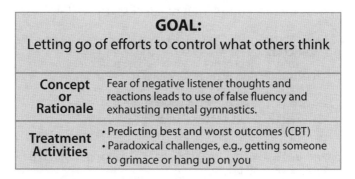

Client: "I never raise my hand in class."

Clinician: If you raise your hand and speak up in class . . . ("Kids will laugh and look at each other"). And that would mean . . . ("They think I'm weird or stupid. I know I'm not, but I don't want to think about that").

Clinician: Can you think of a challenging assignment that you might do, even if you are not ready to do it?

Client: "I guess I can *allow* them to think I am stupid, and be prepared for that. Or, try to make them think I'm stupid! But I am not gonna do that anytime soon!"

Something a little less challenging is a "stop sign" assignment. Similar to automatic thoughts, the client identifies "stop signs" throughout the day, moments when he or she would spontaneously speak, but instead, hold back due to stuttering. Once consistent stop signs are identified, a healthy challenge is to "run a stop sign" by speaking in the face of fear. Below is a list of "stop signs" from a teen client:

- *Hallway hello:* I saw a friend in the hall on the way to class, but I knew the timing would not work out, so I pretended to be looking in my backpack as we passed.
- *Help with math:* The girl next to me asked for help with a math problem because she knows I am good at math. I said I didn't know the answer when I did.
- *Sandwich order:* I was just about to order my sandwich, but there were too many people who could hear. I told my sister to order for me because I needed to go get something.

Assignments that involve planning to "run a stop sign" are usually accomplished with a good deal of pride.

Changing Ideas of Success and Failure (Figure 9–16)

Once engaged in ARTS, there is a gradual shift in perception of success and failure. Prior to therapy, a list of successes might include:

- There is no oral report for this class.
- He finished my sentence and I never showed stuttering.
- The bell rang before it was my turn to read.
- My friend introduced me and I didn't have to say my name.

Successful suppression of stuttering is celebrated, even with an understanding that these successes may increase the fear of show-

GOAL: Changing one's idea of success and failure	
Concept or Rationale	Defining success as "stuttering openly and honestly" builds self-esteem and frees one to enjoy communication.
Treatment Activities	• Identifying the success prior to action • Counting and celebrating successes

Figure 9–16. Sample treatment goal: Changing ideas of personal success and failure.

ing stuttering in the future. Hiding visible stuttering, as well as one's identity as a person who stutters, is the ultimate goal in every interaction. By completing activities to increase tolerance for showing stuttering, desensitization takes place and reactivity is reduced. After intentionally showing stuttering, or allowing themselves to be identified as someone who stutters, clients begin to report feelings of relief: "I felt embarrassed for a few minutes, but I was so relieved that I didn't have to hide." Gradually, a cognitive shift emerges as clients report successes:

- I participated in class.
- I ordered my own food, and I stuttered.
- I decided to go to guitar camp this summer.
- I talked about stuttering with my dad.

While there are no assignments that directly target the cognitive shift that represents a change in the client's definition of success and failure, progress is noted through reports of successes from the week, and self-evaluation of speaking experiences. While a success used to be, "My oral report was good. I didn't stutter very much. I don't think people noticed the disfluencies I had," a success is now, "My oral report went well. I said everything I wanted to say. People seemed to like it."

Enacting the Role of a Person Who Stutters (Figure 9–17)

In an earlier discussion of Role Theory, the notion of "false role behavior" was defined as taking on the role of fluent speaker by using an avoidance behavior or demonstrating an attitude that masks stuttering. This kind of fluency is known as "false fluency" (Sheehan, 1970). By taking on the role of "person who stutters," the act of stuttering results in role congruency. By reducing conflict (wanting to be fluent and realizing you can't), both frequency of stuttering and struggle are reduced.

Self-disclosure as a person who stutters, or "advertising," is an important assignment in the context of many treatment programs (e.g., Breitenfeldt & Lorenz, 1989; Dell, 2000). Some examples include letting others know you have begun speech therapy, bringing up stuttering in a casual conversation, and talking to friends and family about stuttering and ways they can help. Self-disclosure gives oneself permission to stutter, which actually reduces it. The act of taking on the role of a person who stutters is counter to hiding it. However, the benefits of advertising extend far beyond role-taking. Through the process of advertising, clients develop support systems important for change, allow others

GOAL: Taking the role of a person who stutters	
Concept or Rationale	Role enactment prevents false fluency and develops self-advocacy, leading to deeper self-acceptance as a person who stutters.
Treatment Activities	• Self-disclosure (advertising) • Voluntary stuttering, to show oneself as a person who stutters when you don't have to

Figure 9–17. Sample treatment goal: Enacting the role of "person who stutters."

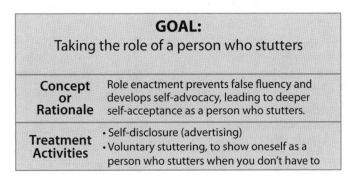

to understand behavior that might not look like "stuttering," and set the tone for trusting relationships. Murphy, Yaruss, and Quesal (2007) describe a case in which self-disclosure resulted in reduced bullying for a school-age child who stuttered.

While important during the early stages of therapy, it is worth noting that for some people, advertising can become a subtle avoidance behavior over time. One client developed a strategy of advertising confidently, adding that she did volunteer work for organizations that advocate for people who stutter. When she realized that her motivation was to protect herself from the potential "pity response" of new acquaintances, she gave herself the assignment *not to advertise*, and to allow others to judge her as they might.

Voluntary stuttering has been used historically as a strategy in stuttering treatment programs. It was first suggested by Bryngelson (1943), as part of an objective attitude toward stuttering, to bring the problem out into the open for the purpose of reducing fear of stuttering (Bloodstein & Ratner, 2008; Hahn, 1943). Dunlap (1942) applied voluntary stuttering as a form of negative practice, that is, to practice a habit in order to reduce it. It has been used in some form in most stuttering modification approaches throughout the years for the purpose of desensitization (Breitenfeldt & Lorenz, 1989; Dell, 2000; Grossman, 2008; Manning, 2010; Van Riper, 1973). Voluntary stuttering, in the context of role-taking, involves showing oneself as a person who stutters when one does not have to (Sheehan, 1975). The value is that it provides an opportunity to be *identified* as a person who stutters, something that would be unthinkable prior to therapy.

Taking Initiative and Responsibility for Change (Figure 9–18)

In reference to what the adult stutterer needs to do, Wendell Johnson wrote, "to recognize his stuttering as behavior, his own behavior, and to take responsibility for it. It is something he himself does—it is not something that somehow happens to him—and if he does not do it, there will be no 'it' at all" (cited in Hahn, 1956, p. 67). Showcasing new advances in understanding the behavioral and physiological basis of stuttering, Smith and Weber (2016, p. 291) lead us to define stuttering as a neurodevelopmental disorder characterized by atypical motor planning and execution networks. However, Johnson's observation of the experience of stuttering reminds us that much of the reactivity in stuttering in older chil-

GOAL: Taking initiative and responsibility for change	
Concept or Rationale	One develops a sense of agency by initiating action and making choices. This promotes self-confidence and resilience.
Treatment Activities	• Standing up to and supporting others • Using language of responsibility • Planning and carrying out assignments

Figure 9–18. Sample treatment goal: Taking responsibility for behavior and initiating change.

dren and adults results from learned behavior (Brutten & Shoemaker, 1967). Clients benefit from exposure to models of language of responsibility and from opportunities to reformulate their own words using the language of responsibility, an exercise that reminds clients they have choices in the way they stutter.

ARTS is an action-oriented treatment that requires the client to "do" in order to change. Assignment development, completion, and report (mentioned earlier) are essential for progress. We encourage clients of all ages to talk about stuttering without apologies or regrets. We turn to excellent resources in dealing with teasing and bullying, as well as exercises to build self-esteem in the process of therapy (Chmela & Reardon, 2001; Langevin & Prasad, 2012; Murphy, Quesal, Reardon-Reeves, & Yaruss, 2013).

OUTCOMES AND SELF-ACCEPTANCE

If I ask a client to provide me with one of his or her current goals in therapy, it is likely that the client will name something related to speech efficiency—for example, reducing blocking behavior. However, when I ask the client to consider the relevance of that goal ("And if you no longer block, what would that mean for you?"), he or she is likely to mention an outcome: "I would be more talkative"; "I would have confidence"; "Social situations would not be so exhausting." These outcomes, and the ones central to ARTS (efficiency, comfort, confidence, and joy in communication) are the by-products of consistent speech work to reduce avoidance and develop role congruency (Sisskin, 2006). Sheehan made it sound so simple when he said that one travels the road to recovery by eliminating every shred of avoidance. However, it isn't so simple. "Recovery" from stuttering may be defined as saying *what* one wants, *when* one wants, *spontaneously, comfortably, efficiently, without worry or anxiety about stuttering*. Clients sometimes ask me why some clients seem to achieve recovery from stuttering and others, while quite satisfied with their outcomes, never get *all the way* there. I believe it may be related to the depth of one's self-acceptance as a person who stutters. Self-acceptance does not happen in a moment of time, rather, it is a process. Those who are involved in the process rarely recognize their progression while in the midst of making it. Progress is recognized retrospectively; as mentioned earlier, we see it through the rearview mirror. A client may note that he showed his stuttering during a meeting at work and didn't really care. Similarly, a child might report that she doesn't care that she stutters when reading in class anymore. It is no coincidence that the form of stuttering also changes to be comfortable and forward-moving.

There is likely a continuum of self-acceptance, varying stages that represent the client's identification with the role of "person who stutters." Initially, the client ***acknowledges*** the behavior of stuttering but works to conceal that identity as much as possible. Soon, the client begins to ***enact*** the role of a person who stutters through "open stuttering" and self-disclosure. There is considerable reactivity at this point due to role conflict. Later, the client ***welcomes*** the role of person who stutters by taking risks and seeking out challenges to reveal that role to others. Feelings of shame diminish through assignments designed to feel them. Eventually the client ***embraces*** the role of person who stutters, as role congruency rarely triggers the desire to conceal it. Finally, the client approaches the zone of ***self-acceptance*** when he or she no longer longs for it. Neutral feelings about one's role of "person who stutters" tend to reduce their importance, and that role joins the ranks of other roles within the identity of the person—for example, wife, daughter, teacher, American, tennis player, person who stutters, etc. With neither negative emotion nor habituated struggle, disfluency exists without reactivity—frequency of disfluency decreases as a by-product.

REFERENCES

ARTS®. (2016). Sisskin Stuttering Center, McLean, VA. Registered, U.S. Patent and Trademark Office.

Bailey, A., Ciarrochi, J., & Hayes, L. (2012). *Get out of your mind and into your life for teens: A guide to living an extraordinary life*. Oakland, CA: New Harbinger.

Beck, A. T. (1997). The past and future of cognitive therapy. *Journal of Psychotherapy Practice and Research, 6*(4), 276.

Beck, J. S. (2011). *Cognitive behavior therapy: Basics and beyond*. New York, NY: Guilford Press.

Buck, M. (2010). Two-factor theory of learning: Application to maladaptive behaviour. *School and Health 21, 2010, Health Education: Contents and Inspiration.*

Bloodstein, O., & Ratner, N. (2008). *A handbook on stuttering*. Clifton Park, NY: Thomson Delmar Learning.

Breitenfeldt, D. H., & Lorenz, D. R. (1989). *Successful stuttering management program*. Cheney, WA: Eastern Washington University School of Health Sciences.

Brutten, E. J., & Shoemaker, D. J. (1967). *The modification of stuttering*. Englewood Cliffs, NJ: Prentice-Hall.

Bryngelson, B. (1943). Stuttering and personality development. *Nervous Child, 2*, 162–171.

Chmela, K., & Reardon, N. (2001). *The school-age child who stutters: Working effectively with attitudes and emotions*. Memphis, TN: Stuttering Foundation of America.

Christensen, R., & Christensen, K. (2009). *Dialectical behavior therapy skills, 101 mindfulness exercises and other fun activities for children and adolescents: A learning supplement*. Bloomington, IL: AuthorHouse.

Conture E. G. (1990). *Stuttering* (2nd ed.). Englewood Cliffs, NJ: Prentice-Hall.

Cooper, E., & Cooper, C. (1985). *Cooper personalized fluency control therapy handbook* (Rev.). Allen, TX: DLM Teaching Resources.

Craig, A. R., Franklin, J. A., & Andrews, G. (1984). A scale to measure locus of control of behaviour. *British Journal of Medical Psychology, 57*(2), 173–180.

Dell, C. W. (2000). *Treating the school-age child who stutters: A guide for clinicians*. Memphis, TN: Stuttering Foundation of America.

Dunlap, K. (1942). The technique of negative practice. *American Journal of Psychology, 55*(2), 270–273.

Fodor, I. E., & Hooker, K. E. (2008). Teaching mindfulness to children. *Gestalt Review, 12*(1), 75–91.

Grossman, H. L. (2008). *Voluntary stuttering: A mixed methods investigation* (Doctoral dissertation). Retrieved from ProQuest. (UMI No. 3343421)

Guitar, B. (2006). *Stuttering: An integrated approach to its nature and treatment*. Baltimore, MD: Lippincott Williams & Wilkins.

Hahn, E. F. (1943). *Stuttering: Significant theories and therapies*. Stanford, CA: Stanford University Press.

Hahn, E. F. (1956). *Stuttering: Significant theories and therapies* (2nd ed.). Stanford, CA: Stanford University Press.

Hayes, S. C. (2005). *Get out of your mind and into your life: The new acceptance and commitment therapy*. Oakland, CA: New Harbinger.

Healey, E. C., Trautman, L. S., & Susca, M. (2004). Clinical applications of a multidimensional approach for the assessment and treatment of stuttering. *Contemporary Issues in Communication Science and Disorders, 31*, 40–48.

Hegde, M. N. (1995). Measurement and explanation of stuttering: A retrospective appreciation of Gene Brutten's contribution. *Journal of Fluency Disorders, 20*(2), 205–230.

Johnson, W. (1946). *People in quandaries: The semantics of personal adjustment*. New York, NY: Harper.

Jones, M. C. (1924). A laboratory study of fear: The case of Peter. *Journal of Genetic Psychology, 31*, 308–315.

Langevin, M., & Prasad, N. N. (2012). A stuttering education and bullying awareness and prevention resource: A feasibility study. *Language, Speech, and Hearing Services in Schools*, *43*(3), 344–358.

Linehan Institute. (2012). *Dialectical behavioral therapy: An informational resource*. Retrieved from http://www.linehaninstitute.org/downloads/NREPP-2012 %20DBTComparitiveEffectivenessResearch.pdf

Logan, K. (2015). *Fluency disorders*. San Diego, CA: Plural.

Manning, W. (2010). *Clinical decision making in fluency disorders*. Clifton Park, NY: Delmar, Cengage Learning.

Menzies, R. G., Onslow, M., Packman, A., & O'Brian, S. (2009). Cognitive behavior therapy for adults who stutter: A tutorial for speech-language pathologists. *Journal of Fluency Disorders*, *34*(3), 187–200.

Miller, N. E. (1944). Personality and the behavior disorders. In J. M. Hunt (Ed.) *Experimental Studies of Conflict*. New York, NY: Ronald.

Mowrer, O. (1947). On the dual nature of learning—a re-interpretation of "conditioning" and "problem-solving." *Harvard Educational Review*, *17*, 102–148.

Murphy, W. P., Quesal, R. W., Reardon-Reeves, N., & Yaruss, J. S. (2013). *Minimizing bullying for children who stutter: A guide for SLPs*. McKinney, TX: Stuttering Therapy Resources.

Murphy, W. P., Yaruss, J. S., & Quesal, R. W. (2007). Enhancing treatment for school-age children who stutter: I. Reducing negative reactions through desensitization and cognitive restructuring. *Journal of Fluency Disorders*, *32*(2), 121–138.

Oberg, K. (1960). Cultural shock: Adjustment to new cultural environments. *Practical Anthropology*, *7*(4), 177–182.

Prochaska, J. O., DiClemente, C. C., & Norcross, J. C. (1992). In search of how people change: Applications to addictive behaviors. *American Psychologist*, *47*(9), 1102.

Quesal, R. W., & Yaruss, J. S. (2000). Historical perspectives on stuttering treatment: Dean Williams. *Contemporary Issues in Communication Science and Disorders*, *27*, 178–187.

Rotter, J. (1966). Generalized expectancies for internal versus external control of reinforcements. *Psychological Monographs*, *80*, Whole No. 609.

Sarbin, T. R. (1943). The concept of role-taking. *Sociometry*, *6*(3), 273–285.

Semple, R. J., & Lee, J. (2011). *Mindfulness-based cognitive therapy for anxious children: A manual for treating childhood anxiety*. Oakland, CA: New Harbinger.

Sheehan, J. G. (1953). Theory and treatment of stuttering as an approach-avoidance conflict. *Journal of Psychology*, *36*(1), 27–49.

Sheehan, J. G. (1970). *Stuttering: Research and treatment*. New York, NY: Harper & Row.

Sheehan, J. (1975). Conflict theory and avoidance-reduction therapy. In J. Eisenson (Ed.), *Stuttering: A second symposium* (pp. 97–198). New York, NY: Harper & Row.

Sheehan, J. G., & Sheehan, V. M., (1984). Avoidance reduction therapy: A response-suppression hypothesis. In B. P. Ryan & W. H. Perkins (Eds.), *Stuttering disorders*. New York, NY: Thieme-Stratton.

Sheehan, V. M., & Sisskin, V. (2001). The creative process in avoidance reduction therapy for stuttering. *SIG 4 Perspectives on Fluency and Fluency Disorders*, *11*(1), 7–11.

Sisskin, V. D. (2006, November). *Group therapy for stuttering: Outcomes for an avoidance reduction model*. Poster session presented at the Annual Convention of the American Speech-Language-Hearing Association (ASHA), Miami, FL.

Smith, A. (1999). Stuttering: A unified approach to a multifactorial, dynamic disorder. In C. Healy & N. Bernstein-Ratner (Eds.), *Research and treatment of fluency disorders: Bridging the gap*. Mahwah, NJ: Erlbaum.

Smith, A., & Cooper, J. A. (1990). Factors in the etiology of stuttering. *American Speech-Language-Hearing Association Reports, Research Needs in Stuttering: Roadblocks and Future Directions*, *18*, 39–47.

Smith, A., & Weber, C. (2016). Where are we and where are we going? *Seminars in Speech and Language*, *37*, 291–297.

Stallard, P. (2003). *Think good–feel good: A cognitive behaviour therapy workbook for children and young people*. Chichester, UK: Wiley.

Starkweather, C. W. (1987). *Fluency and stuttering.* Englewood Cliffs, NJ: Prentice-Hall.

Starkweather, C. W., Gottwald, S. R., & Halfond, M. M. (1990). *Stuttering prevention: A clinical method.* Englewood Cliffs, NJ: Prentice-Hall.

Van Riper, C. (1937). The growth of the stuttering spasm. *Quarterly Journal of Speech, 23*(1), 70–73.

Van Riper, C. (1973). *The treatment of stuttering.* Englewood Cliffs, NJ: Prentice-Hall.

Watson, J. B., & Rayner, R. (1920). Conditioned emotional reactions. *Journal of Experimental Psychology, 3*(1), 1.

Williams, D. E. (1957). A point of view about stuttering. *Journal of Speech and Hearing Disorders, 22*(3), 390.

Williams, D. E. (1971). Stuttering therapy for children. In L. E. Travis (Ed.), *Handbook of speech pathology and audiology* (pp. 1073–1093). New York, NY: Appleton-Century-Crofts.

Williams, D. E. (1979). A perspective on approaches to stuttering therapy. In H. Gregory (Ed.), *Controversies about stuttering therapy* (pp. 253–268). Baltimore, MD: University Park Press.

Winkelman, M. (1994). Cultural shock and adaptation. *Journal of Counseling and Development: JCD, 73*(2), 121–126.

Wolpe, J. (1958). *Psychotherapy by reciprocal inhibition.* Stanford, CA: Stanford University Press.

Yaruss, J. S. (2007). Application of the ICF in fluency disorders. *Seminars in Speech and Language, 28*, 312–322.

CHAPTER 10

Peer Support for People Who Stutter

History, Benefits, and Accessibility

Mitchell Trichon and Erik X. Raj

INTRODUCTION

As one of the authors of this chapter, I would like to share some thoughts about my early experiences with self-help activities described in this chapter because they continue to be such a useful and now increasingly accessible resource for me and so many other people who stutter (PWS).

It had been many years since I participated in a self-help group, although I enjoyed meeting other PWS. I was fortunate enough to know quite a few, including some who are related to me. But that year was different. I had returned to school to study speech-language pathology while unknowingly seeking some answers in my own stuttering journey. I knew I needed to further explore "self-acceptance," despite having previously associated this idea with waving the white surrender flag for controlling my speech. As a result, I started a local self-help group and participated in a couple of national self-help conferences. These experiences made me realize their value, to me and to the stuttering community.

At these events, I listened to the stories as well as the varieties of stuttered speech of many people who became my friends. I was inspired at my core by the courage of many who struggled to say their name or to tell their story to me or to hundreds, and by the leadership of those who have built bridges for so many others who stutter. I realized that there was much to learn about being among other PWS. It helped me realize that it wasn't stuttering itself that was limiting my potential; it was how I thought about my stuttering, and fortunately that was malleable.

Self-help activities are beneficial to PWS and can serve as a valuable supplement to speech therapy. They help people who stutter connect in important and meaningful ways.

As authors of this chapter, we hope it helps readers to understand the importance of considering self-help activities as a potential piece of the stuttering management puzzle.

– Mitchell Trichon

People often seek speech-language therapy for stuttering, but more and more people are using peer support as an additional way to help manage their communication disorder. Today, the Internet is a beacon of hope for individuals who want to connect with others who are dealing with the same struggles. Some people are fortunate enough to find information about peer support or "self-help" organizations, or Internet-based self-help activities (see list at the end of this chapter). Through these types of channels, people who stutter are able to be a part of a caring and helpful community where members actively grow together toward better understanding the complexity of stuttering.

The word *self-help* could be considered a misnomer. *Self-help* usually refers to an individual's interaction with others with the same condition for the benefit of the individuals who participate. *Self-help* can also refer to the actions of individuals to improve themselves in a specific way. In the realm of stuttering, this often means reading literature or watching videos about stuttering in order to gain knowledge for one's own benefit. In this chapter the term *self-help* refers to peer interaction for the purposes of support.

Self-help groups have been defined in multiple ways. One of the more popular definitions, by Katz and Bender (1976), reads:

> Self-help groups are voluntary, small group structures for mutual aid and the accomplishment of a special purpose. They are usually formed by peers who have come together for mutual assistance in satisfying a common need, overcoming a common handicap or life-disrupting problem and bringing about desired social and/or personal change. (p. 9)

Richardson and Goodman (1983) define *self-help groups* as "groups of people who feel they have a common problem and have joined together to do something about it" (p. 2).

Regardless of how *self-help groups* are defined, the concept of sharing experiential knowledge to benefit one another has expanded well beyond the smaller-size, traditional, self-help groups. In fact, it has grown beyond the boundaries of an in-person interaction. Before further exploring the origins of self-help in the United States and a variety of self-help activities, differentiations between self-help groups and other related terms are provided.

Borkman (1999) looks to the manager of the group to decipher classification. She believes that *support groups* are managed by professionals, while *self-help groups* and *mutual-aid groups* are not directly managed by professionals. Furthermore, she considers *self-help groups* to be a type of *mutual-aid group* in which individuals help themselves and draw on "latent internal resources and healing powers within the context of his or her lived experience with an issue or predicament" (p. 4).

To simplify terminology, Yaruss, Quesal, and Reeves (2007) deemphasize the importance of who manages the group and refers to all the groups described above as *self-help groups* or *mutual-aid groups*. They do, however, make the distinction between groups that were founded by or "originated" from professionals who are "associated" with a particular stuttering treatment. Such groups should be referred to as *therapy groups* or *maintenance groups*. Professionals can create *self-help groups* that are associated with a self-help organization, as long as they follow guidelines of the organization and the ethics of their profession (Trichon, 2010). However, a further distinction must be made regarding groups that are affiliated with professional therapy services and if those services are required or optional. If therapy services are required, the group should be considered a therapy group or maintenance group. However, if therapy services are not required for group involvement, it is still a self-help group because it includes non-clients. The group would be related to but run independently of the therapy services provided.

It should also be noted that self-help groups can differ in their primary focus. Some self-help groups may focus on discussing experiences and challenges associated with stuttering, while other self-help groups focus on the exchange of feedback about the use of speech skills to help manage their stuttered speech (Carlisle, 1987; Ramig, 1993). Groups that place emphasis on giving each other feedback about the use of one or more methods of speech therapy are called *practice groups* and can be led by either professionals or non-professionals.

As one can see, differentiating between the various types of groups can be a challenge (Hunt, 1987), so for the purpose of clarity for this chapter, the terms *self-help* and *self-help groups*, as described by Yaruss, Quesal, and Reeves (2007), will be used with the exception that *self-help groups* can also be created by professionals as long as they follow the guidelines of the organization and ethics of their profession.

SELF-HELP IN THE UNITED STATES

Human communication allows individuals to share their needs and experiences with each other. People listen to the experiences of others and decide if they are relevant or important to them. People in similar situations or with similar conditions tend to value each other's experiences if and when they communicate and it usually results in mutual support.

The self-help movement in the United States emerged from immigration in the mid-1800s. This created ethnic communities that turned to each other to face the challenges of adjusting to their new lives in America (Katz & Bender, 1976). Alcoholics Anonymous (AA), however, was one of the first nationally known self-help organizations in the United States (Alcoholics Anonymous, n.d.). The self-help movement grew into the realms of physical and mental disorders by the mid-1950s and early 1960s but used organizational and operational models instead (Reeves, 2006). In the mid-1960s, the growth of consumerism propelled the growth of the self-help movement (Hunt, 1987; Ramig, 1993), which, however, was understood to be a social movement rather than a medical phenomenon (Adamsen & Rasmussen, 2001; Emerick, 1996; Vattano, 1972).

The health care system further influenced the self-help movement. By the 1970s the health care system in the United States had become less patient centered (Borkman, 1999; Damen, Mortelmans, & Van Hove, 2000), resulting in frustration from those seeking professional help. During this same period there was expansion in the self-help movement. There seemed to be a partition between people offering professional help and those who were supporters of self-help groups. This divide was highlighted by the U.S. Surgeon General, Dr. C. Everett Koop, in the foreword to *The Self-Help Way: Mutual Aid and Health*: "Many professionals still believe that … transformation, change, and healing are the prerogative of an elite who possess knowledge and techniques bestowed by specialized training institutions" (Romeder, 1990, Foreword).

In the 1980s, Dr. Koop helped influence an attitudinal shift from "mutual disrespect" to more collaboration, by sponsoring a National Workshop on Self-Help and Public Health for both consumers and professionals (Borkman, 1999; Surgeon General Workshop, 1988). People were starting to realize that health care providers alone were not able to reduce the suffering experienced by people who were physically or mentally ill. Koop later wrote, "Consumers are becoming more interested in taking charge of their own lives. Professionals need to recognize this trend and acknowledge the potential benefits of self-help". (Diggs, 1990, p. 33) This brought about more open-minded professionals in the late 1980s. Professionals helped promote self-help organizations without feeling the need to control them (Borkman, 1999).

In the next decade, literature indicates that professionals became more relatable to the public. The 1990s saw professionals revealing their vulnerabilities and their affiliations with self-help groups. This helped to give more credibility to the benefits of self-help groups and to change the negative stereotypes of a self-helper to one that has "strengths, resources, capabilities, and special knowledge to contribute to [his/her] own and [his/her] peers' recovery" (Borkman, 1999, p. 78). Research during this time included the consideration of both professional and self-help outlets as a part of treatment. This is partially due to the professionals' dual role as professionals and as leaders or proponents in the self-help community (Medvene, Wituk, & Luke, 1999).

By 2000, self-help groups existed for every condition and/or disorder recognized by the World Health Organization (Banks, 2000), equaling over a half million self-help groups for over 60 million participants (Riessman, 2000). The Internet and advances in technology and its applications contributed to the creation, exposure, and growth of self-help at the local and organizational levels (Trichon, 2010). Organizations found the benefits of having an Internet presence (i.e., a website with useful information about the given organization) to attract people. Search engines play a major role in this by guiding people to websites of interest, based on an individual's search commands. Social networking websites have also become instrumental in connecting and reconnecting people, especially with the formation of specialized groups that have been created for special purposes, including illnesses and disorders. There is little doubt that the Internet has been an invaluable resource for helping people to find both in-person and Internet-based self-help resources, especially for people with conditions that might be considered embarrassing or socially stigmatizing, such as alcoholism, cancer, acquired immunodeficiency syndrome (AIDS), depression, or diabetes (Davison, Pennebaker, & Dickerson, 2000).

Having some background knowledge of the development and expansion of the self-help movement within the United States makes it easier to understand the development and expansion of self-help for people who stutter in the United States and beyond. To review this history, it is important to describe the ways that self-help organizations have adapted and why others have been created to meet the needs of people. It is evident that self-help has become more accessible to those who seek it. In the next section, self-help activities will be described in the following two major categories: in-person self-help activities and Internet-based self-help activities. This is not meant to be an exhaustive list but it does present many of the popular modes of accessing self-help today, especially within the stuttering community. Descriptions of each activity are based on what is known within the stuttering community.

IN-PERSON SELF-HELP ACTIVITIES

There are three major categories of in-person self-help activities: *self-help groups*, *self-help workshops*, and *self-help conferences*. These three forms of in-person self-help activities vary in many ways, including length of time, frequency, number of attendees, variability of location, and amount of effort needed to host the activity. Regardless of the type of in-person self-help activity, an increase in the amount of research has come into existence to support their utility in the realm of stuttering (Boyle, 2013; Gathman, 1986; Hunt, 1987; Klein, Jackson, & Caggiano, 2015; Krauss-Lehrman & Reeves, 1989; Plexico, Manning, & DiLollo, 2005; Ramig, 1993; Tetnowski &

Azios, 2013; Tetnowski & McClure, 2009; Trichon, 2010; Trichon & Tetnowski, 2011; Trichon, Tetnowski, & De Nardo, 2016; Trichon, Tetnowski, & Rentschler, 2007; Yaruss, Quesal, Reeves et al., 2002).

Self-Help Groups

Self-help groups or *self-help group meetings* are the most common and most basic form of an in-person self-help activity. Meeting sizes usually range from 2 to 20 people and they typically meet once or twice a month. Meetings usually range from 1 to 2 hours in length and can be formal, with preplanned topics and activities, or informal. They are usually attended by people who live relatively close to the meeting location and are hosted by one or two facilitators.

In the realm of self-help groups for PWS, there are several studies that provide evidence supporting the value of self-help groups. One such study was Gathman's (1986) unpublished work which was later discussed by Ramig (1993). Ramig noted that there was high motivation to attend groups and that group attendance improved self-concept and attitude, and reduced anxiety. Group participants reported an increase or maintenance of fluency. An increase in fluency was also supported by Starkweather and Givens-Ackerman (1997) and Bloom and Cooperman (1999).

Krauss-Lehrman and Reeves's (1989) study, which surveyed 141 attendees of the self-help group meetings of the National Stuttering Project (NSP, now known as the National Stuttering Association), revealed the rankings of the most important focus of self-help groups to be: (1) sharing feelings and experiences, (2) providing a nonthreatening place to talk, (3) helping self-image, (4) meeting other stutterers, (5) learning more about stuttering, and (6) providing adjunct support to speech therapy. Ramig (1993) noted that the results were consistent with the NSP culture, which is more socially focused and less fluency focused.

Trichon, Tetnowski, and Rentschler (2007) used a qualitative approach to understand the experiences of six participants who attended self-help meetings for PWS and found that they attended meetings to gain more education, more fluency, and self-awareness. However, what they valued most about the groups was the encouragement, safe environment, shared feelings, sense of community, and exposure to other PWS.

Boyle (2013) surveyed 279 adults who had support group involvement—they experienced lower internalized stigma, were more likely to believe they would continue to stutter, and did not view fluency as highly or moderately important when talking to others compared with participants with no support group experience. In addition, individuals who joined support groups to help others to feel better about themselves described having higher self-esteem, self-efficacy, and life satisfaction, while decreasing internalized stigma and perceived stuttering severity, compared with individuals with no support group experience.

Self-Help Workshops

Self-help workshops are organized events that usually last one day and are therefore often referred to as *one-day workshops, local workshops,* or *one-day conferences*. Self-help workshops will often have an opening and closing general session for all participants. The time between is often filled with sessions on various topics. Sessions can be for all the participants to attend at the same time or they can be break-out sessions, in which participants will choose the sessions that interest them most or be assigned to the session that best suits them based on age, gender, whether a person has the condition or is a supporter, or other factors. Self-help workshops may also include keynote speakers and/or open-microphone sessions in which anyone attending the conference can share his/her thoughts with the audience. Most attendees of the workshops are from the region, hence these are often called *self-help regional workshops*. To avoid confusion, it is also important to note that the term *workshop* is also commonly used at self-help conferences to refer to the individual sessions, therefore, "workshop" should be understood in the context in which it is being used (Trichon, 2010).

Attendance at self-help workshops is typically larger than self-help group meetings. Size will depend on the organization and hosts of the event, who are usually individuals from the local group or chapter. The scheduling of self-help workshops may be sporadic, while others may be more regularly scheduled, usually on an annual basis. Locations may be kept the same for the regularly scheduled ones, while others may vary in location.

Self-Help Conferences

Self-help conferences typically vary between 2½ to 4 days in length. Like self-help workshops, self-help conferences usually have opening and closing general sessions for all participants to attend, but may also have other general sessions which may be dedicated to special events such as one or more keynote speakers or open microphone. Break-out sessions or conference workshops (including those on self-help topics) can be either assigned to participants based on their demographics or chosen by the participants based on their interests. This may include sessions for professional training. Self-help conferences also have scheduled social events, which may include going bowling, attending a sporting event, or visiting a tourist attraction in the host city. Informal social events also emerge from the participants naturally socializing with each other (e.g., dinner outings or meetings at a hotel restaurant, bar, or pool). To help fund the organization conferences and activities, there is usually a fundraising event in the form of a live auction, silent auction, raffle, or a combination of the three. The fundraising event usually concludes with a banquet, which features music and dancing.

Self-help conferences are organized by national organizations and are usually held annually, while international organizations are usually held biennially or triennially. The number of participants are typically larger than a self-help workshop and vary by organization and from year to year, but attendance at such conferences have been trending upward. Since there has been an increase in the attendance of self-help conferences, *regional conferences* or *annual regional conferences* have come into existence over the last few years (National Stuttering Association, n.d.-*b*). These conferences begin in the evening and conclude the morning after one full day (spanning three days). These conferences are smaller in scale and serve as a supplement to the regular annual self-help conference to meet the demands for more conferences, to provide greater accessibility to conferences by varying the dates and location from the regular annual conference, and to offer a conference experience at a lower cost (National Stuttering Association, n.d.-*b*).

Experiences at Self-Help Conferences

Trichon (2010) interviewed 12 adults who attended self-help conferences for PWS to learn about their lived experiences at the conference. Several major themes emerged from the semi-structured interviews. Participants valued the socializing opportunities with other PWS and affiliations with each other.

Participants also found that their perceived roles had shifted from needing help to offering help and that they experienced a positive change of emotions. Lastly, participants also found that they were redefining themselves and being more open and self-disclosing about their stuttering after the conference (Trichon & Tetnowski, 2011).

Trichon, Tetnowski, and De Nardo (2016) surveyed 117 participants both before and 4 to 6 months after a self-help conference using the Overall Assessment of the Speaker's Experience of Stuttering (OASES; Yaruss & Quesal, 2007) to determine if there was a correlation between attending conferences and reducing the negative impact that stuttering has on individuals. Results indicated that stuttering had less of a negative impact on people who attend more conferences. Preliminary results of similar studies by Trichon (2017) that focus on first-time attendees who are adults, teens, and school age also reflect the benefits of attending self-help conferences for PWS.

Klein, Jackson, and Caggiano (2015) surveyed 45 children who stutter (CWS) at a self-help conference or "convention" for CWS. They found that parents who attended self-help conferences were more comfortable discussing stuttering with their children, their teachers, relatives, friends, and speech therapists. However, parents were not comfortable with someone interrupting their child while he/she was stuttering.

McClure, D'Amico, and Tetnowski's (2009) survey of 1,235 people who are "active participants" in the National Stuttering Association (self-help groups and self-help conferences) lends additional support to the utility of in-person self-help activities for people who stutter. They found that active participants in the last three years, who included 686 adults who stutter and 31 teens who stutter, were less likely to avoid speaking situations, less likely to say their stuttering interferes with work or school, and more likely to talk about stuttering with family members, friends, and/or coworkers.

ORGANIZATIONS FOR PEOPLE WHO STUTTER IN THE UNITED STATES

It is natural for PWS to look for ways of coping or managing their stuttering problem. This may include efforts at trying to become more fluent or reducing the negative impact that stuttering can have. People who have had such success and are moved by people who continue to struggle may want to help others who still suffer. These are the roots of organizations that help people who stutter in the United States. Below are several of these organizations that have existed or still exist in the United States.

Kingsley Clubs

The *Kingsley Clubs* are the oldest known stuttering groups in the United States. The first of the groups originated in Philadelphia, Pennsylvania in 1921 ("Stammerers deliver," 1929) and then expanded to multiple groups in New York City, commencing in 1923 ("Stammerers' club," 1926). The original Kingsley Clubs in both cities were founded by J. Stanley Smith ("Stammerers Hold Dinner," 1930), lawyer and philanthropist, and were named after the English priest, professor, social reformer, and novelist Charles Kingsley (Leff, 2008). Smith established the organization with four other charter members with the goal of helping stammerers to speak confidently and easily ("Stammerers Deliver," 1929) and to correct their mental attitude about communication ("Stammerers Hold Dinner," 1930). What they found was a sympathetic fellowship and encouragement in each other. Additional members often preferred to meet with Smith privately before joining the monthly group. Smith's speech training predated the speech-language pathology profession, which was officially established in 1925 with the formation of what is known today as the American Speech-Language Hearing Association (ASHA, 2017).

The meetings focused on respiration, vocalization, and articulation to fellow members ("Stammerers deliver," 1929). It was probably because of this additional speech training that the group and the "school" together was referred to as the Smith School for the Correction of Stammering and Stuttering, which embodied or was affiliated with the Kingsley Club (Smith, 1925). It can be debated that the Kingsley Club of Philadelphia is the earliest documented self-help group for PWS in the United States

The Kingsley Clubs' banquet or "Dinner and Club Night" also began in 1921. It is the first known self-help banquet for people who stutter. This is significant, since banquets are one of the key elements of a self-help conference for people who stutter. Some may make the claim that it is the first known self-help workshop for people who stutter, since they plan for many participants to give speeches ("Stammerers deliver," 1929).

Stuttering Foundation

The *Stuttering Foundation* (SF) was founded in 1947, by businessman, philanthropist, and member of the Kingsley Club, Malcolm Fraser. A young Fraser became Smith's private secretary from 1925 to 1927. He helped Smith manage the Kingsley Clubs (The Stuttering Foundation, n.d.-*a*). The influence of Smith and/or the Kingsley Club may have inspired Fraser—with his later business success in co-founding and developing the Genuine Parts Company, specializing in automotive replacement parts—to found the *Speech Foundation of America* (now known as the Stuttering Foundation [n.d.-*a*]). In addition, Fraser donated money for what is now known as the National Stuttering Association (NSA) (The Stuttering Foundation, n.d.-*a*).

The Stuttering Foundation is not a self-help organization (Yaruss, Quesal, & Reeves, 2007), but it is recognized as "the first and largest nonprofit charitable organization in the world working toward the prevention and improved treatment of stuttering" (The Stuttering Foundation, n.d.-*b*, para. 3). It provides many helpful resources to people who stutter, their parents, and professionals about treatment and related research. Among their more notable resources are free brochures, e-books, videos, blog posts, and newsletters. The e-book *Self-Therapy for the Stutterer* is now in its eleventh edition (Fraser, 1978, 2010) and has been one of the foundation's most popular books/e-books. For professionals, the foundation hosts and funds workshops that focus on improving professional skills, improving the academic training of future clinicians, and supporting stuttering research. It also has an online store in which one can order from the foundation's library of affordable books and DVDs. It has had over 57 million webpage visits since it was launched (The Stuttering Foundation, n.d.-*b*). The *Stuttering Foundation* is widely considered to be one of the most useful resources for PWS today.

Council of Adult Stutterers, National Council on Stuttering

In 1965, the first nationally recognized self-help group for stuttering was formed at Catholic University in Washington, DC. The *Council of Adult Stutterers* was formed with the assistance of a speech-language pathologist, Eugene Walle (Yaruss, Quesal, & Reeves,

2007). One of the founders, Michael Heffron, communicated that he wanted to form or join a group in which "members want to help themselves and to help other stutterers. . . . I would seek to make stutterers proud, not that they stutter, for only a fool can take pride in affliction, but that they are doing something to help themselves" (as cited in Van Riper, 1973, p. 169).

Other groups formed in other states, including North Carolina, Georgia, Florida (Reeves, 2006), New York, Missouri, Michigan, and Illinois (Bloodstein, 1993). Michael Hartford, a member of the *Council of Adult Stutterers,* took the advice of Walle to form an umbrella organization for all the groups, and so the *National Council on Stuttering* (NCOS) was formed in 1966 (Reeves, 2006). As a unified organization, it distributed newsletters (Bloodstein, 1993) and held annual conferences (Bloodstein, 1993; Reeves, 2006). The groups were a safe place to discuss stuttering-related experiences and reflect a positive attitude about speech and self-concepts. Eventually, the NCOS memberships declined and the organization disbanded (Reeves, 2006).

Speak Easy International

In 1977, *Speak Easy International,* a nonprofit organization, was founded to empower PWS by providing a forum for mutual aid and support for one another while raising awareness about stuttering. Bob Gathman, the founder and a person who stutters, with the help of his wife, Antoinette Gathman, envisioned the Speak Easy organization (not to be confused with the in-the-ear fluency device, the SpeechEasy) as a network of self-help groups. The organization was successful in expanding from New Jersey to having groups in New York, Connecticut, and Arizona (Bloodstein, 1993), but none outside of the United States (as the full name of the organization may suggest).

Speak Easy has been hosting annual self-help conferences or "symposia" since 1981 in New Jersey. The 2½-day conferences include workshops, keynote speakers, open microphone sessions, and a banquet. The Paramus, New Jersey chapter is the only remaining active chapter. It has a website and social network group page on Facebook. Its membership consists primarily of adults.

National Stuttering Association

The National Stuttering Project, now known as the *National Stuttering Association* (NSA) is a non-profit organization that was formed to provide a forum for mutual aid and support for one another while advocating for others who stutter. It was founded in 1977 by Michael Sugarman and Bob Goldman, both PWS (Manning, 2010; Sugarman, 1999; Yaruss, Quesal, & Reeves, 2007). The organization aims to serve PWS of all ages, their family members, and the professionals that serve them.

The NSA has a website with educational information about stuttering for PWS of various ages, family of PWS, speech-language pathologists and other professionals. The website also has newsletters, past and present, including *Letting Go.* Furthermore, the website provides free printable brochures and has an online store and many other valuable resources.

The NSA has various local chapters specifically for adults, teens, and children. Today it has "nearly 200 chapters" throughout the United States (National Stuttering Association, n.d.-*a*). It also hosts self-help workshops or local workshops in various areas of the country which focus on PWS but may also have professional training workshops that may be planned the day before or as part of the workshop itself. The organization has produced an annual conference since 1984. This 3-day event includes workshops, keynote speakers, open microphone sessions, and planned social activities and finishes with an evening banquet. In recent years, this event has attracted approximately 750 to 1,000 participants per conference. Recently the NSA has offered a 2-day research symposium for professionals before its annual conference. Regional self-help conferences have also come into existence in recent years. These are options that are shorter and less expensive and offer location and time options for attendance.

In addition to the many ways that the NSA includes professionals in its self-help activities and hosts training programs for them, it also has been facilitating more interaction between PWS and professionals. It created the National Stuttering Association Research Committee (NSARC) in 1999. This committee helps to support stuttering research while protecting its members who stutter. In 2002, it also hosted a joint symposium for scientists and PWS to recognize research needs and facilitate collaboration (Yaruss & Reeves, 2002).

First Amendment, International Foundation for Stutterers

The *First Amendment* was named after the part of the U.S. Bill of Rights that addresses the rights of "freedom of speech." The group was founded in New Jersey by Elliot Dennis, a PWS, in 1980 (Berger, n.d.). This organization was originally a practice group for a fluency shaping program (Lanman, 1984). The *International Foundation for Stutterers, Inc.* (IFS) (WebMD, n.d.) was formed with the help of Edward Riordan and Mark Cosman, both PWS. The goal of the organization was to create a network of self-help practice groups. It succeeded in creating 16 groups (International Foundation for Stutterers, 1984) in the United States. Groups were independent of each other and focused on either fluency shaping programs including the Precision Fluency Shaping Program or the Air-Flow Program. As one member said, "We come here to speak fluently, not to stutter. . . . When someone has a block and is not flowing right, they get stopped" (as cited in Lanman, 1984, p. Dl).

IFS published a quarterly newsletter to keep members abreast of the news in other groups. Some groups had annual dinners, but the IFS as a whole did not have annual self-help conferences. The organization's groups were most active during the 1980s. Today there is one active group in Princeton, New Jersey (E. Dennis, personal communication, March 3, 2017).

Friends: The National Association of Young People Who Stutter

Friends—The National Association of Young People Who Stutter was founded in 1997, by John Ahlbach, former executive director of the NSA and a PWS, and Lee Caggiano, a speech-language pathologist and mother of a child who stutters. Friends is a non-profit, volunteer organization that aims to provide and foster a network of support and education for young people who stutter, including children, teenagers, and young adults, their families, and professionals who work with them.

Friends hosts nearly a dozen one-day workshops annually throughout the United States. Workshops include general sessions, break-out sessions that focus on age or relation to the PWS, and open microphones. It also hosts an annual self-help conference or "convention." Conventions are 2½-day events that include all of the same activities as the workshops but also a keynote address, planned evening activities, and a closing banquet.

The Friends website provides various forms of supporting material for young PWS family members and professionals who work with PWS. It also includes a mentoring program, in which children get support from teens who stutter. Past issues of its newsletter, *Reaching Out* (discontinued) are also available on their website.

Stuttering Association for the Young

The *Stuttering Association for the Young* (SAY) (formerly known as *Our Time Theatre Company*) was founded in New York City in 2001 by Taro Alexander, a professional actor and PWS. It is a non-profit organization that creates unique programs to provide accepting environments to help empower children who stutter to communicate their messages. It has various programs including Camp SAY, Confident Voices, and SAY Storytellers (The Stuttering Association for the Young, n.d.).

INTERNATIONAL ORGANIZATIONS FOR PEOPLE WHO STUTTER

The *International Stuttering Association* (ISA) is an umbrella organization for the world's national and international self-help organizations for PWS. This not-for-profit organization has nearly 50 registered organizations. It seeks to improve the conditions of all those whose lives are affected by stuttering in all countries in various ways, which include: sharing experiences of self-help and therapies, developing self-help movement in countries all over the world, and educating the public about stuttering (International Stuttering Association, n.d.-*a*).

The ISA has strived to develop the relationship between PWS and professionals (Manning, 2010; Yaruss & Reeves, 2002). The organization's roots can be traced back to the World Congresses of People Who Stutter. The inaugural World Congress in 1986 was held in Osaka, Japan. The conference was attended by more than 300 participants and included "speeches, symposia, workshops, laughter, singing, partying, and fun" (Bloodstein, 1993, p. 170). A declaration was adopted that called on researchers, clinicians, and PWS to broaden the communication network through publications and international conferences to help solve the problem of stuttering (Bloodstein, 1993). In 1995, during the 4th World Congress in Linkoping, Sweden, the ISA was officially founded (Pill et al., 2001). The ISA publishes a newsletter called *One Voice*, which includes information about the various self-help organizations all over the world. In 2000, the ISA in partnership with the *International Fluency Association* (IFA), sponsored the creation of the *Bill of Rights and Responsibilities of People Who Stutter* to build "a more humane, just, and compassionate world for the millions of people who stutter" (International Stuttering Association, n.d.-*b*, para. 1).

The ISA also hosts the World Congress of People Who Stutter as a triennial conference. This self-help conference is 4 days long and is attended mainly by people from the self-help community. They include workshops, keynote speakers, open microphone sessions, planned social activities, and a "Gala Dinner" or evening banquet (J. Eckardt, personal communication, July 31, 2010; M. Hoffman personal communication, July 31, 2010).

International Fluency Association

The IFA, founded in 1989, is a not-for-profit organization devoted to an "interdisciplinary approach" (IFA, 1991) "to the understanding and management of fluency disorders, and to the improvement in the quality of life for persons with fluency disorders" (IFA, n.d.).

The IFA has also played a role in improving relationships between PWS in the self-help community and the professionals who serve them (Manning, 2010; Yaruss & Reeves, 2002; Reeves, 2006). The IFA is not a self-help organization, but its membership includes professionals and PWS from the self-help community (Starkweather, as cited in De Nil, 1995; Reeves, 2006). A recent trend has shown more collaboration between the ISA and the IFA, including a joint conference with the International Cluttering Association (ICA) (International Cluttering Association, n.d.).

OBSTACLES OF IN-PERSON SELF-HELP ACTIVITIES

The self-help community for PWS has been steadily increasing over the last couple of decades. There are more organizations and more ways to connect to other PWS and more evidence to show the benefits of self-help activities for PWS. However, there is only a small percentage of PWS who take advantage of in-person self-help activities. Trichon, Tetnowski, and De Nardo (2016) list some of the likely reasons why people do not attend such activities (Table 10–1).

Table 10–1. Reasons People Do Not Attend In-Person Self-Help Activities for PWS

Lack of	Examples
Knowledge of their existence	People who stutter
	Professionals
	Parents
Willingness to attend	Resistance to self-acceptance
	Self-perception of surrendering
	Avoidance of others who stutter
	Potential utility not understood
Referrals from professionals	Knowledge of their existence
	Narrow focus on fluency
	Scarcity of research
Accessibility	Transportation time
	Transportation cost

Source: Adapted from Trichon, M., Tetnowski, J., & De Nardo, T. (2016, November). *Self-help conferences for people who stutter and the change in the speaker's experience of stuttering: Clinical implications.* Poster presented at annual conference of the American Speech-Language-Hearing Association, Philadelphia, PA.

INTERNET-BASED SELF-HELP ACTIVITIES FOR PWS

Recent data reveals that 84% of Americans use the Internet (Perrin & Duggan, 2015). With such a large number of Internet users, it is somewhat difficult to remember a time when the Internet was not as popular as it is today. This is presumably because an overwhelming majority of individuals within the United States have embraced the Internet as a valid distributor of digital content and an efficient facilitator of communication. As an ever-present part of people's daily lives, the Internet allows all of its users to access the World Wide Web for constantly evolving purposes such as education, entertainment, and everything in between.

Arguably one of the biggest highlights of the Internet is the fact that it knows no distance, in regard to miles or kilometers. Regardless of geographic location, the Internet has acted as a wide and sturdy bridge for PWS to digitally come together to meet and converse with other PWS from all over the world (Kuster, 2002; Kuster & Bowen, 2002). The ability to partake in these types of digital opportunities that allow stuttering experiences and knowledge to be easily shared with individuals, at a distance, could be considered valid proof that "the technological age is upon us and the possibilities it offers [PWS] are indeed exciting" (Packman & Meredith, 2011, p. 83).

As long as a PWS has access to an Internet connection and an Internet-enabled device such as a personal computer or a smartphone, that individual is able to start to contribute to online conversations about stuttering with peers who share that diagnosis in ways that have never been easier. This instantaneous ability to use the Internet to digitally befriend and supportively correspond with others who also stutter has been found to decrease loneliness and increase confidence (Fuse & Lanham, 2016; Raj & Daniels, 2017; Stoudt & Ouellette, 2004). PWS should consider the pros and cons of accessing Internet-based self-help activities versus accessing in-person self-help activities for PWS (Table 10–2).

Email Lists and Discussion Groups

PWS, and those interested in the subject of stuttering, have long begun to embrace the Internet as a means for obtaining information about stuttering and digitally connecting and sharing with others who stutter, in a supportive manner (Fuse & Lanham, 2016; Kuster, 1998, 2002, 2012, 2015; Kuster & Bowen, 2002; Meredith, Miller, & Simmons, 2012; Packman & Meredith, 2011; Raj & Daniels, 2017; Reitzes & Snyder 2009; Shields, 2000; Stoudt & Ouellette, 2004; Snyder, Reitzes, & Jackson, 2009; Tellis, Gabel, Smith, & Tellis, 2002). Email lists are one of the easiest ways to digitally connect and share with others on the Internet. By joining a given email list that focuses on stuttering, subscribers are able to actively participate in ongoing discussions or passively watch as discussions expand from continuous online conversations. This subscription-based digital form of peer support started to gain popularity in the later part of the 1980s and well into the 1990s. Notable email lists from that time that focused on stuttering were STUTT-L (started by C. Woodruff Starkweather), STUT-HLP (started by Robert Quesal), and STUTT-X (started by Donald Mowrer) (Kuster, 1998, 2015).

Stoudt and Ouellette (2004) were among the first researchers to subscribe to an email list that was devoted to stuttering, in an effort to better understand digital support spaces. In their analysis of over a month's worth of archival email postings (365 messages total),

Table 10–2. Pros and Cons of Internet-Based vs. In-Person Self-Help Activities for PWS

Pros	Cons
General	
No travel costs	Need Internet connection
No travel time	Need proper equipment
Variety of people (e.g. location, culture)	Difficult to meet in person
Videoconferencing	
Choose safe, quiet environment	Need to find safe, quiet location
More speaking opportunity (limited slots)	No guaranteed slot (limited slots)
More meeting times	Potential technical difficulties
Partial meetings are acceptable	

Source: Adapted from Trichon, M. (2012, November). *Stutter Social: Video chat support group.* Poster presented at annual conference of the American Speech-Language-Hearing Association, Atlanta, GA.

they found that the stuttering community within that particular email list often posted stuttering-related questions to one another as to how best to navigate the sometimes difficult speaking situations in which PWS occasionally find themselves. More often than not, the members of that online community empathetically responded to such inquiries with caring thoughts, practical advice, and other beneficial words that communicated to the person that he or she was also "in the same boat" and knew "how hard it is to face people" [during certain speaking situations]" (p. 183). Through the peer support process of digitally connecting and sharing, members of the observed email list seemed to enjoy the consistent reminder that "other people are facing the same problems" (p. 185) and that each member of the digital support group is not alone in his or her journey as a PWS.

Another online environment where PWS were able to digitally connect and share with others was through discussion groups. Sometimes referred to as "newsgroups," these online locations gained recognition around the same time as email lists. As described by Kuster (1998, 2015), this digital medium did not require people to have a subscription to it in order to be able to access the back-and-forth peer connecting and information sharing that happens within it. All one had to do was log onto a specific discussion group and that person could instantly gain access to view the stuttering-related discussions within it and could choose to add to the conversation.

The Stuttering Homepage and Key Pals

In 1995, Judith Kuster (in consultation with John Harrison, then the program director of the National Stuttering Project) launched The Stuttering Homepage (http://www.mnsu.edu/comdis/kuster/stutter.html), and it is maintained through Minnesota State University, Mankato, by Judith Kuster, professor emerita in the Department of Speech, Hearing, and Rehabilitation Services. The Stuttering Homepage was the first known website dedicated exclusively to the subject of stuttering. This public digital location, which does not require one to subscribe to it, features an impressive collection of stuttering information that is useful for people of all ages who stutter, as well as people who do not stutter but have an interest in the communication disorder (Raj & Daniels, 2017). Examples of sections that could be found on The Stuttering Homepage are direct links to some of the most popular stuttering-related email lists and discussion groups, as well as stuttering-related articles and Internet resources. Most of the content within The Stuttering Homepage is for adults to explore and consume. However, it also features sections that are specifically for young persons who stutter, which are appropriately titled *Just for Kids* and *Just for Teens* (Tellis et al., 2002).

In 1997, The Stuttering Homepage started to experiment with different ways in which PWS were able to digitally connect and share with one another for supportive purposes. One discontinued section of the website that made asynchronous support-based communication between children who stutter possible was a Web-based email directory that was titled *Key Pals*. Started in 1997 and concluded in 2012, the Key Pals page featured the first names and brief descriptions of children who stutter who were interested in engaging in email-based correspondences with other children who stutter. After signing a permission slip, with the help of a child's parent(s) and/or speech-language pathologist, children were able to submit their contact information to The Stuttering Homepage for approval to be added to the Key Pals page. Once a child's contact information was approved and live on the email directory, he or she might receive an email message from another child who stutters, and that potential support-based correspondence could be seen as "helpful for children learning to cope with stuttering, working on therapy, or simply trying to find new friends who understand what it is like to stutter" (Kuster, 2012).

The Stuttering Homepage and Chat Rooms

Another part of The Stuttering Homepage that also was started in 1997 was the chat rooms section (Kuster, 2002). Within this public online space, PWS were able to digitally connect and share with other PWS through instant messaging in real time (Shields, 2000). This synchronous support-based communication between peers who stutter was different from the Key Pals approach in that communicating to one another through email was not a real-time experience, whereas communicating to one another through the use of chat rooms was instantaneous. Tellis and colleagues (2002) highlighted a few of the chat rooms that were a part of The Stuttering Homepage. One chat room was exclusively for school-aged students who stutter to simultaneously communicate with their peers about their experiences with stuttering. Additionally, another chat room was geared more toward the parents of children who stutter. This chat room allowed for a digital support group to exist where caregivers could engage in real-time stuttering-related conversations about the children who stutter in their lives.

International Stuttering Awareness Day Online Conference

A section of The Stuttering Homepage that allows for asynchronous communication about stuttering during designated dates in October is the International Stuttering Awareness Day Online Conference. Started by Judith Kuster in 1998 and a part of The Stuttering Homepage until 2012 (now run by and a part of The International Stuttering Association), this continuous online event has been digitally bringing together PWS (and professionals) from all across the globe on an annual basis for over 15 years. Also, the online event allows PWS to digitally connect and share with professionals within the field of communication sciences and disorders. From this international meeting of the minds, new ideas and collaborations may be explored that directly relate to continuously improving the treatment of stuttering.

One of the most convenient aspects of the International Stuttering Awareness Day Online Conference is the fact that it is asynchronous in nature. The conscious decision to have the online conference be an asynchronous one came from the realization that with so many different time zones throughout the world, real-time discussions, similar to those found within the chat rooms of the late 1990s, did not seem like an optimal way to allow for stuttering-related dialogues to unfold during this event (Kuster, 2002). With currently just under two decades worth of text-based panel discussions, essays, and forums where online conference participants were encouraged to ask stuttering-related questions to their hand-picked stuttering experts through the use of online commenting, the International Stuttering Awareness Day Online Conference could be seen as one of the first and longest running online support communities for PWS.

Blogs

Around the turn of the 21st century, weblogs, more commonly known as "blogs," started to become prevalent. Blogs are personal websites that typically revolve around a central topic and are usually run by a sole individual. Blogs allow those on the Internet to be able to write informal commentary on whatever the chosen topic is in a way where each entry is date-stamped and appears in reverse chronological order. Through blogging, which is the act of continuously writing on a personal blog, writers can publish their thoughts and feelings online in a public manner as a way to digitally connect and share with an audience of like-minded readers at any point in time (Embrey, 2002). Digitally connecting and sharing on a personal blog is different from the experience of being a part of the International Stuttering Awareness Day Online Conference because a personal blog usually has an ongoing writing schedule and is not limited to a writing schedule that only occurs during a single month.

The growth of blogging was so apparent in the earlier part of the 2000s that the Merriam-Webster dictionary declared the word "blog" its "Word of the Year" in 2004, and by 2009, roughly 1 out of every 10 adult Internet users had a personal blog (Lenhart, Purcell, Smith, & Zickuhr, 2010). With this substantial number of people on the Internet choosing to start blogs, it only makes sense that PWS would adopt blogging as a way to gain support by digitally connecting and sharing with others who also stutter, through the process of writing online. For many PWS, online writing is seen as a valuable experience that often allows them to be able to communicate freely without any perceived judgment (Stoudt & Ouellette, 2004). A list of stuttering-related blogs is included in Table 10–3.

One trait that all of the highlighted stuttering-related blogs have in common is that they contain writings that are honest and down-to-earth. Each of the authors, in his or her specific style of writing, shares stories about growing up as a PWS and how stuttering has had an impact on the lives they live. The writing of the bloggers is often seen as courageous because of their willingness to share a great deal about their communication successes and setbacks. Through writing in their respective blogs, they are able to chronicle their journeys in an authentic way.

Generally speaking, starting blogs and consuming the writings within blogs could be seen as a useful and supportive exercise because it allows both writers and readers the opportunity to reflect on published thoughts and feelings on the Internet (Ferdig & Trammell, 2004). For example, from those reflections, supportive conversations could occur within a blog's public comments section. Additionally, a less public and more private one-on-one supportive conversation could transpire between a reader and a writer because readers

Table 10–3. Stuttering-Related Blogs

Blog Name	Blog Link
Stuttering Is Cool	http://stutteringiscool.com/
Stutter Rock Star	http://stutterrockstar.com/
The Stuttering Foundation's Blog	http://stutteringhelp.org/blog
The Stuttering Brain	http://thestutteringbrain.blogspot.ie/
Katherine Preston's Blog	http://katherinepreston.com/blog/
Stuttering Student	http://stutteringstudent.blogspot.ie/

typically have the option to digitally connect and share with writers via email to further comment and converse about a given piece of writing that appears on a blog. For PWS, actively writing on the Internet for everyone to see, and reflecting on those writings, might prove to help them to be better able to define and/or redefine what stuttering means to them and how it has played a role in shaping their lives.

Podcasts

As the first decade of the 2000s progressed and PWS kept on blogging, the Internet continued to expand as a supportive space that allowed for any and all individuals to digitally connect and share with each other in ways other than writing. Audio-based blogging, most commonly known as "podcasting," allows a person's voice, in the form of an audio file, to be front and center during an instance of sharing that occurs on the World Wide Web. An audio podcast is a user-created audio file that is made available for download on the Internet (Beamish & Brown, 2012). Podcasting dates back to around 2004 and the word "podcast" is a neologism derived from the words "pod" and "broadcast," as in iPod, the line of portable media players designed and marketed by Apple Inc. (Hobson, 2012). Since 2008, there has been a steady increase in Americans who listen to podcasts (Vogt, 2016).

Thanks to audio podcasting, PWS are able to realize that digitally connecting and sharing on the Internet does not necessarily have to be an exclusively visual experience that centers solely on written words. Spoken words can be the focus. Because of increased Internet speeds, improved computer operating systems, newly invented media and mobile devices, and more affordable computer equipment, a number of PWS are choosing to digitally share online, not just by typing their words on a keyboard, but by using their own voice to speak their words directly into a microphone during an audio podcasting recording session. Regardless of their stuttering severity, a number of PWS are digitally creating and sharing audio files in an effort to distribute stuttering information to the masses (Snyder et al., 2009). Audio podcasting is one of the ways that PWS are able to use the Internet to actively talk about talking through the use of their own talking voice.

One of the most popular stuttering podcasts on the Internet is StutterTalk (http://www.stuttertalk.com/). This podcast was started in 2007 by Peter Reitzes, Eric Jackson, and Greg Snyder and has since published more than 600 episodes. It frequently highlights in-depth interviews with PWS, researchers, speech-language pathologists, leaders in the self-help community, and others (StutterTalk, n.d.). Examples of StutterTalk episodes include discussion on topics such as voluntary stuttering, covert stuttering, speaking strategies, acceptance, the role of religion in therapy, talking to parents about stuttering, and more. As described by the creators of StutterTalk, "listeners hear us stutter and hear us talking about stuttering from healthy, open, and honest perspectives" (Snyder et al., 2009, p. 89).

It is often mentioned throughout episodes of StutterTalk how listeners can leave comments or reviews about the audio podcast, as well as send any questions to the hosts of StutterTalk. Additionally, PWS have the ability to leave a voicemail message at any point in time by visiting a link in the contact section of the StutterTalk website. Sometimes, these voicemail messages are played on the show and bits of content within the voicemail message are used to start a new episode topic. These are examples of how PWS are able to digitally connect and share with other individuals who are a part of the StutterTalk community, in whatever way they feel most comfortable (Reitzes & Snyder, 2009).

Arguably because of audio podcasts such as StutterTalk, others have emerged to increase the number of stuttering-related audio podcasts and the overall variety of these audio-driven programs focused on discussions about communication. Two such examples are the *Stuttering Is Cool* podcast by Daniele Rossi (http://www.stutteringiscool.com/stuttering-is-cool-podcast/) and the *Women Who Stutter* podcast by Pamela Mertz (http://www.stutterrockstar.com/), which both exist on their own designated websites. These audio podcasts have created a valid support space online where PWS are encouraged to digitally connect and share with the hosts and guests through the use of commenting on the specific website that the audio podcast is featuring and emailing the hosts and guests with any feedback.

Vlogs

Video blogging, sometimes referred to as "vlogging," is similar to podcasting, in that they both allow people to use their own voices to speak about something and share that message with peers through the use of the Internet. However, vlogging differs because it goes beyond audio and includes a visual channel that allows an online audience to not only hear the voice of the speaker, but also see the face. Because of the multiple sensory channels that are in place within a video, a greater feeling of social contact and presence might be attached to the overall experience (Harley & Fitzpatrick, 2009). Audio podcasters usually just utilize their microphones to highlight their voices as means to deliver their chosen topics of conversation, but those who participate in vlogging go one step further by turning on a video camera not only to record their verbal output, but also to capture all of the visual suprasegmental aspects of speech that are in the camera frame. With this in mind, the audio-visual vlogging experience could be considered to be a more rich form of Internet-based communication, compared with audio podcasting or text-based blogging.

For over a decade since its launch in 2005, YouTube has been the premier video-sharing social media website that is currently the second most visited destination on the Internet, globally (Alexa Internet, 2017). With over a billion users, which are equal to almost one-third of all people on the Internet, individuals from all over the world are spending countless hours discovering, watching, and sharing user-created videos (YouTube, n.d.). Specific YouTube user videos that could be of interest for PWS to explore are by The Stuttering Foundation (https://www.youtube.com/user/stutteringfdn) and the National Stuttering Association (https://www.youtube.com/user/NSAsitevideos). Both of these YouTube user accounts are attached to large non-profit organizations that are exclusively dedicated to helping PWS through support, education, advocacy, and research. The videos that can be found within both users' accounts feature a variety of PWS who speak candidly about their experiences with stuttering.

YouTube contains numerous ways that easily allow all of its users to digitally connect and share with one another. Viewers can post open text–based or video comments onto a video's page as a public response to it. Viewers can also post closed text–based messages to the person who posted the video as a private response. In all of these instances, the commenting feature allows users to directly communicate to the individual who has uploaded the given video. Presumably, if a person who stutters views a video of another person who stutters that is sharing information about his or her stuttering journey, both people could directly communicate to one another through comments to ask questions and further expand thoughts and ideas that were within the initially viewed video.

Social Media Websites

Another feature that YouTube has in place is the ability to easily share a YouTube video through a handful of direct share links to some of the most popular social media websites that a user might also be a part of (e.g., Facebook, Twitter, LinkedIn). This is a key option to have in place because 65% of adult Internet users in the United States actively use social networking websites (Perrin, 2015). Similarly, about 76% of PWS actively participate in stuttering communities online that exist within social media websites (Raj & Daniels, 2017), and over 50% of PWS stated that they did so several times a day (Fuse & Lanham, 2016; Raj & Daniels, 2017). This major adoption of social media by PWS begins to paint the picture that there seems to be something special about coming together, as PWS, within a social media website to digitally connect and share with other PWS.

Changes in PWS as a Result of Engaging in Social Media Websites

In one of the first research studies that looked specifically at 42 PWS and their thoughts about digitally connecting and sharing within social media websites with other PWS, Raj and Daniels (2016) were able to discover a number of positive findings. For one, the self-esteem levels of PWS were significantly higher after being a part of an online community for PWS. Participants from that study went from feeling fearful to fearless and they transitioned from feeling helpless to helpful. Additionally, the PWS were able to communicate how their levels of support significantly spiked after being a part of a stuttering-focused online community. Those individuals went from feeling insecure to confident and went from experiencing loneliness to camaraderie.

Similar findings were revealed in work done by Fuse and Lanham (2016) that looked at the impact of social media website usage on the quality of life of 96 PWS. One-third of the participants from that study agreed or strongly agreed with the statement "social media has improved my overall confidence." Additionally, a majority of participants agreed or strongly agreed that digitally connecting and sharing with other PWS via social media websites has been a positive and helpful experience. These findings begin to suggest that social media websites, and the intentional communication that comes as a result of being a part of the communities that are within those websites, may play a substantial role in the lives of some PWS.

Videoconferencing Communities

Videoconferencing communities provide a structure for virtual meetings, including schedules and hosts. In this medium, a videoconferencing platform is used to connect PWS in which users may see and hear each other synchronously. Users need a computer or mobile device with a webcam and a microphone to participate. Participants can remain anonymous by turning off their video and/or audio. Links to the scheduled virtual meeting can be posted on the community's website or on social networking groups (Trichon, in press).

Stutter Social is a videoconferencing community that was conceptualized and brought to life by Mitchell Trichon, David Resnick, and Daniele Rossi in 2011 (Stutter Social, n.d.). About a year after it was conceptualized and tested on a Skype platform, Google, Inc. released Google+, a social networking platform which allowed for, among other tools, a multi-person instant messaging, text, and video chat platform called *Hangouts*, which allowed for simultaneous one-on-one video chats or group video chats for up to 10 people (Erkollar & Obeyer, 2011; Gundotra, 2011; Lytle, 2013). In 2015, Stutter Social also introduced a stand-alone private social network application. PWS need to request access online (bit.ly/getstuttersocial).

Stutter Social's video conference meetings are facilitated by volunteer hosts who have demonstrated some form of leadership in one or more mediums of self-help for PWS (Stutter Social, n.d.). Meetings vary from talking about stuttering-related topics to having everyday conversations not related to stuttering (Stutter Social, n.d.). Despite being at a distance and being digital, this type of interaction has similarities to non-digital, face-to-face self-help group meetings (Trichon & Tetnowski, 2011; Yaruss et al., 2002).

As described by Trichon and Tetnowski (2011), similarities between non-digital, face-to-face self-help groups and digital ones can be found in both of the experiences' abilities to allow PWS to converse and build friendships with other PWS. As described by one member who partakes in both non-digital and digital self-help experiences, it was mentioned that "it's so beneficial to be able to reach out to someone else who stutters [either in-person or online] when I've had a difficult day and just need to vent. I know they will understand." (Luckman, 2015) Additionally, PWS are finding benefit in being affiliated with both non-digital and digital self-help groups. Members of both types of communities have confessed that they look forward to being a part of them and that, with digital self-help groups, they "religiously read every post" (Trichon & Tetnowski, 2011, p. 292).

Virtual Reality Environments

Videoconferencing is not the only way that like-minded individuals can digitally come together, via the Internet, to synchronously talk about a topic of interest. Digital communities that exist within online virtual reality spaces are starting to gain traction and seem to show promise as locations where PWS can digitally connect and share with one another. Virtual reality has been described as a "tantalizing communication medium whose essence challenges our most deeply held notions of what communication is or can be" (Biocca & Levy, 1995, p. vii). Those who choose to take part in virtual reality experiences are willingly putting themselves into a computer-simulated world for a portion of their day to form and foster relationships with others, through various forms of communication.

It has been found that the lives of PWS were enhanced after participating within an Internet-based, three-dimensional virtual environment (Brundage, 2007), such as Second Life (Meredith et al., 2012; Packman & Meredith, 2011). Second Life is one of the leading virtual reality–centered websites. It started in 2003 and is described as a free online, computer-simulated environment where millions of people are represented by avatars online (Stewart, Hansen, & Carey, 2010). As described by Meredith et al. (2012), an avatar is a digital depiction of a user that can enable a person to interact and synchronously communicate with other Second Life members in a simulated, real-world environment. Communication in this virtual world can range from text to graphical icons, to visual gestures and voice.

Through the described three-dimensional experience that virtual reality environments allow, PWS can communicate with other PWS without leaving the physical location that they are in (Packman & Meredith, 2011). Meredith and colleagues (2012) described two ways in which PWS could benefit from virtual reality environments. Simulation and support group experiences were described as a pair of valid ways for at-a-distance interactions between PWS to take place. Within a simulation experience, a person who stutters could verbally practice numerous speaking techniques with others during a virtual role-playing session that may help the individual feel more confident and comfortable as a communicator, as well as possibly decrease a communicator's anxiety (Walkom, 2016) and distress levels (Brundage, Brinton, & Hancock, 2016). Examples of role-playing sessions that have been explored within a three-dimensional medium include answering questions at a job interview, ordering food at a restaurant, and speaking on the telephone. Through the intentional role-playing within the digital world, desensitization of commonly feared physical world situations could start to find its way into the minds and hearts of some PWS.

After simulation scenarios are attempted, PWS are able to engage in a support group experience to digitally discuss their perceptions of how they did. As mentioned by Meredith and colleagues (2012), the self-support structures that allow for support group experiences within Second Life include digital meeting rooms. Digital meeting rooms are equipped with interactive whiteboards (potentially for writing out thoughts and feelings that relate to being a person who stutters) and World Wide Web capabilities (potentially for referencing a specific website or streaming an online video that relates to stuttering). This description of how a digital support group could operate within a three-dimensional medium is yet another example that illustrates the new and exciting ways that PWS can gain stuttering support from other PWS through the use of the Internet.

CHALLENGES ASSOCIATED WITH DIGITALLY CONNECTING AND SHARING ONLINE

Research unrelated to PWS has shown that individuals who use the Internet to digitally connect and share with others have reported occasionally using fake usernames in the past or admitted to impersonating someone else on a given website (Wang, Norice, & Cranor, 2011). Also, electronic aggression, or online cyberbullying, seems to be a growing trend among school-aged children (Law, Shapka, Hymel, Olson, & Waterhouse, 2012). These instances raise concern for individuals' safety while interacting and digitally sharing thoughts, feelings, experiences, and information on the Internet. Ideally, websites used by PWS who are looking to digitally connect, befriend, and share with others who may or may not stutter should have restricted access and be monitored to ensure that all individuals truly are who they say they are (Packman & Meredith, 2011). Security measures might prove to be important because one could imagine how a virtual trespasser or "troll" may pose a threat to the safe environment provided by the participants. This could certainly compromise the self-help forum.

An unexpected situation might arise and harm a person who stutters because it could cause feelings of betrayal and trigger other negative emotions and situations. However, because the Internet is generally an open-access area, proper verification of all Internet users to ensure safety could prove difficult. One must practice good judgment and learn to be cautious when consuming content found on the Internet and interacting with others online (Kuster & Bowen, 2002). It is critical that "newbies" to online communities use caution while becoming more accustomed to this type of digital environment.

In addition to safety, people should consider the credibility of the online locations and/or people when exploring the Internet and digitally connecting and sharing with others who stutter. These individuals must be aware that not all thoughts are helpful, and can even be harmful, and that not all information digitally shared online is accurate. For example, sometimes PWS are brought up in a certain type of culture and might have been exposed to false information, or myths, about stuttering (Kuster, 1999; Robinson & Crowe, 1998) and may distribute this false information unintentionally. However, some individuals may deliberately deceive or scam those with various medical conditions or disorders by falsely promoting a "miracle" cure (Wahlberg, 2007). Therefore, it is imperative that new users of the Internet and online communities investigate the stuttering information being shared before fully committing to its authenticity. PWS should be encouraged to consult speech-language pathologists who hold a Certificate of Clinical Competence from the American Speech-Language-Hearing Association about any claims that are being posted about stuttering theories, information, and treatment (Tellis et al., 2002).

Lastly, as the world continues to welcome the Internet with open arms, it is not uncommon to hear of individuals who have developed unhealthy addictions to the Internet. There are only so many hours in a day, and some individuals tend to spend too much time online. Time spent on "digital life" activities, such as surfing the Internet or constantly checking Internet messages, can detract from "real-life" activities. This could be the start of a habit that leads to numerous non-beneficial situations. As Barnes (1996) mentioned, workers could begin to neglect their jobs, students could fall behind on assignments, and romantic partners could start to ignore each other. Individuals who develop this type of addiction "spend enormous amounts of time on the net inventing personas and establishing what appears to be electronic friendships. But in reality, the technology becomes a dysfunctional codependency" (p. 35). Like all things in life, moderation is key, and it is essential that PWS who use the Internet to digitally connect and share with other PWS be aware of the possibilities of becoming addicted to the Internet.

In short, the Internet brings a new dimension to the world of self-help and should be explored with curiosity and caution. Because of the Internet, "even the smallest subpopulation [PWS] has instant access to digitized content that directly serves their interests and needs" (Reitzes & Snyder, 2009, p. 33). Thankfully, it contains a myriad of online self-help and support resources for PWS. It allows them to connect and collaborate in ways that directly impact the way they view themselves and their quality of life. As the Internet and related digital technologies continue to evolve, it can further advance the self-help experience of PWS, making it more beneficial for the stuttering community.

CONCLUSION

The purpose of this chapter was to highlight the history and benefits of a wide variety of self-help organizations and Internet-based self-help activities that PWS have engaged in over the years. Because of the accessibility of these types of peer-support experiences, PWS are now able to see, with clarity, that they are not alone. As stated by a member of the stuttering community who is involved in both in-person and Internet-based self-help experiences, "we show up for each other . . . for shame cannot live in the light of day, in the warmth of empathy, of someone saying, 'Me too.'" (Najman, 2015) This ability to truly see and understand the power of a supportive community helps the overall quality of life of PWS. Whether a person who stutters chooses to start conversations during an organized meeting, where all parties involved are physically in the same location, or whether a person who stutters chooses to start conversations within an Internet-based location where all parties involved are worldwide, the one thing that remains constant is the communication in general. Conversations are being started by PWS and through those conversations, individuals are able to turn to their peers for support during any and all life moments that relate to stuttering specifically, and life in general.

In no way are we suggesting that peer support should take the place of speech-language therapy for stuttering. On the contrary, the self-help organizations and Internet-based self-help activities described throughout this chapter are best explored in tandem with speech-language therapy. There is a positive correlation between peer support and the successes achieved in speech-language therapy for stuttering, in that PWS who are active in peer-support activities are more likely to consider therapy successful (McClure, 2009). The evidence for peer support shows that it is valid in its intention to positively impact those who take part in it. Therefore, it is recommended that clinicians make a conscious decision to assist their clients who stutter in becoming more aware of the numerous self-help and peer-support possibilities that are available to them.

RESOURCES FOR PEOPLE WHO STUTTER

Refer to Table 10–4.

Table 10–4. Resources for People Who Stutter

Organization Name	Website Address
National Stuttering Association (NSA)	westutter.org
Friends	friendswhostutter.org
Stuttering Association for the Young (SAY)	say.org
The Stuttering Foundation	stutteringhelp.org
Stutter Social	stuttersocial.com
International Stuttering Association	isastutter.org
The Stuttering Homepage	stutteringhomepage.com
Stutter Talk	stuttertalk.com

REFERENCES

Adamsen, L., & Rasmussen, J. M. (2001). Sociological perspectives on self-help groups: Reflections on conceptualization and social processes. *Journal of Advanced Nursing*, *35*(6), 909–917.

Alcoholics Anonymous. (n.d.). *Historical data: The birth of A.A. and its growth in the U.S. and Canada.* Retrieved from http://www.aa.org/pages/en_US/historical-data-the-birth-of-aa-and-its-growth-in-the-uscanada

Alexa Internet. (2017). The top 500 sites on the web—February 12. *Alexa Internet.* Retrieved February 26, 2017 from http://www.alexa.com/topsites/global

American Speech-Language-Hearing Association. (2017). *History of ASHA.* Retrieved from http://www.asha.org/about/history.htm

Banks, E. (2000, Summer). Self-help and the new health agenda. Self-help 2000. *The Newsletter of the National Self-Help Clearinghouse.*

Barnes, S. B. (1996). Internet relationships: The bright and the dark sides of cyber-friendship. *Telektronikk*, *96*(1), 26–39.

Beamish, P., & Brown, J. (2012). Podcasting in the classroom: A case study. *TEACH Journal of Christian Education*, *2*(2), 21–23.

Berger, A. (n.d.). Support members share knowledge and experience. *News Tribune*, Freehold, NJ. East Norriton, PA: International Foundation for Stutterers Archives.

Biocca, F., & Levy, M. R. (Eds) (1995). *Communication in the age of virtual reality.* Hillsdale, NJ: Erlbaum.

Bloodstein, O. (1993). *Stuttering: The search for a cause and cure.* Boston, MA: Allyn & Bacon.

Bloom, C., & Cooperman, D. (1999). *Synergistic stuttering therapy: A holistic approach.* Woburn, MA: Butterworth-Heinemann.

Borkman, T. (1999). *Understanding self-help/mutual aid: Experiential learning in the commons.* New Brunswick, NJ: Rutgers University Press.

Boyle, M. P. (2013). Psychological characteristics and perceptions of stuttering of adults who stutter with and without support group experience. *Journal of Fluency Disorders 38*(4), 368–381.

Brundage, S. B. (2007). Virtual reality augmentation for functional assessment and treatment of stuttering. *Topics in Language Disorders, 27*(3), 254–271.

Brundage, S. B., Brinton, J. M., & Hancock, A. B. (2016). Utility of virtual reality environments to examine physiological reactivity and subjective distress in adults who stutter. *Journal of Fluency Disorders, 50,* 85–95.

Carlisle, J. (1987). Self-help groups and client perception. *Human Communication Canada, 3,* 23–27.

Damen, S., Mortelmans, D., & Van Hove, E. (2000). Self-help groups in Belgium: Their place in the care network. *Sociology of Health and Illness, 22,* 331–348.

Davison, K. P., Pennebaker, J. W., & Dickerson, S. S. (2000). Who talks? The social psychology of illness support groups. *American Psychologist, 55*(2), 205–217.

De Nil, L. F. (1995). Interview with Dr. C. Woodruff Starkweather, fifth president-elect of the International Fluency Association. *Journal of Fluency Disorders, 20*(3), 303–313.

Diggs, C. C. (1990). Self-help for communication disorders. *ASHA, 32*(1), 32–34.

Education: Ex-stammerers. (1938, May 16). *Time, 31*(21). Retrieved from http://content.time.com/time/subscriber/article/0,33009,759702,00.html

Embrey, T. R. (2002). You blog, we blog: A guide to how teacher-librarians can use weblogs to build communication and research skills. *Teacher Librarian, 30*(2), 7–9.

Emerick, R. E. (1996). Mad liberation: The sociology of knowledge and the ultimate civil rights movement. *Journal of Mind and Behavior, 17*(2), 135–159.

Erkollar, A., & Oberer, B. (2011, December). Trends in social media application: The potential of Google+ for education shown in the example of a Bachelor's degree course on marketing. In *International Conference on Advanced Software Engineering and Its Applications* (pp. 569–578). Berlin/Heidelberg, Germany: Springer.

Ferdig, R. E., & Trammell, K. D. (2004). Content delivery in the 'Blogosphere'. *T.H.E. Journal Online: Technological Horizons in Education, 31*(7), 12–20.

Fraser, M. (1978). *Self-therapy for the stutterer* (1st ed.). Memphis, TN: Stuttering Foundation of America. Publication 0012.

Fraser, M. (2010). *Self-therapy for the stutterer* (11th ed.). Memphis, TN: Stuttering Foundation of America. Publication 0012. Retrieved from http://www.stutteringhelp.org/sites/default/files/Migrate/book0012_11th_ed.pdf

Fuse, A., & Lanham, E. A. (2016). Impact of social media and quality life of people who stutter. *Journal of Fluency Disorders, 50,* 59–71.

Gathman, B. (1986). Clarifying the focus and function of self-help. *The Speak Easy Newsletter, 6,* 5–6.

Gundotra, V. (June 28, 2011). *Introducing the Google+ project: Real-life sharing, rethought for the Web.* Google Official Blog. Google.

Hale, P. J. (2012). Darwin's other bulldog: Charles Kingsley and the popularization of evolution in Victorian England. *Science & Education, 21*(7), 977–1014. doi:10.1007/s11191-011-9414-8

Harley, D., & Fitzpatrick, G. (2009). Creating a conversational context through video blogging: A case study of Geriatric1927. *Computers in Human Behavior, 25*(3), 679–689.

Hobson, J. (2012). How I use it: Podcasts. *Occupational Medicine, 62*(5), 394.

Hunt, B. (1987). Self-help for stutterers—experience in Britain. In L. Rustin, H. Purser, & D. Rowley (Eds.), *Progress in the treatment of fluency disorders* (pp. 198–214). London, UK: Taylor & Francis.

International Cluttering Association. (n.d.). *Revised mission.* Retrieved from http://associations.missouristate.edu/ICA/

International Fluency Association. (n.d.). *Our mission*. Retrieved from http://www.theifa.org/

International Fluency Association. (1991). International Fluency Association founding articles, *Journal of Fluency Disorders*, *76*(1), 79–84.

International Foundation for Stutterers, Inc. (1984). I.F.S. self-help speech groups. *Look Who's Talking 1*(2), p. 2.

International Stuttering Association. (n.d.-*a*). Retrieved February 26, 2017 from http://www.isastutter.org/

International Stuttering Association. (n.d.-*b*). *Bill of rights and responsibilities of people who stutter*. Retrieved February 26, 2017 from http://www.isastutter.org/bill-of-rights-and-responsibilities

Katz, A. H., & Bender, E. I. (1976). Self-help groups in western society—history and prospects. *Journal of Applied Behavioral Science*, *12*(3), 265–282.

Klein, J. P., Jackson, E. S., & Caggiano, L. (2015). A questionnaire for parents of children who stutter attending a self-help convention. *Perspectives on Fluency and Fluency Disorders 25*, 10–21.

Kuster, J. (1998). Internet resources about stuttering. *The Stuttering Homepage*. Retrieved February 26, 2017 from http://www.mnsu.edu/comdis/isad/papers/kuster.html

Kuster, J. (1999). Folk myths about stuttering. *The Stuttering Homepage*. Retrieved from http://www.mnsu.edu/comdis/kuster/Infostuttering/folkmyths.html

Kuster, J. (2002). Online conferences: A new way to reach out and around the world. *ACQuiring Knowledge in Speech, Language and Hearing*, *4*(2), 86–89.

Kuster, J. (2012). Key pals. *The Stuttering Homepage*. Retrieved February 26, 2017 from http://www.mnsu.edu/comdis/kuster/kids/keypals.html

Kuster, J. (2015). Discussion forums. *The Stuttering Homepage*. Retrieved February 26, 2017, from http://www.mnsu.edu/comdis/kuster/Internet/Listserv.html

Kuster, J., & Bowen, C. (2002). Fluency and fluency disorders on the Web. *ACQuiring Knowledge in Speech, Language and Hearing*, *4*(2), 75–77.

Lanman, S. (1984, October 23). Stutterers lead life of nightmare and frustration. *The Home*. News, p. ID.

Law, D. M., Shapka, J. D., Hymel, S., Olson, B. F., & Waterhouse, T. (2012). The changing face of bullying: An empirical comparison between traditional and Internet bullying and victimization. *Computers in Human Behavior*, *28*(1), 226–232.

Leff, D. (2008). *AboutDarwin.com: Dedicated to the life and times of Charles Darwin*. Retrieved from https://www.aboutdarwin.com/about_01.html

Lenhart, A., Purcell, K., Smith, A., & Zickuhr, K. (2010). Social media and young adults. *Pew Internet & American Life Project*. Retrieved from http://www.pewinternet.org/2010/02/03/social-media-and-young-adults/

Luckman, C. (2015). *The real me*. Retrieved from http://isad.isastutter.org/isad-2015/papers-presented-by-2015/stories-and-experiences-with-stuttering-by-pws/the-real-me/

Lytle, R. (2013). *The beginner's guide to Google+*. New York, NY: Mashable.

Manning, W. H. (2010). *Clinical decision making in fluency disorders* (3rd ed.). Clifton Park, NY: Delmar Cengage Learning.

McClure, J. (2009). *The experience of people who stutter: A survey by the National Stuttering Association*. Retrieved from http://www.mnsu.edu/comdis/isad12/papers/mcclure12.html

McClure, J., D'Amico, R., & Tetnowski, J. (2009). *The experience of people who stutter: A survey by the National Stuttering Association*. Retrieved from http://www.WeStutter.org

Medvene, L. J., Wituk, S., & Luke, D. A. (1999). Characteristics of self-help group leaders: The significance of professional and founder statuses. *International Journal of Self Help and Self Care*, *7*(1), 91–105.

Meredith, G., Miller, C., & Simmons, G. (2012). Stuttering support and nursing education. In R. Hinrichs & C. Wankel (Eds.), *Engaging the avatar: New frontiers in immersive education* (pp. 217–254). Charlotte, NC: Information Age.

Merriam-Webster. (2004). *2004 word of the year*. Press release. Retrieved from https://www.merriam-webster.com/press-release/2004-word-of-the-year

Najman, H. (2015). *Streets of shame*. Retrieved from http://isad.isastutter.org/isad-2015/papers-presented-by-2015/stories-and-experiences-with-stuttering-by-pws/streets-of-shame/

National Stuttering Association. (n.d.-*a*). Homepage. Retrieved from http://www.westutter.org

National Stuttering Association. (n.d.-*b*). *NSA fall retreat*. Retrieved from http://www.westutter.org/nsa-fall-retreat/

Packman, A., & Meredith, G. (2011). Technology and the evolution of clinical methods for stuttering. *Journal of Fluency Disorders, 36*, 75–85.

Perrin, A. (2015). *Social media usage: 2005–2015. Pew Research Center: Internet, Science & Tech.* Retrieved from http://www.pewinternet.org/2015/10/08/social-networking-usage-2005–2015/

Perrin, A., & Duggan, M. (2015). *Americans' Internet Access: 2000-2015. Pew Research Center: Internet, Science & Tech.* Retrieved from http://www.pewinternet.org/2015/06/26/americans-internet-access-2000-2015/

Pill, J., Ravid, B., Irwin, M., Hoffmann, S., De Vloed, M., Krall, T., & Hoffman, M. (2001). *International Stuttering Association*. Paper presented at the International Stuttering Awareness Day Online Conference, 2001. Retrieved from http://www.mnsu.edu/comdis/isad4/papers/pill.html

Plexico, L., Manning, W. H., & DiLollo, A. (2005). A phenomenological understanding of successful stuttering management. *Journal of Fluency Disorders, 30*(1), 1–22.

Ramig, P. (1993). The impact of self-help groups on persons who stutter: A call for research. *Journal of Fluency Disorders, 18*, 351–361.

Raj, E. X., & Daniels, D. E. (2017). Psychosocial support for adults who stutter: Exploring the role of online communities. *Speech, Language, and Hearing, 20*(3), 144–153.

Reeves, L. (2006). The role of self-help/mutual aid in addressing the needs of individuals who stutter. In N. B. Ratner & J. A. Tetnowski (Eds.), *Current issues in stuttering research and practice* (pp. 255–278). Mahwah, NJ: Erlbaum.

Reitzes, P., & Snyder, G. (2009). The infusion of interactive digital media with self-help and stuttering treatment. *SIG 4 Perspectives on Fluency and Fluency Disorders, 19*(1), 28–38.

Richardson, A., & Goodman, M. (1983). *Self-help and social care: Mutual aid organisations in practice.* London, UK: Policy Studies Institute.

Riessman, F. (2000). Self-help comes of age. *Social Policy, 30*, 47–49.

Robinson, T. L., & Crowe, T. A. (1998). Culture-based considerations in programming for stuttering intervention with African American clients and their families. *Language, Speech, and Hearing Sciences in Schools, 29*, 172–179.

Romeder, J.-M. (1990). *The self-help way: Mutual aid and health.* Ottawa, Canada: Canadian Council on Social Development.

Shields, L. (2000). Using the Internet with children who stutter. *The Stuttering Homepage.* Retrieved from http://www.mnsu.edu/comdis/ISAD3/papers/shields2.html

Smith, J. S. (1925). *J. S. Smith School for Stuttering.* Memphis, TN: Malcolm Fraser Archives at the Stuttering Foundation.

Snyder, G., Reitzes, P., & Jackson, E. (2009). Digital audio and self-help for people who stutter. *Journal of Stuttering Therapy, Advocacy & Research, 3*, 88–89.

Stammering (1925, April 24). [Advertisement]. *The Evening Journal.* Wilmington, DE. p. 26

Stammerers' club is branching out. (1926, April 4). *The Philadelphia Record.*

Stammerers deliver fluent after-dinner speeches here. (1929, December 26). *Evening Bulletin*, p. 33.

Stammerers hold dinner: Kingsley club members all make speeches at gathering here. (1930, February 9). *New York Times*, p. N7.

Starkweather, C. W., & Givens-Ackerman, J. (1997). *Stuttering.* Austin, TX.: ProEd.

Stoudt, B. G., & Ouellette, S. C. (2004). Making room for words: People who stutter on the Internet. *Qualitative Research in Psychology, 1*(3), 175–194.

Stuttering Association for the Young (n.d.). Homepage. Retrieved from http://www.say.org/

Stuttering Foundation. (n.d.-*a*). *The early years Malcolm Fraser: One person can make a difference* [PowerPoint Slides]. Retrieved from http://www.stutteringhelp.org/sites/default/files/OnePersonMadeADifference.pdf

Stuttering Foundation. (n.d.-*b*). *Mission statement.* Retrieved from http://www.stutteringhelp.org/mission-statement

StutterTalk. (n.d.). *About.* Retrieved from http://stuttertalk.com/about/

Stutter Social. (n.d.). *About.* Retrieved from http://stuttersocial.com/about.php

Sugarman, M. (1999). *Overview and brief history of the National Stuttering Association.* Retrieved from http://www.mnsu.edu/comdis/isad2/papers/sugarman2.html

Surgeon General Workshop on Self-Help and Public Health. (1988). U.S. Department of Health and Human Services, Public Health Services, Health Resources and Service Administration, Bureau of Maternal Health and Child Health and Resources Development Publication no. 224–250. Washington, DC: U.S. Government Printing Office.

Tellis, G. M., Gabel, R. M., Smith, D., & Tellis, C. M. (2002). Information about stuttering on the Internet: A resource for school speech-language pathologists. *Contemporary Issues in Communication Science and Disorders, 29,* 165–172.

Tetnowski, J., & Azios, M. & (2013, November). *The impact of self-help: A parental perspective.* An oral session presented at the American Speech and Hearing Association annual conference, Chicago, IL.

Tetnowski, J. A., & McClure, J. A. (2009). *Executive summary of 2009 Survey.* Seminar presented at the annual conference of the National Stuttering Association, Phoenix, AZ.

Trichon, M. (2010). *Self-help conferences for people who stutter: An interpretive phenomenological analysis* (Doctoral dissertation). Retrieved from http://gradworks.umi.com/3446333.pdf

Trichon, M. (2012, November). *Stutter social: Video chat support group.* Poster presented at annual conference of the American Speech-Language-Hearing Association, Atlanta, GA.

Trichon, M. (in press). Self-help groups. In J. S. Damico & M. J. Ball (Eds.), *Encyclopedia of human communication sciences and disorders.* Thousand Oaks, CA: Sage.

Trichon, M. (2017). Self-help conferences for people who stutter: First-timers and the change in the speaker's experience of stuttering for adults, teens, and school-age children—OASES data (unpublished raw data).

Trichon, M., & Tetnowski, J. (2011). Self-help conferences for people who stutter: A qualitative investigation. *Journal of Fluency Disorders, 36,* 290–295.

Trichon, M., Tetnowski, J., & De Nardo, T. (2016, November). *Self-help conferences for people who stutter and the change in the speaker's experience of stuttering: Clinical implications.* Workshop conducted at annual conference of the American Speech-Language-Hearing Association, Philadelphia, PA.

Trichon, M., Tetnowski, J., & Rentschler G. (2007). Perspectives of participants of self-help groups for people who stutter. In J. Au-Yeung & M. M. Leahy (Ed.), *Research, Treatment, and Self-help in Fluency Disorders: New Horizons. Proceedings of the Fifth World Congress on Fluency Disorders, 25–28 July, 2006, Dublin, Ireland.* (pp. 171–176). The International Fluency Association.

Vattano, A. J. (1972). Power to the people: Self-help groups. *Social Work, 17,* 7–17.

Van Riper, C. (1973). *The treatment of stuttering.* Englewood Cliffs, NJ: Prentice-Hall.

Vogt, N. (2016). Podcasting: Fact sheet. *State of the News Media 2016.* Retrieved from http://www.journalism.org/2016/06/15/podcasting-fact-sheet/

Wahlberg, A. (2007). A quackery with a difference—new medical pluralism and the problem of "dangerous practitioners" in the United Kingdom. *Social Science & Medicine, 65*(11), 2307–2316.

Walkom, G. (2016, October). Virtual reality exposure therapy: To benefit those who stutter and treat social anxiety. In Interactive Technologies and Games (iTAG), *2016 International Conference on Interactive Technologies and Games* (pp. 36–41). IEEE. Retrieved from http://ieeexplore.ieee.org/xpl/mostRecentIssue.jsp?reload=true&punumber=7782003

Wang, Y., Norice, G., & Cranor, L. F. (2011). Who is concerned about what? A study of American, Chinese and Indian users' privacy concerns on social network sites. *Lecture Notes in Computer Science, 6740,* 146–153.

WebMD. (n.d.). *Brain and nervous system health center: Speech and stuttering.* Retrieved from http://www.webmd.com/brain/speech-stuttering

Yaruss, J. S., & Quesal, R. W. (2008). *Overall assessment of the speaker's experience of stuttering.* Minneapolis, MN: NCS Pearson.

Yaruss, J. S., Quesal, R. W., & Reeves, L. (2007). Self-help and mutual aid groups as an adjunct to stuttering therapy. In E. G. Conture & R. F. (Eds.), *Stuttering and related disorders of fluency* (3rd ed.; pp. 256–276). New York, NY: Thieme.

Yaruss, J. S., Quesal, R. W., Reeves, L., Molt, L. F., Kluetz, B., Caruso, A. J., . . . Lewis, F. (2002). Speech treatment and support group experiences of people who participate in the National Stuttering Association. *Journal of Fluency Disorders, 27*(2), 115–134.

Yaruss, J. S., & Reeves, L. (2002). *Pioneering stuttering in the 21st century: The first joint symposium for scientists and consumers (Summary report and proceedings).* Anaheim, CA: National Stuttering Association.

YouTube. (2017). *Statistics.* Retrieved from https://www.youtube.com/yt/press/statistics.html

CHAPTER 11

Community-Centered Assessment and Treatment

Targeting the Social, Emotional, and Cognitive Aspects of Stuttering in Children

Craig Coleman

INTRODUCTION

The concept of community-centered health care has gained much traction over the last decade (Fanjiang, Grossman, Compton, & Reid, 2005; Johnson, Abraham, Conway, Simmons, Edgman-Levitan, Sodomka, & Ford, 2008). It has marked the next step in the evolution of care that has transitioned over the years from clinician-centered to patient-centered to family-centered, and now to community-centered. This evolution has occurred as health care professionals have identified the importance of involving the patient and family in the assessment and treatment process.

In stuttering, there has been much emphasis placed on the importance of involving parents in the treatment process (de Sonneville-Koedoot, Stolk, Rietveld, & Franken, 2015; Millard, Nicholas, & Cook, 2008; Yaruss, Coleman, & Hammer, 2006). While parents and other family members are often a central part of a child's life, the family-centered model falls short of allowing the speech-language pathologist (SLP) the opportunity to assess and treat the child in the context of a larger community, where many of their day-to-day activities and communication occur.

The purpose of this chapter is to describe a model of community-centered care in stuttering assessment and treatment. By the end of the chapter, readers will be able to describe the model and identify specific assessment and treatment concepts to support the model. Use of the model for both preschool and school-age/adolescent children will be discussed, as it is important to encourage positive social emotional behavior and cognitive reactions to stuttering at all ages. The importance of using the model to improve carry-over to settings outside the clinic will also be discussed.

STUTTERING AND COMMUNITY-CENTERED CARE

Stuttering is a complex disorder that involves disruptions in the forward flow of speech, which can take many forms (repetitions, prolongations, blocks). Stuttering may also include physical tension, secondary behaviors (hand-tapping, head-nodding, etc.), negative thoughts and emotions related to speaking, and reduced overall communication (ASHA, 1993; Yaruss, 1998, 2004). Stuttering is very different from disfluency, which is merely a disruption in the flow of speech that all speakers experience.

Many SLPs have reported decreased comfort and knowledge with stuttering (Coleman & Weidner, 2014; Tellis, Bressler, & Emerick, 2008), despite the fact that most graduate programs offer coursework in assessment and treatment of the disorder (Coleman, Miller, & Gambill, 2016). When considering the varying viewpoints of stuttering that have been presented over the last century, it is not surprising that SLPs, and the general public, have a difficult time with knowledge, perceptions, and comfort level. For example, stuttering has been viewed as an emotional disorder, a learned behavior, and a genetic/neurophysiological disorder, all in the last century. The goal of community-centered care is not only to treat the child in the context of the family, but to treat the child in the context of the larger community so that lack of knowledge, lack of comfort, and false perceptions of stuttering do not become insurmountable obstacles in the therapy process.

Identifying the Community

The term "community" is often used to describe a group of people who live in the same area, share similar interests, or engage in similar activities. For the purposes of this chapter, the term "community" will be used to describe the social or educational context in which a child who stutters communicates with others (Coleman, 2013). As such, a child's community may include family, neighbors, peers, teachers, coaches, instructors, SLPs, waiters/waitresses, check-out clerks, and so forth. The size of the community depends on the child, the varying degree of his/her interactions, how often the child participates in activities, and so forth. When defining a child's community, there is no simple answer or procedural rule to follow. This process must be individualized to the child and it can be a great starting point in the therapy process, as clinicians can work with the child to determine with whom the child communicates on a consistent basis, and which interactions cause the child's comfort level to change. Children can be encouraged to make a list of people they interact with frequently, situations that are more or less difficult for them, and people they wished knew more about stuttering.

The Community-Centered Care Model for Stuttering

The community-centered care model for stuttering (Coleman, 2013) has five primary components: Assessment/Consultation, Treatment, Support, Follow-up, and Education. The model is shown in Figure 11–1.

Rather than being a purely hierarchical model, this model represents the interaction that exists between the various components, with education being the center of the model, because it overlaps with all other components. The circular aspect of the model highlights the non-linear process. Children who stutter, particularly those older than the preschool stage, may go through stages of this model at multiple times during their lives. For example, formal treatment may be needed for short

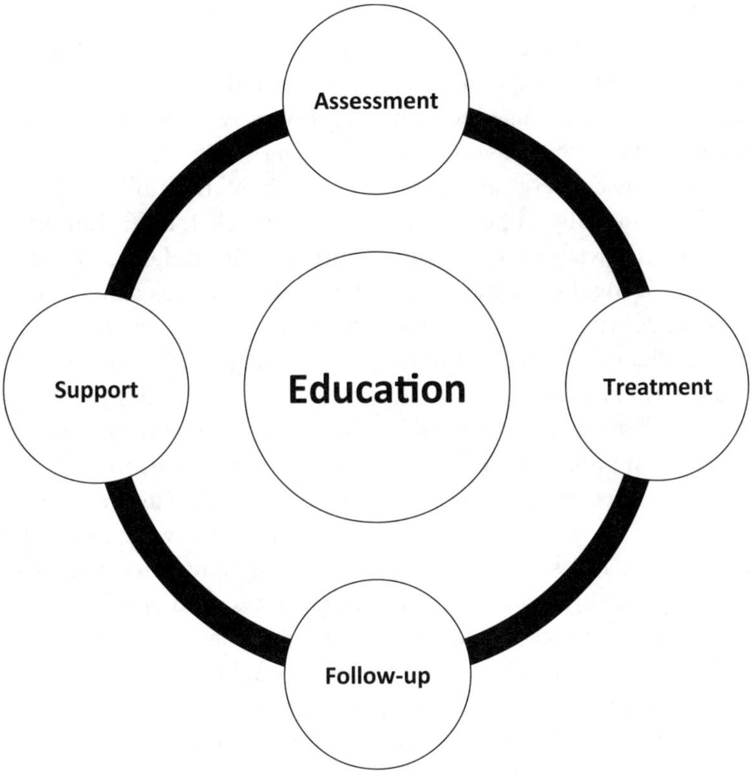

Figure 11–1. The community-centered care model for stuttering.

intervals throughout a child's life, while support is more of a continual process. Looking at the model this way can also eliminate the concept of "relapse" in stuttering. Oftentimes, the term "relapse" is used to describe persons who stutter when they are experiencing more disfluencies in their speech. This term is problematic for chronic conditions, such as stuttering, because the condition does not go away and return. People may experience various levels of severity throughout their lives, but stuttering typically does not completely "go away" after the preschool/early school-age years.

Education

For children who stutter, education has been utilized as part of the treatment process for the preschool population (Yaruss, Coleman, & Hammer, 2006), as well as school-age and adolescent children (Yaruss, Coleman, & Quesal, 2012). In addition, the importance of educating family members during the treatment process has been described (Yaruss, Coleman, & Hammer, 2006). Still, the need for education appears to permeate much further than the child and family.

For example, a study by Coleman and Weidner (2014), reported that many SLPs were not able to accurately define the term "stuttering." In addition, SLPs have reported a general lack of comfort in their knowledge of stuttering and treating people who stutter (Coleman & Weidner, 2014; Tellis, Bressler, & Emerick, 2008). Thus, education should begin with professionals to make sure children are being assessed and treated by an SLP with knowledge about stuttering. SLPs can utilize resources such as the American Board on Fluency Disorders (http://www.stutteringspecialists.org) to find colleagues who specialize in stuttering. In addition, continuing education opportunities are available to SLPs to help them stay current on assessment and treatment trends. This is especially important in stuttering because there have been significant shifts in perceptions of the disorder, and recognition about its underlying causes, over the last 30 years. The traditional forms of continuing education, such as journals, conventions, and workshops are still available to clinicians looking for improved training. Additionally, webinars have allowed even further access to experts in the field.

Education must also focus on improving knowledge and perceptions of stuttering in the child's community. For example, a child who stutters may participate in activities such as sports, band, dance, and so on, where there are coaches, instructors, or others who may have limited knowledge of stuttering. Thus, it is equally important for those individuals to have accurate information about stuttering so they know how to best respond when the child stutters or experiences negative reactions.

For many children, the most important groups of people in their lives, outside of their family, are their teachers and peers. Because stuttering is a relatively low-incidence disorder (with approximately 1% of the population), classroom teachers and other children may only encounter a very limited number of children who stutter. As such, helping teachers to better understand stuttering and helping children who stutter educate their peers about stuttering can be an extremely powerful tool in preventing misconceptions about stuttering and limiting teasing and bullying in the school setting. In addition, teachers may be of further assistance by having classroom discussions about individual differences in general to highlight the uniqueness of each individual in the class. These discussions may ultimately help children who stutter by allowing the class to celebrate individual differences rather than single out children in a negative way when they present with unique characteristics.

It is highly unlikely that teachers will receive much formal training on stuttering during their academic preparation. A study by Barney and Coleman (2014) revealed that student teachers had very limited knowledge of stuttering or how to help children who stutter who may someday be in their classroom. Still, these same student teachers generally had positive perceptions of children who stutter. For example, they indicated that children who stutter would have the same level of intelligence, the same attention span, and similar behaviors as children who did not stutter. The only area where they suspected children who stutter would be different was in overall social performance.

When education is discussed in the context of the family, it is important for all family members who interact with the child on a consistent basis to be knowledgeable about stuttering, and not just the parents. To highlight the importance of this concept, consider a child who spends several hours a day with his grandparents while his parents are at work. In a case such as this, it is equally important for the grandparents to have accurate knowledge and perceptions of stuttering. Otherwise, parents may spend their limited time with the child each day working on appropriate activities related to stuttering, but the child may be receiving contradictory information during a significant part of each day when with his grandparents.

Ultimately, SLPs must decide what we want the child, family, and community to know about stuttering. First, it is important for people to understand the underlying factors that contribute to the cause of stuttering. Many recent studies have indicated genetic (Drayna & Kang, 2011) and neurophysiological (Chang, 2014; Chang, Erickson, Ambrose, Hasegawa-Johnson, & Ludlow, 2008; Chang & Zhu, 2013) differences between people who stutter and people who do not stutter. Having these discussions about genetics and neurophysiology allows others to view stuttering as a health condition rather than a perceived nervous or anxiety disorder. It allows people to move away from thinking about stuttering as a learned behavior or something they can "catch" from others. When children have a better understanding of the underlying causes of stuttering, they are better able to answer questions from their peers about why they stutter. For example, if other children ask why they stutter, children who stutter may often be instructed to simply ignore the question or walk away. While this practice does not escalate the event further, it also does not answer the question. If children can respond to such questions by simply stating, "Stuttering is just part of who I am. It's not something I do on purpose and it doesn't mean that there is anything wrong with me," they can help other children to better understand stuttering while also being advocates for themselves.

Second, as children get older, into the school-age years, it becomes important for those around them to understand that stuttering will likely not be cured. Instead, stuttering must be viewed as a condition that can be successfully managed. In this manner, stuttering is analogous to conditions such as asthma, allergies, and diabetes. While those conditions are not typically cured, they can be successfully managed with the right intervention and support. Viewing stuttering in this way also allows others to move away from offering simple advice such as telling children to slow down, think about what they want to say, or just try harder to use their strategies. Typically, simple suggestions are not productive for a complex condition such as stuttering.

Third, it can be very empowering for children who stutter to learn about other famous or successful people who stutter. This can also be useful for the child's peers to see that stuttering is not a condition to be feared and that many people who stutter can be very successful in all walks of life.

Fourth, the child, family, and community should be aware of basic facts related to stuttering. Basic stuttering trivia games can be used to help children learn about stuttering and compete against others to help spread their knowledge about stuttering.

Finally, some education needs are specific to various individuals. For example, teachers need to understand how to interact with children in the classroom. When children who stutter give oral presentations, time limit adjustments may be necessary. In addition, modifications may need to be made to oral reading activities so that a child's reading ability is not measured based only on speech fluency. Children who stutter may also find oral reading more difficult when teachers utilize down-the-row reading to have everyone in the class participate. In general, teachers can utilize similar strategies as family members do when interacting with children who stutter. This includes giving the child as much time as necessary to finish an utterance and focusing on the content of the child's speech rather than simply how fluent the child happens to be at that moment. Teachers can be instrumental in helping a child deal with bullying in the classroom by promoting individual differences and by maintaining an atmosphere where children feel comfortable expressing their concerns, thoughts, and feelings.

When working with children who stutter, there are key differences in preschool children, school-age children, and adolescents. Education is one area where those differences exist. For preschool children, parents will need to be educated on the risk factors associated with chronic stuttering versus normal speech disfluency that many children experience in their language development. Family members at this stage may also be taught indirect strategies to help improve the child's fluency. These include helping parents learn a slower rate of speech, modifying questions, and using recasting and rephrasing to model fluent speech and higher-level language (Yaruss, Coleman, & Hammer, 2006). Understanding the differences between indirect therapy, direct therapy, and operant conditioning is also important at this stage because of the variety of treatment approaches available to young children who stutter.

Various treatment approaches have been demonstrated to be effective for preschool children who stutter (de Sonneville-Koedoot, Stolk, Rietveld, & Franken, 2015; Jones et al., 2005; Millard, Nicholas, & Cook, 2008; Yaruss, Coleman, & Hammer, 2006). Each of these approaches heavily relies on parent involvement in the treatment process, highlighting the need for family education at this stage.

Assessment

A speech fluency assessment is likely to include both formal and informal components. For children of all ages, the evaluation process may begin with a thorough case history form that allows the parents, or other members of the family, to report on medical history, general development, and speech and language development. In addition, this is the place where parents can start to express their concerns about their child's stuttering. While the case history form typically serves as a good starting point, a formal interview with the parents, or other family members, usually takes place at the beginning of an evaluation.

For a preschool child, clinicians may then move to observing the child interacting with the parents to determine the child's disfluency rate in a setting with familiar communication partners. The clinician may then interact more directly with the child while placing various levels of communication pressure on the child to determine how those levels impact speech fluency. For example, the clinician may begin interacting with the child using a very slow pace, not asking many direct questions, and giving the child more than enough time to respond. The clinician may then move to assessing speech fluency while placing more demands on the child, such as increasing rate of speech, getting the child more excited, interrupting the child, or asking many direct questions. The clinician can then compare the child's disfluency rate in these situations to determine how fluent the child can be when there is little communication pressure and if his stuttering increases when that pressure is increased. It is important to note that clinicians may not need to engage in high-pressure situations with the child if the child exhibits a high disfluency rate in low-pressure situations.

Clinicians may also have the child engage in picture description activities, reading activities (when age appropriate), or communication with siblings or peers to determine the child's level of stuttering in various communication situations.

In addition to looking at frequency and type of stuttering, clinicians will also look for levels of physical tension and presence of secondary behaviors during stuttering episodes. Assessment of these indicators gives the clinician a good picture of the child's surface-level stuttering. Clinicians can use a formal assessment tool such as the *Stuttering Severity Instrument–4* (SSI-4; Riley, 2009) to report on surface-level characteristics of stuttering. Because of the variability of stuttering at the preschool ages, clinicians will want to check with parents to determine if the evaluation was representative of the child's typical speech fluency in everyday situations. If the parents feel that the evaluation is not representative of the child's speech fluency that they typically observe at home, clinicians may ask the parents to provide video samples of the child's speech outside of the clinic.

Assessing reactions of the child can be difficult for preschool children, as they may have difficulty verbalizing their reactions and emotions related to stuttering. While some formal assessment tools are available, clinicians can also look for avoidance of words and speaking situations, physical tension, secondary behaviors, and other indicators of negative reactions. For example, children at this stage may exhibit increased loudness and pitch during stuttering episodes, which indicates some level of awareness of stuttering.

Some clinicians use children's books (Coleman & Weidner, 2012) to help assess reactions of the child. Children may have an easier time verbalizing their own reactions if they can see another character experiencing similar characteristics and reactions.

When assessing older children in the school-age and adolescent years, clinicians will still look at surface-level characteristics of stuttering by having the child engage in conversations, reading tasks, and picture descriptions with various communication partners. Clinicians can still utilize the SSI-4 to evaluate observable characteristics.

As children get older, it becomes increasingly important to get their input on their stuttering. Clinicians can utilize a formal assessment tool such as the *Overall Assessment of the Speaker's Experience of Stuttering* (OASES; Yaruss & Quesal, 2006) to assess the child's emotions and thoughts related to stuttering. In addition to providing a severity level across different areas of impact, the OASES allows clinicians to begin having discussions with the child on specific activities that the child may view as difficult as a person who stutters. These discussions are typically used to help identify treatment goals. For example, if a child reports that talking in front of a group of people is more difficult, that should be a goal during therapy.

If the goal of assessment is to evaluate the child in the context of the community, other measures need to be utilized to gauge the perceptions of the child's family, teachers, and others therein.

The *Community-Centered Stuttering Assessment* (CCSA) (Coleman, Miller, & Dowler, 2015) protocol was developed to assess the perceptions of parents, teachers, and SLPs for the child who stutters. The CCSA is a set of questionnaires that allows parents, teachers, and SLPs to rate the child's speech fluency, physical tension, secondary behaviors, and overall severity through both quantitative ratings and qualitative reports at home, in school, and in the clinic. The CCSA serves as a complement to the OASES to allow clinicians to compare the child's responses on the OASES with the responses of others in the child's family and community.

The CCSA also contains a questionnaire on bullying related to stuttering. This can also be a good starting point in discussions to provide support to the child and education on how to handle bullying for the family and school if necessary. The entire CCSA protocol is available at www.stutteringu.com

When formal assessment has been completed, clinicians often utilize a wrap-up session to go over results and determine a treatment plan. For older children, this is a good point to start a discussion on the goals of therapy. Both children and parents can be asked to provide goals they would like to target in therapy. In many cases, they may report wanting to work on eliminating the child's stuttering. For school-age and adolescent children, a complete elimination of stuttering is not likely. Instead, clinicians can begin discussing the treatment goals that will be targeted to focus on successful management of stuttering.

In conclusion, the primary difference between a traditional speech fluency assessment and a community-centered assessment is obtaining information from multiple sources and ensuring that children who stutter are evaluated not only in the context of their interaction with the clinician, but in the context of their everyday interactions with family members, peers, and others in the community.

Treatment

Treatment for preschool children may involve components of indirect therapy, direct therapy, operant therapy, or some combination of the three. Yaruss, Coleman, and Hammer (2006) described a family-focused treatment approach that incorporates components of both indirect treatment and direct treatment to target improved fluency, improved reactions, improved education, and improved overall communication. The approach utilized in the community-centered model is adapted from the family-focused model.

In the community-centered model, treatment for preschool children begins with parent education. Generally, for the first two sessions the bulk of treatment is spent on educating the parents about stuttering as well as reevaluating the child's speech fluency in various situations. This allows the clinician to begin parent education while gaining a better perspective of the child's speech fluency over time, rather than the one snapshot opportunity at the diagnostic evaluation.

During the next three to four sessions, parents are able to watch the clinician model fluency enhancing strategies with the child and then practice the strategies themselves while the clinician observes and gives feedback. These strategies include using a reduced communication rate, modifying questions, limiting verbal interruptions, reducing competition for talking time, and using recasting and rephrasing. The strategies were laid out in detail in a previous report by Yaruss, Coleman, and Hammer (2006).

For some children, these first several sessions may be enough to facilitate significant changes in the child's speech fluency. Still, other children will need to move on to more direct intervention. For these children, direct treatment may target use of a slower speaking rate through increased pauses, reducing physical tension, direct discussion of negative reactions associated with stuttering, and direct work on overall communication so that the child is not avoiding words or speaking situations.

A significant focus of treatment in the community-centered model is to incorporate siblings and peers in the therapy process as much as possible. This not only helps target generalization but also helps children to interact with other children with whom they share real-life experiences on a day-to-day basis. In addition, a significant focus is placed on having the child participate in therapy outside of the clinic room. For example, children can talk to others in the clinic, take therapy outside, and bring others into the therapy process.

For school-age and adolescent children who stutter, the child and family should be heavily involved in the selection of treatment goals and selection of activities that can be utilized to target those objectives. The child and family should be made aware very early on in the treatment process that stuttering is not likely to be cured, and the overall goal of treatment is effective management.

When considering whether or not treatment should be carried out, a major consideration must be the child's level of motivation for making changes in his or her speech and reactions to stuttering. Stuttering treatment involves a lot of risk-taking, as children are often asked to participate in activities that they may fear. Children who are not motivated to come to therapy are much less likely to engage in difficult activities such as pseudostuttering, role-playing difficult communication situations, and entering new communication environments that they may have previously avoided. It is important to remember that many people who stutter will want treatment at some point in their lives. If they are forced into treatment when they are not yet ready, the chances of a successful outcome are greatly reduced. In addition, when they are later ready for therapy, they may only have negative experiences with treatment in their past.

Support

Support can be a critical part of the treatment process for both preschool children and older children. For preschool children, parents may benefit from meeting other parents of young children who stutter, or from meeting parents of children who have been able to successfully manage their stuttering. For older children, support groups serve as an important piece of the treatment puzzle. Through support groups, children have the opportunity to meet other peers who are experiencing similar circumstances. They also have an opportunity to discuss challenging situations and obstacles that they have been able to overcome with others who can appreciate these circumstances.

Support groups are different from treatment groups in that treatment groups often have specific goals that the children are working toward meeting. For support groups, the goals are often geared toward having the child improve his or her communication and gain comfort with stuttering. This may mean that support groups can take on unique characteristics based on the individuals who participate in the groups. Studies have indicated that support groups are effective as a piece of overall treatment for both children (Coleman & Weidner, 2013) and adults (Yaruss, Quesal, & Reeves, 2007) who stutter.

In some settings, it can be difficult to have a large support group for children who stutter. For example, clinicians working in the schools may find it difficult to have these support groups if only one child on their caseload stutters. In cases such as these, clinicians may work with others until they have enough children to offer a combined support group or they can utilize virtual support groups (Coleman & Weidner, 2013) where children meet online with clinicians serving as facilitators.

Over the past several years, many summer programs have also become available to children who stutter and their families (Byrd et al., 2016; Coleman & Weidner, 2014). These programs typically contain a support aspect that allows children and families to connect with each other. Having children participate in these programs also allows clinicians to move away from providing clinical services only in the treatment room and get the child out into other real-world settings.

Support groups serve as a key piece to the community-centered model, as they allow a much smoother transition for children to step back into roles in their community during and after treatment. For example, support groups do not always need to contain only children who stutter. Clinicians may also incorporate friends and siblings who do not stutter into the support group so that they are better able to understand stuttering, and a child who stutters is able to work on generalization activities with the clinician present.

Follow-Up

Like many other health conditions that are managed, stuttering treatment does not end on the last therapy session. As children who stutter go through various stages in their lives, it is quite possible then that they will need to return to therapy periodically. This expectation can be set early in the therapy process so that the child does not feel like he is failing if he needs treatment in the future. In fact, for most chronic conditions, some form of ongoing follow-up with a health care provider is typical. For example, those being treated for diabetes do not visit the doctor for a three-month period and never return. Similarly, children who stutter should not be expected to manage their stuttering on their own for the rest of their lives after a brief period of speech therapy. Historically, the term "relapse" has been used as a label when children who stutter need to return to speech therapy. However, the term "relapse" is very misleading when discussing a chronic condition, because the condition never fully goes away.

Follow-up is necessary for children of all ages and can take many forms. Parents may follow-up with the clinician through periodic phone calls or emails to inform the clinician on the child's progress and challenges related to their stuttering. In addition, more formal follow-up can be scheduled through periodic visits to the clinician to reassess speech fluency and impact of stuttering on the child's life.

No matter what form follow-up takes, children and parents should be aware that success in therapy does not mean that they no longer need to communicate with the clinician. Forming a successful therapeutic relationship has been shown to be an important piece of the treatment process when working with people who stutter (Plexico, Manning, & DiLollo, 2010). Part of building an effective therapeutic alliance is helping children and families understand that the partnership will continue long past the final speech therapy session.

Case Studies

For the remainder of this chapter, two hypothetical case studies will be utilized to demonstrate how community-centered stuttering treatment can be implemented for preschool children and school-age children.

Preschool

Johnny is a 4-year-old boy who began stuttering approximately one year ago. He has a family history of stuttering, as his father continues to stutter as an adult. There are no other speech and language concerns. He is aware of his stuttering and is starting to exhibit negative reactions. For example, Johnny will say, "I can't talk right" when he begins to stutter. In addition, he is beginning to exhibit avoidance of words and speaking situations, and his utterance length has decreased as he has become aware of his stuttering. He exhibits a disfluency rate of 15% with repetitions, prolongations, and blocks.

Johnny exhibits moderate physical tension, including pitch and loudness changes during stuttering episodes. He also exhibits secondary behaviors such as eye-blinking and head-moving during stuttering moments. During his assessment, he exhibited an SSI-4 rating of moderate to severe. Johnny has two siblings, ages 8 and 10. He attends weekly swimming lessons.

For Johnny, treatment would begin with family education at the diagnostic session. This allows parents to begin implementing changes in the home environment immediately rather than waiting until the treatment phase formally begins. Because Johnny is experiencing negative reactions to stuttering, parents will need to learn how to respond to those reactions. In some cases, simply letting the child know that it is okay to stutter or have bumpy speech is enough to begin to ease his worries about speaking. Johnny's parents may also be encouraged to have disfluencies themselves and point them out to him to let him know that they also have some bumpy speech and that is okay.

During the education portion of the process, Johnny's parents and the clinician can also begin discussing factors in the environment and Johnny's temperament. While both environment and temperament do not likely cause children to begin stuttering, they can play a role in reactions to stuttering. We also need to identify those in the family and community who interact with the child on a consistent basis to provide information to them as well. Information handouts can be utilized so that parents, family members, and others in the community begin to learn about stuttering. Some possible sources of information are as follows:

http://www.stutteringu.com

http://www.westutter.org

http://www.stutteringhelp.org

http://www.stutteringhomepage.com

http://www.friendswhostutter.org

http://www.stuttertalk.com

For Johnny, risk factors associated with stuttering that should be discussed with the parents include family history of stuttering, male gender, stuttering for over one year, negative reactions toward stuttering, and the presence of physical tension and secondary behaviors. Clinicians can refer to Yairi and Ambrose (2013) for a complete review of risk factors associated with stuttering.

Since Johnny also attends weekly swimming lessons, information on stuttering should also be provided to the swimming instructor. This may help the instructor react in an appropriate way when Johnny stutters.

Formal treatment with Johnny may begin by targeting reactions to stuttering, since he is currently avoiding speaking situations and exhibiting physical tension and secondary behaviors. Clinicians can encourage him to play with his stuttering through purposeful stuttering activities in therapy, at home, and with his peers. To that end, it is important for clinicians and parents to demonstrate a willingness to play with stuttering themselves in a comfortable manner.

Treatment may also include targeting reduction in physical tension and secondary behaviors. Johnny can begin by discriminating between hard stuttering and easy stuttering, with and without physical tension and secondary behaviors. Once he is able to discriminate between the two, his clinician can then have him move toward using various types of stuttering in more structured (then less structured) situations and activities.

Stuttering modification strategies (Van Riper, 1973) can also be incorporated into the therapy process to reduce the amount of tension and modify stuttering. Examples of these strategies may include easing-out, pull-outs, and cancellations. Clinicians may use different terminology when working with a young child who stutters. For example, clinicians may use terms such as "easy bumps" and "hard bumps" to describe stuttering that includes less tension and more tension, respectively.

Speech modification strategies (Bothe, 2002) can be utilized to target a reduction in the disfluency rate. Johnny may begin by discriminating between fluent (smooth) and disfluent (bumpy) speech. He can then learn other modification strategies such as easy starts, increased use of pauses, prolonged speech, etc. One term that children who stutter identify with easily is "turtle talk." Turtle talk refers to a slower rate of speech that is achieved by breaking up sentences into smaller parts and using pauses between phrases.

Throughout treatment, Johnny will also need to work on activities and objectives that target improved overall communication. This will include discussion of avoidance of words and speaking situations and the impact these can have on the child's ability to interact with others. In addition, Johnny may need to work on other aspects of communication such as eye contact, turn-taking, topic maintenance, and initiating conversations with others.

Since Johnny has two siblings, they also need to be incorporated into the therapy sessions part of the time. Incorporating the siblings into the therapy process can help with generalization, and in this case it can also be used to target avoidance of speaking situations by having the siblings participate in challenging communication environments. One time each month, Johnny can participate in a group session with other children who stutter while their parents are participating in support groups geared toward improving their knowledge and acceptance of stuttering.

This case is a good example of when support and education overlap. Not only should Johnny's siblings be a part of the therapy process, but peers should be as well. Recognizing the need to mitigate negative attitudes among young children who do not stutter, Weidner (2015) developed the *Attitude Change and Tolerance Program* (*InterACT*). The *InterACT* program is designed to educate young children about stuttering within the larger context of human differences. It is implemented over the course of two 30-minute lessons, which each comprise an educational video featuring lifelike puppets, a small group discussion, and an activity coloring book. The storyline features a young boy who stutters and his four friends (one of whom is in a wheelchair). The characters talk about their own unique differences while emphasizing the nature of stuttering and how to interact with a person who stutters. The underlying theme of the program is "everyone is different and everyone's the same," which seeks to raise children's awareness and tolerance of human differences, including stuttering.

In a recent study, Weidner and St. Louis (2016) used their instrument, the *Public Opinion Survey on Human Attributes—Stuttering/Child* to measure the extent to which preschool children's stuttering attitudes changed before and after the program. Specifically, they investigated children's beliefs about stuttering and people who stutter, and their self-reactions toward their peers who stutter. Results showed that children's stuttering attitudes significantly improved following the *InterACT* program. The participants were able to define stuttering, identify its causes, and report sensitive interactions with children who stutter. For example, they were significantly less likely to indicate that they would tell stuttering peers to "slow down," finish their words, or laugh at a stutterer. Perhaps most importantly, children's perceptions of the traits of peers who stutter markedly improved. They were less likely to describe stuttering peers as being shy, nervous, or having a bad problem. Based on the results of that study, the *InterACT* program has shown promise for being an effective educational tool for young, non-stuttering children. Incorporating the *InterACT* program for Johnny may be helpful in educating his peers about stuttering.

When weekly individual sessions are no longer needed for Johnny, treatment may be scaled back to once every other week and then one time per month to ensure that he is maintaining and generalizing improved speech fluency, improved overall communication, and improved reactions to stuttering.

School-Age

Tyrone is a 10-year-old child with a family history of stuttering. His father and brother continue to stutter. Tyrone exhibits a disfluency rate of 22% in conversational speech and 35% in reading activities. He exhibits secondary behaviors such as eye-blinking and hand-tapping during stuttering episodes. He also exhibits severe physical tension, and nearly all of his disfluencies are blocks. He exhibits avoidance behaviors and has limited his utterance length to two or three words per sentence. Tyrone has an SSI-4 rating of severe and overall OASES-S (for school-age children 7 to 12) rating of severe. On CCSA measures, Tyrone's participation at home and at school is significantly affected by his stuttering. Tyrone reports that bullying related to his stuttering occurs frequently. He has two older siblings and plays youth football.

Once again, the treatment process can begin with education. In this case, education should begin with Tyrone to help make him the expert on his stuttering. Initial activities can include having him learn about famous people who stutter, how his speech system works, types of stuttering, speech modification and stuttering modification strategies, and other basic facts about stuttering. As Tyrone begins to learn about stuttering, he can educate others in his family about stuttering. Then, as he begins to gain some comfort with his stuttering, he can move on to educating others in his environment.

From a treatment perspective, it is very tempting in a case like this to begin by using strategies to help Tyrone become more fluent; other people around him, such as parents, teachers, and peers also want him to be fluent. Tyrone too wants to be more fluent, but it is also important that he wants to change the impact of stuttering and reduce the amount of effort required to speak.

When speaking requires a great deal of effort, the child is less likely to engage and talk. As such, one of the primary goals of therapy in the early stages should be to reduce the amount of effort and frustration associated with speaking. One of the first skills learned can be stuttering modification strategies designed to help a child speak with less tension and struggle. These strategies can also target desensitization, as the child needs to be stuttering to utilize the strategies. Stuttering modification strategies can also be useful in helping a child talk about his or her stuttering. A discussion with the child should also take place about what is viewed as more effortful: use of strategies or stuttering. Typically, children will have much more motivation to use strategies and techniques when they reduce the effort required to speak.

For Tyrone, pseudostuttering in various communication situations, such as the clinic, in school, on the phone, or at restaurants, can also be helpful in targeting desensitization as well as teaching him what it feels like to stutter when he is in control. When avoidance of speaking situations is present for a child, one of the goals of therapy should be to have the child enter a new speaking situation each week. In these activities, the use of strategies and the disfluency rate do not matter, since the goal is to improve the child's participation rather than focus only on fluency. In fact, as children begin to improve their reactions and decrease their avoidance of speaking situations, an increase in surface-level stuttering may be noted. Clinicians and parents should be aware of this, as it is not a negative sign of progress in speech therapy, but can be expected as children speak more. Activities such as journaling can be utilized so that parents, clinicians, teachers, and others in the community can track and comment on the child's participation levels in various situations.

Because Tyrone reported that bullying occurs frequently due to his stuttering, helping him develop appropriate reactions to bullies should also be part of the therapy process. Educating him about stuttering will help him be able to better respond to others' questions and comments about stuttering. Role-playing specific situations related to bullying can also help him feel better able to respond to the bullies. Both clinicians and teachers who lack experience in working with children who stutter may feel less comfortable addressing bullying. Collaboration between professionals may be necessary, as bullying can be a very threatening situation to a child.

One of the final treatment targets for Tyrone may be improved speech fluency. If fluency shaping strategies are targeted too early in the therapy process, he may continue to avoid words and situations and place too much emphasis on being fluent. Another consideration, making this a later target, is that by this point the clinician will know how much the child is actually stuttering rather than using avoidance strategies to hide his or her stuttering.

For this case, we can expand the treatment circle by bringing siblings into the therapy sessions periodically and by providing Tyrone's football coach with information on stuttering and stuttering management strategies that are specific to that context.

Tyrone can participate in an in-person support group or a virtual support group where he has the opportunity to meet other children who stutter. For children this age, we may also recommend that they attend a summer program for children who stutter. For example, we offer a stuttering summer program at Marshall University, Stuttering U. (Coleman & Weidner, 2014). This program allows children to meet and interact with other children who stutter, while their parents participate in educational sessions to learn more about stuttering and meet other parents of children who stutter.

Children in the school-age years can continue to participate in support groups following the completion of formal treatment. They can also be seen for follow-up sessions through tele-therapy, which is becoming an increasingly utilized format of providing speech therapy services. In fact, tele-therapy allows many more children who stutter to have access to a specialist. It also allows children who may live in rural areas to have a wider variety of options for treatment.

CONCLUSIONS

Community-centered stuttering therapy builds on traditional speech therapy by extending the treatment circle to include others in the community. In addition, assessment and treatment are built on the belief that input from everyone involved in the child's life is important. Treatment is not viewed as a short-term prospect, but a lifelong journey to successful management. Goals of therapy are structured so that the child not only improves in the treatment room, but is also able to generalize treatment progress to other communication situations within his/her everyday community.

REFERENCES

American Speech-Language-Hearing Association. (1993). *Definitions of communication disorders and variations* [Relevant paper]. Retrieved from www.asha.org/policy

Barney, E., & Coleman, C. (2014, November). *Pre-service teachers' knowledge and perceptions of stuttering.* Poster presented at the annual convention of the American Speech-Language-Hearing Association, Orlando, FL.

Bothe, A. K. (2002). Speech modification approaches to stuttering treatment in schools. *Seminars in Speech and Language, 23*(3), 181–186.

Byrd, C., Chmela, K., Coleman, C., Weidner, M., Kelly, E., Reichhardt, R., & Irani, F. (2016). An introduction to camps for children who stutter: What they are and how they can help. *Perspectives of the ASHA Special Interest Groups, 1*(4), 55–69.

Chang, S. E. (2014). Research updates in neuroimaging studies of children who stutter. *Seminars in Speech and Language, 35*, 67–79.

Chang, S. E., Erickson, K. I., Ambrose, N. G., Hasegawa-Johnson, M. A., & Ludlow, C. L. (2008). Brain anatomy differences in childhood stuttering. *Neuroimage, 39*(3), 1333–1344.

Chang, S. E., & Zhu, D. C. (2013). Neural network connectivity differences in children who stutter. *Brain, 136* (Pt. 12), 3709–3726.

Coleman, C. (2013, November). *Community-centered stuttering intervention: Widening the treatment circle.* Poster presented at the annual convention of the American Speech-Language-Hearing Association, Chicago, IL.

Coleman, C., Miller, L., & Dowler, K. (2015, November). *Community-centered stuttering assessment: Questionnaires for clinical practice.*

Poster presented at the Annual Conference of the American Speech-Language-Hearing Association, Denver, CO.

Coleman, C., Miller, L., & Gambill, J. (2016, November). *Update on graduate coursework in stuttering.* Poster presented at the Annual Conference of the American Speech-Language-Hearing Association, Philadelphia, PA.

Coleman, C., & Weidner, M. (2012, November). *Using stories in stuttering treatment.* Poster presented at the annual convention of the American Speech-Language-Hearing Association, Atlanta, GA.

Coleman, C., & Weidner, M. (2013, November). *Impact of support groups for children who stutter.* Poster presented at the annual convention of the American Speech-Language-Hearing Association, Chicago, IL.

Coleman C., & Weidner, M. (2014, November) *Stuttering U: A summer camp for children who stutter and their families.* Poster presented at the annual convention of the American Speech-Language-Hearing Association, Orlando, FL.

de Sonneville-Koedoot, C., Stolk, E., Rietveld, T., & Franken, M. C. (2015). Direct versus indirect treatment for preschool children who stutter: The RESTART randomized trial. *PloS One, 10*(7), e0133758.

Drayna, D., & Kang, C. (2011). Genetic approaches to understanding the causes of stuttering. *Journal of Neurodevelopmental Disorders, 3*(4), 374–380.

Fanjiang, G., Grossman, J. H., Compton, W. D., & Reid, P. P. (Eds.). (2005). *Building a better delivery system: A new engineering/health care partnership.* Washington, DC: National Academies Press.

Johnson, B., Abraham, M., Conway, J., Simmons, L., Edgman-Levitan, S., Sodomka, P., & Ford, D. (2008). *Partnering with patients and families to design a patient- and family-centered health care system.* Bethesda MD: Institute for Family-Centered Care.

Jones, M., Onslow, M., Packman, A., Williams, S., Ormond, T., Schwarz, I., & Gebski, V. (2005). Randomised controlled trial of the Lidcombe programme of early stuttering intervention. *British Medical Journal, 331*(7518), 659.

Millard, S. K., Nicholas, A., & Cook, F. M. (2008). Is parent–child interaction therapy effective in reducing stuttering? *Journal of Speech, Language, and Hearing Research, 51*(3), 636–650.

Plexico, L. W., Manning, W. H., & DiLollo, A. (2010). Client perceptions of effective and ineffective therapeutic alliances during treatment for stuttering. *Journal of Fluency Disorders, 35*(4), 333–354.

Riley, G. (2009). *Stuttering Severity Instrument for children and adults.* Austin, TX: Pro-Ed.

Tellis, G. M., Bressler, L., & Emerick, K. (2008). An exploration of clinicians' views about assessment and treatment of stuttering. *SIG 4 Perspectives on Fluency and Fluency Disorders, 18*(1), 16–23.

Van Riper, C. (1973). *The treatment of stuttering.* Englewood Cliffs, NJ: Prentice-Hall.

Weidner, M. E. (2015). *InterACT Program.* Morgantown, WV: MC Speech Books.

Weidner, M. E., & St. Louis, K. O. (2016). *Improving children's stuttering attitudes.* Poster presented at the American Speech-Language-Hearing Association, Philadelphia, PA.

Yairi, E., & Ambrose, N. (2013). Epidemiology of stuttering: 21st century advances. *Journal of Fluency Disorders, 38*(2), 66–87.

Yaruss, J. S. (1998). Describing the consequences of disorders: Stuttering and the International Classification of Impairments, Disabilities, and Handicaps. *Journal of Speech, Language, and Hearing Research, 49,* 249–257.

Yaruss, J. S. (2004). Speech disfluency and stuttering in children. In R. D. Kent (Ed.), *The MIT encyclopedia of communication disorders* (pp. 180–183). Cambridge, MA: MIT Press.

Yaruss, J. S., Coleman, C., & Hammer, D. (2006). Treating preschool children who stutter: Description and preliminary evaluation of a family-focused treatment approach. *Language, Speech, and Hearing Services in Schools, 37*(2), 118–136.

Yaruss, J. S., Coleman, C. E., & Quesal, R. W. (2012). Stuttering in school-age children: A comprehensive approach to treatment. *Language, Speech, and Hearing Services in Schools, 43*(4), 536–548.

Yaruss, J. S., & Quesal, R. W. (2006). Overall Assessment of the Speaker's Experience of

Stuttering (OASES): Documenting multiple outcomes in stuttering treatment. *Journal of Fluency Disorders, 31*(2), 90–115.

Yaruss, J. S., Quesal, R. W., & Reeves, L. (2007). Self-help and mutual aid groups. In E. G. Conture & R. F. Curlee (Eds.), *Stuttering and related disorders of fluency* (pp. 256–276). New York, NY: Thieme.

CHAPTER 12

Final Thoughts

Barbara J. Amster and Evelyn R. Klein

As clinicians, we do not always know the long-term impact that we have had on our clients' lives. Recently, after visiting a dedication and naming of a treatment program for children who stutter, we were impressed by the donor who funded the project and how his experience in speech therapy changed his life. A person who stutters, he donated the funds with the stipulation that the program be named after his former speech-language pathologist, Dr. Woody Starkweather, who is also an author of a chapter in this book. Dr. Starkweather's focus was not only on speech production but also on helping him to build self-esteem and self-acceptance. The donor gave a heartfelt speech about his former speech-language pathologist and how much he helped him. All the while he stuttered. Nevertheless, what a wonderful communicator he was! As he reflected on his treatment, which began at age 16, he remarked that for the first time he began to feel comfortable in his own skin. Prior to that he was always running away from the stuttering, avoiding or trying to control it. Now, approaching middle age, a success in his field, with a family of his own, he accepts his stuttering as a part of himself. What relates to this book is the message that speech fluency should not be the only goal of good therapy. Being comfortable with yourself, being authentic, and communicating freely are what matter. We hope that this book serves as a guide to help your clients become true to themselves and find their own path to a fulfilling life. Stuttering does not have to define them!

Index

Note: Page numbers in **bold** reference non-text material.

B

C

D

E

F

G

H

I

Q

R

S

T